Psychotherapy
With Cardiac Patients

Psychotherapy With Cardiac Patients

BEHAVIORAL CARDIOLOGY IN PRACTICE

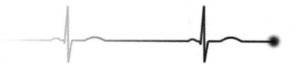

Ellen A. Dornelas

AMERICAN PSYCHOLOGICAL ASSOCIATION

WASHINGTON, DC

Published by
American Psychological Association
750 First Street, NE
Washington, DC 20002
www.apa.org

To order
APA Order Department
P.O. Box 92984
Washington, DC 20090-2984
Tel: (800) 374-2721; Direct: (202) 336-5510
Fax: (202) 336-5502; TDD/TTY: (202) 336-6123
Online: www.apa.org/books/
E-mail: order@apa.org

In the U.K., Europe, Africa, and the Middle East, copies may be ordered from
American Psychological Association
3 Henrietta Street
Covent Garden, London
WC2E 8LU England

Typeset in Goudy by Stephen McDougal, Mechanicsville, MD

Printer: Book-mart Press, North Bergen, NJ
Cover Designer: Berg Design, Albany, NY
Technical/Production Editor: Tiffany L. Klaff

The opinions and statements published are the responsibility of the authors, and such opinions and statements do not necessarily represent the policies of the American Psychological Association.

Library of Congress Cataloging-in-Publication Data

Dornelas, Ellen A.
    Psychotherapy with cardiac patients : behavioral cardiology in practice / Ellen A. Dornelas. — 1st ed.
        p. ; cm.
    Includes bibliographical references and index.
    ISBN-13: 978-1-4338-0356-7
    ISBN-10: 1-4338-0356-9
    1. Heart—Diseases—Patients—Mental health. 2. Cardiology—Psychological aspects.
3. Psychotherapy. I. American Psychological Association. II. Title.
    [DNLM: 1. Heart Diseases—psychology. 2. Behavioral Medicine—methods.
3. Heart Diseases—therapy. 4. Psychotherapy—methods. WG 210 D713p 2008]

    RC682.D69 2008
    616.1'20651—dc22   2007050836

British Library Cataloguing-in-Publication Data
A CIP record is available from the British Library.

Printed in the United States of America
First Edition

To Dilton, with all my love

CONTENTS

ACKNOWLEDGMENTS

My deepest appreciation goes to the cardiac patients I have treated, who have taught me much of what I know about the psychological complexities of living with heart disease. In different ways, you have truly affected my growth as a clinician and a human being, and I am profoundly grateful for having had the opportunity to work with you. Additionally, I am extremely humbled by the opportunity to summarize the work of so many behavioral cardiology scientists who have paved the way with many decades of research for a book for the clinical readership.

In writing this book, the support of my colleague and friend, Paul D. Thompson, chief of cardiology at Hartford Hospital, has been invaluable. I am also appreciative of the time and support of my colleagues who have read drafts of the manuscript in its early stages, writer Garret Condon; cardiologist Jeffrey Kluger; and psychologists Jennifer Ferrand, Roxanne Stepnowski, Ed Fischer, and Terry DiLorenzo. Special appreciation and thanks are also due to many colleagues, including Jeremy Barbagallo, my partner in the delivery of services at Hartford Hospital. I am thankful for the opportunities I have had to work with and learn from Matt Burg, whose breadth of knowledge in behavioral cardiology is impressive. I am also very grateful to Sam Sears, who helped to advance my knowledge about the complexity of living with an implantable cardioverter defibrillator. To David Waters, the cardiologist who originally hired me to work in the division of cardiology at Hartford Hospital, thanks for opening the door! The input of psychiatrist Eric Chamberlin, who reviewed the chapter on medications for this book, was extremely helpful. Leigh McCullough, a gifted theorist and clinician, has helped me to advance my technical skills and is owed a big thank you. I am also grateful to several early mentors at Albert Einstein College of Medicine, who helped set me on a path to working with cardiac patients: Charlie Swencionis, Judy Wylie-Rosett, and Gil Levin. Jeffrey Magnavita has been a valued colleague who has given me support from the beginning and provided critical feedback on the initial proposal, helped me to find a publisher, and offered encouragement throughout the process. Special thanks to Susan Reynolds, Phuong Huynh, and Tiffany Klaff at the American Psychological Association for their superb editorial guidance. To the anonymous reviewers of the manuscript and the initial proposal, I am indebted and only wish I could give you my thanks in person.

Authorship of this book would not have been possible without the support of my family. The encouragement, love, and confidence of Dilton, my husband of 20 years, have been instrumental in my personal and career development. I am incredibly grateful for the love and trust of my children, Katie and Julia, who have been very patient through many manuscript revisions and lost weekends. My parents, Tom and Anita Anderson, as well as my late mother, Carole Anderson, my two amazing siblings Heidi and Eric, and my wonderful niece Siobhan have provided support in both my personal life and writing.

Like most, my family has been touched by cardiovascular illness, and it is my hope that this book will honor the memories of loved ones who have died from heart disease.

Psychotherapy
With Cardiac Patients

INTRODUCTION

Heart disease is the leading cause of death in the United States. Every 26 seconds an American suffers a coronary event (American Heart Association, 2005). There is a wide range of psychological sequelae from cardiac events, yet surprisingly few books teach psychotherapy practitioners how to tailor their approaches to meet the needs of this patient population. This book provides clinicians with a framework to integrate the broad fields of cardiology and psychotherapy and describes a wide variety of psychotherapeutic approaches that are appropriate for cardiac patients.

As the U.S. population ages, the incidence of heart disease will increase. By 2010, the U.S. Census estimates that there will be more than 40 million people over the age of 65 in the United States. With the aging of the baby boom generation, there is an unprecedented opportunity for mental health professionals to extend their services to meet the needs of the medically ill. For example, when the 58-year-old President Bill Clinton received cardiac bypass surgery, a *Time* magazine editorial from Lance Morrow advised him, "You may find yourself falling into illogical depression and inexplicable rage. We all should be grateful for this gift of time but for some reason the operation lays one emotionally low" (Morrow, 2004, p. 84). Because heart disease is so prevalent, therapists in general practice often unknowingly encounter clients whose depression or anxiety may have been precipitated by a cardiac event or whose presenting problem may be complicated by cardiovascular disease. At the same time, a growing number of mental health providers have obtained training in health psychology and have specific interest in treating people with cardiac illness. The growth of practitioners in this area is partly attributable to a quantum leap forward over the past decade in understanding the relationship between emotions and cardiovascular functioning, as well as an increased demand for psychotherapy services from a well-educated lay public who understands that there is a relationship between quality of life and physical health. Although psychotherapy practitioners commonly encounter some of the psychological difficulties that follow cardiac disease (e.g., depression), cardiac patients often require a different approach from nonmedical patients. Depression that follows a heart attack has different prognostic significance and treatment implications from depression that follows, for example, a diagnosis of cancer. Therapists who have a good understanding about problems of the heart are not only more credible as practitioners but are also at an advantage in their ability to tailor treatment to the unique needs of the client with cardiac disease.

WHAT IS BEHAVIORAL CARDIOLOGY?

Behavioral cardiology applies the theories and principles of the behavioral sciences to the psychological and behavioral aspects of cardiac disease. Many people intuitively understand that psychological factors are important, both as precipitants and consequences of cardiac events, but few therapists feel confident enough in their knowledge of heart disease to target therapy for this patient population. Many other names are used to refer to this field of study, including cardiac psychology, psychocardiology, medical psychology, psychosomatic medicine, health psychology, and behavioral medicine. Also, innumerable practitioners who work with cardiac patients are not psychologists, and a descriptor that applies to all clinicians who might work in this field holds appeal. In medical settings and nonmedical settings, the root word *psych* brings up feelings of stigmatization, fear, and avoidance in patients as well as medical practitioners. So, in selecting the term *behavioral cardiology*, this volume follows in a path set by others (Das & O'Keefe, 2006; Pickering, Clemow, Davidson, & Gerin, 2003; Rozanski, Blumenthal, Davidson, Saab, & Kubzansky, 2005). Given the breadth of the field, there will no doubt be even more heterogeneity in the future in the language used to describe the work of the clinician who works with people who have heart disease.

Similarly, the terms *patient* and *client* are used interchangeably in this book. More often than not, in medical settings, people who seek treatment are referred to as *patients*, and the use of the word *client* sets the clinician apart from other medical providers. In this context, the pejorative sense of stigmatization associated with the word *patient* that might occur in a psychiatric hospital does not occur; in fact, people with heart disease usually refer to themselves as patients, which seems to underscore that they perceive their cardiac disease to be related to their psychological well-being.

SEMINAL WORKS IN THE FIELD

Several seminal works have laid the groundwork for this book. *Heart and Mind: The Practice of Cardiac Psychology* (Allan & Scheidt, 1996) was the first such edited book published by the American Psychological Association (APA). Edited by a psychologist and a cardiologist, this weighty volume was aimed at researchers and clinical professionals in the fields of both psychology and medicine. Writers who published on this topic in the years to follow are indebted to Allan and Scheidt for providing one of the first organizational frameworks to integrate these two vast fields. At about the same time, psychologist Wayne Sotile (1996) published *Psychosocial Interventions for Cardiopulmonary Patients: A Guide for Health Professionals*, a book that was far ahead of the curve in terms of recognizing the psychological needs of cardiac patients. Although Sotile did not target the book for mental health professionals, his was the first cohesive, clinically relevant book from a single practitioner working in the field. At the time of this writing, one of the most recent books in this field is titled *Clinical Psychology and Heart Disease* (Molinari, Compare, & Parati, 2006). This well-written, comprehensive book has chapter contributors from many countries, and consequently it provides a much-needed global perspective on this field. Skala, Freedland, and Carney (2005) are leaders in the field of behavioral cardiology who wrote the book *Heart Disease*, for the Advances in Psychotherapy: Evidence-Based Practice series. Clinicians who need a compact reference book on the topic will find this volume helpful.

Psychotherapy With Cardiac Patients: Behavioral Cardiology in Practice is different from these other works in a number of ways. There has long been a need for a clinically useful book that would encompass the broad spectrum of cardiac disease encountered in clinical practice and provide guidance for how to intervene. In contrast to earlier works in the field, this book emphasizes clinical examples from patients in the medical setting, integrated with summaries of the empirical literature. This book also makes use of interviews with selected leaders in this field, including psychologists Samuel Sears and Matthew Burg and nationally known cardiologist David Waters, as well as a leader in psychology who has written about his personal struggles with heart disease, past president of the APA Ronald Levant. Our intent is that the inclusion of this interview material will help to illustrate key points without exhausting the reader. *Psychotherapy With Cardiac Patients* advances the organizational framework that ties the two broad and disparate fields of cardiology and psychotherapy together. As a single-author volume, the book is written in such a way as to provide an integrated method and rationale for systematically applying psychotherapy expertise to the treatment of the person with heart disease.

LIMITATIONS

There are several limitations to this book that deserve mention. Regrettably, the topic of ethnicity and race is not emphasized as much as I would have liked. There are dramatic differences in risk for heart disease among Blacks, Whites, Hispanics, Asian Americans, and Native/Alaskan Americans. As Mexicans, Cubans, Central Americans, South Americans, and Asian Americans acculturate to U.S. society, their risk for heart disease as well as mental health problems increases sharply. Additionally, psychotherapeutic strategies are underused for ethnic minority populations. This topic is not specifically addressed because so little has been written on it, making it difficult to speculate on approaches to psychotherapeutic treatment of ethnic and racial minorities who have heart disease. Too often, racial or ethnic status is confounded with socioeconomic status and educational level. Many of the racial and ethnic differences noted in heart and mental health research vanish among highly educated racial and ethnic minority subgroups (B. B. Brown, 1978). To the extent that literature on this topic is available, as is the case with one of the major clinical trials testing cognitive behavior therapy for cardiac patients (Berkman et al., 2003; Schneiderman et al., 2004), it has been incorporated into the book. However, there is wide heterogeneity in the ethnicity of the patients presented in clinical examples, reflective of my own experience in treating the kinds of ethnic minority clients who live in the Northeast United States, primarily African Americans, Caribbean Americans, South Americans, and Puerto Ricans. This volume has made every effort to recognize cultural differences, within the bounds of the currently available empirical literature.

Other topics are important but beyond the scope of the book, such as discussion of the many types of diagnostic tests for cardiology or classes of medications used to treat cardiovascular disease. Atherosclerotic-based diseases such as stroke and cerebrovascular disease are mentioned only in a cursory way. The decision to omit discussion of stroke was made primarily because psychotherapy with patients who have suffered stroke is qualitatively different from those with heart dysfunction, and stroke is not the focus of the book. This book only covers treatment of adults. In so doing, it follows the path of most health psychology texts in that pediatric behavioral cardiology is considered its own distinct field. Thus, the primary limitations of this book concern the necessary omission of topics that are related and important but are left out either because there is little scientific literature available or because the topic is beyond the scope of this volume.

MANY PSYCHOTHERAPEUTIC APPROACHES ARE USEFUL

Psychotherapy for Cardiac Patients does not advocate one model of psychotherapy over another. Psychotherapy research has repeatedly demonstrated that no one approach is markedly superior to another (Elkin et al., 1989) and that common factors account for the greatest amount of variance in therapy outcome across many treatment contexts (Horvath & Luborsky, 1993). In this volume, the primary theoretical orientations that guide treatment stem from the myriad commonly practiced models of psychotherapy, such as cognitive behavioral, interpersonal, and psychodynamic psychotherapy. Many other forms of therapy are also incorporated, including marital therapy, grief therapy, motivational interviewing, relational psychotherapy, stress management and relaxation therapies, and experiential approaches that center primarily on affect expression. Although most research tends to focus on the difference in theoretical orientation between psychotherapy models, this emphasis is very limiting and seems to lead to less rather than more understanding of what works in therapy. Consequently, this book presents strategies that are viable for the treatment of psychological problems commonly encountered in patients with cardiovascular disease when applied by therapists with excellent general clinical skills. Case examples and clinical recommendations are presented to facilitate the integration of the knowledge about heart disease, psychosocial factors related to cardiac illness, and psychotherapeutic techniques. In other words, this book teaches good therapists to apply what they already know about psychotherapy to the care of this important and often undertreated patient population.

PSYCHOTHERAPY IS NOT FOR EVERYONE

Although the burden of psychological distress on the cardiac population is quite high and the risk posed by failing to treat distressed patients is substantial, psychotherapy is not the only treatment for psychological distress. Moreover, psychotherapy is not the right treatment for every distressed person with heart disease. Some of these patients respond well to medication and support. Some patients may be too physically disabled or lack the psychological-mindedness necessary to make use of psychotherapeutic approaches. Future studies of psychotherapy as a treatment for this patient population will help to identify those subgroups of patients who derive benefit from psychotherapy and identify other treatments that will be useful to those who are not helped by this treatment modality. More research and clinical practice perspectives will further enhance the practice of behavioral cardiology.

THE IMPORTANCE OF THE ABILITY
TO GENERALIZE ACROSS DOMAINS

This book assumes that clinicians who understand the importance of each psychological factor to cardiac health will be able to generalize that information, regardless of the cardiac diagnosis. For example, depression may occur following heart attack or while awaiting transplant. The variation in the context helps the clinician to guide psychotherapy. There is a burgeoning number of scientific articles that point out that negative emotions tend to cluster together and may work additively or synergistically to influence cardiac prognosis (Frasure-Smith et al., 2002; Williams et al., 1997). Although there has been substantive progress in understanding the link between psychological health and cardiac illness, there have been very few major clinical trials of psychotherapy for cardiac patients funded by the National Institutes of Health. Traditionally, behavioral cardiology researchers have often been more interested in behavioral intervention to modify cardiac outcomes rather than to alleviate psychological distress. It has been implied, although not proven, that with respect to alleviation of psychological symptoms, cardiac patients are not different from other populations and that standard psychotherapies that work well in noncardiac populations will be equally effective for the treatment of the patient with heart disease.

In fact, it is difficult to examine the differences in how cardiac patients respond to therapy as compared with other populations. Psychotherapy trials themselves are difficult to conduct because scientific rigor leads to an artificial environment in which to conduct therapy. The typical research study patient must meet rigorous inclusion and exclusion criteria. Therefore, the sample is reduced to a homogeneous sample of people experiencing a single circumscribed problem who are willing to participate in a research study. By definition, psychotherapy research is highly structured, involves a great deal of assessment, and bears little resemblance to the actual practice of psychotherapy. This has made the results of randomized controlled trials testing psychotherapy interventions for cardiac patients particularly challenging to interpret (Berkman et al., 2003; Lesperance et al., 2007).

In reading this book, one may find it helpful to bear these principles in mind—that multiple therapeutic approaches are useful, psychotherapy is not for everyone, and it is important to be able to generalize across domains. These axioms are meant to help the reader integrate the wide variety of contradictory and competing perspectives from the empirical literature with the abstract and inherently complex nature of clinical practice.

ORGANIZATION OF THE BOOK

The practice of behavioral cardiology has evolved from a convergence of separate but parallel theoretical lines of behavioral cardiology and psychotherapy research. The most difficult aspect of integrating the broad areas of psychotherapy and behavioral cardiology involves decisions on how to organize and integrate the material. This volume cannot be comprehensive because both fields are so vast; instead, there is a selective emphasis on a broad spectrum of different psychological dysfunctions and cardiac illnesses. For example, all of the chapters that include therapeutic approaches in this book also include a section on assessment. Selected assessment tools are reviewed for clinical use because it is time consuming and laborious for clinicians to comb the empirical literature and weigh the various merits of one measure over another. Suggestions and examples of how these tools might be incorporated into clinical practice are also provided. Types of psychological dysfunction (e.g., depression, anxiety) are paired with particular therapeutic approaches that are conceptually related. There is an infinite number of permutations in how psychological clinical syndromes, personality traits, cardiac diseases, and cardiac interventions might be organized. So although certain psychological problems, cardiac conditions, and psychotherapeutic strategies are emphasized in each chapter of this book, the evidence presented is expected to contribute to the reader's fund of knowledge such that it can be generalized and applied across the spectrum of cardiac conditions.

The book is organized in three parts. Part I, "Understanding Behavioral Cardiology," provides a broad overview of the field of behavioral cardiology. In chapter 1, "Exploring the Heart," the anatomy and functioning of the heart, major categories of cardiac disease, and some of the common diagnostic procedures and treatments for such problems are described. Chapter 2, "Risk Factors and Perceptions of Risk for Cardiovascular Disease," discusses the modifiable and nonmodifiable risk factors for heart disease and provides information about how people make health behavior changes. Chapter 3, "Emotions and the Heart," is a compact chapter that provides an overview of the neurobiological research connecting emotions and cardiovascular disease and introduces the clinical material in Part II: "Psychosocial Factors and Cardiovascular Disease."

Chapter 4, "Depression," is the first chapter in Part II and discusses the voluminous literature on the occurrence of depression prior to and following a cardiac diagnosis. Two major clinical trials that tested cognitive behavioral and interpersonal psychotherapy interventions for cardiac patients with depression are discussed in this chapter. Chapter 5, "Anxiety," addresses anxiety and stress, with attention to the presentation of panic disorder and noncardiac chest pain in clinical practice and the special needs of people who have implantable cardioverter defibrillators. Cognitive techniques to reduce anxiety, many types of relaxation methods, and biofeedback are discussed in this chapter. Chapter 6, "Anger and Hostility," reviews literature on these topics and delineates how practitioners can address these problems in clinical practice. This topic is complex in that it does not focus on symptom constellations, as is the case with depression and anxiety, but instead on emotional states and personality traits. Chapter 7, "Interpersonal Relationships and Social Support," describes how social relationships can have both a positive and negative impact on the heart. This chapter moves away from individual therapy to focus on other modalities such as support groups, family systems therapy, and emotionally focused couples therapy. Chapter 8, "Coping With Chronic Heart Disease," examines the needs of the chronically ill cardiac patient, with a focus on the rapidly growing population of people living with congestive heart disease. Caregiver burden and the difficulties of dealing with prognostic uncertainty with respect to heart disease are discussed in detail in this chapter. Medical family therapy and intervention approaches with nonadherent patients are the psychotherapeutic focus. Chapter 9, "Existential Issues, Heart Transplant, and End-Stage Cardiac Disease," highlights the life and death concerns of people with end-stage heart disease. To some degree, most cardiac patients weigh existential issues after a diagnosis of heart disease, so this topic is relevant for nearly all patients, although it is most prominent in people dealing with end-of-life issues. Humanistic–existential therapy and expressive writing are presented as psychotherapeutic strategies. Additionally, a section titled "The Good Death" in this chapter provides some guidance on how to facilitate discussion of how a patient wants to die. The chapter concludes the section on psychosocial factors and heart health as well as the in-depth description of psychotherapeutic approaches.

Part III: "Special Topics in Behavioral Cardiology Care," covers issues that are frequently encountered in clinical practice with a cardiac population. Chapter 10, "Addictions to Cocaine, Alcohol, or Cigarettes," considers the treatment of cardiac patients who have addictions to one or more of these substances. Therapeutic approaches that include motivational interviewing, supportive 12-step groups, Internet education, and support and telephone hotlines are presented. Chapter 11, "Morbid Obesity," focuses on working with cardiac patients who are extremely overweight. The dramatic growth of the field of bariatric surgery over the past decade has created an influx of morbidly obese patients who seek psychotherapy for depression, anxiety, body image issues, and motivational problems that undermine their weight loss efforts. Binge-eating disorder, night-eating disorder, and the complex challenges of working with candidates for bariatric surgery are discussed in this chapter. Chapter 12, "Psychotropic Medications," gives the reader a basic understanding of the medications often prescribed to cardiac patients (e.g., antidepressants, anxiolytics) and thus commonly encountered by behavioral cardiology clinicians. Considerations about the use of psychotropic medication in conjunction with psychotherapy are explored. Chapter 13,

"Sex Differences," reviews the literature on sex factors that influence risk for and treatment of heart disease. The mitigating influence of attitudes, beliefs, and social factors is addressed in this chapter. In contrast to standard outpatient psychotherapy practices, the majority of referrals for behavioral cardiology psychotherapists are men rather than women. Therefore, this chapter incorporates considerations as to how psychotherapy can be specifically tailored for men. "The Practice of Behavioral Cardiology" is the concluding chapter of the book and summarizes how a clinician might develop a behavioral cardiology practice devoted to the treatment of patients with heart disease. Training issues, choice of practice settings, and the rewards and pitfalls of clinical practice in the field of behavioral cardiology are discussed.

James Bugental, the existential–humanistic psychologist, once said in an interview, "At a time when I was most productive, I was always trying to storm the wall of 'psychological science' " (V. Yalom, 2000, n.p.). Similarly, after 50 years of research in behavioral cardiology, the time has probably come for clinicians to storm the wall—to begin to apply the best of what psychological science offers—to the care of people with heart disease.

I

UNDERSTANDING BEHAVIORAL CARDIOLOGY

1

EXPLORING THE HEART

The heart is a complex organ. Clinicians unfamiliar with heart disease often wish for a quick and easy reference tool. This chapter presents such a guide. Laypeople think of the heart as a pump. Heart disease, broadly speaking, involves damage to the pump's casing (heart muscle), its power source (the heart's electrical system), or its valves (the heart has four). The heart muscle is threatened if the arteries that feed it are blocked. A failure of the heart's complex electrical system can be fatal. And when one or more of the valves do not operate properly, the heart's pumping power is compromised.

BASIC ANATOMY AND PHYSIOLOGY OF THE HEART

The heart is about the size of a fist and has four chambers (see Figure 1.1). The upper chambers are called the right and left atria, and the lower chambers are called the right and left ventricles. The atria collect blood and pass it on to the ventricles; the ventricles pump blood out of the heart. The right side of the heart pumps to the lungs, whereas the left side of the heart pumps to the rest of the body. So it is no surprise that the left side of the heart has to work much harder than the right side. The atria are separated from the

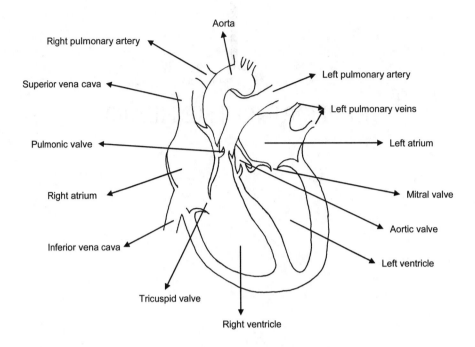

Figure 1.1. Diagram of the heart (illustration by Marisa Scarnati).

ventricles, and the ventricles are separated from their exit blood vessels by valves that ensure that blood flows in one direction.

The contraction of the atria and ventricles is controlled by an electrical conduction system. Blood is pushed out of each chamber as the heart muscle contracts during what is called *systole*. The chambers fill during relaxation or *diastole*. At rest, the heart muscle contracts about 72 times a minute. Contraction of the heart is initiated by the sinoatrial (SA) node, a cluster of electrically more active cells called pacemaker cells located at the top of the right atrium. These cells leak potassium from the inside to the outside, and when the walls of the cells reach a specific electrical charge, sodium rushes in and potassium rushes out, creating something similar to an electrical "spark" that travels down the electrical conduction system and causes the muscle cells to contract. The electrical impulses spread from the SA node to the rest of the atria and to the atrioventricular (AV) node. The AV node slows down the electrical impulse before it reaches the ventricles. Muscle fibers in the conduction pathways distribute the impulse across the ventricles, and this impulse causes the ventricles to contract.

The cardiac cycle is the sequence of events that occur in a complete beat of the heart. Each contraction causes deoxygenated blood from the head and upper body to flow into the superior vena cava, while deoxygenated blood from the rest of the body flows into the inferior vena cava, both of which empty into the right atrium of the heart. The tricuspid valve opens to allow blood to flow from the right atrium to the right ventricle. Valves have flaps (leaflets) that allow blood to flow in and then to close completely so that blood does not leak backward (regurgitation). As the right ventricle contracts, the tricuspid valve closes and the pulmonic valve opens so that blood is forced into the pulmonary artery toward the lungs. The pulmonary vein transports oxygen-rich blood from the lungs back to the heart and the left atrium. When the left atrial muscle is activated by the electrical system, it contracts, which opens the mitral valve, allowing blood to flow to the left ventricle. The left ventricle, when electrically activated, contracts, which closes the mitral valve and opens the aortic valve, forcing blood to flow into the aorta and the body. This cycle is repeated with each heartbeat, about 60 to 80 times a minute for most people at rest.

The heart itself is a muscle that requires oxygen. As the blood exits the heart through the aorta, some is immediately directed into the left and right coronary arteries. The coronary arteries are so named because they sit on the outside of the heart like a crown or corona. The coronary arteries branch into progressively smaller vessels. The left coronary artery divides into the left anterior descending artery and circumflex branch, which supplies blood primarily to the left ventricle's front and side and to the left atrium. The right coronary artery divides into vessels that supply blood to the back of the left ventricle and to the right ventricle, right atrium, and SA node. If the heart needs to increase the amount of oxygen to the body (e.g., during physical exertion), it does so by increasing the amount of blood ejected with each contraction and increasing the number of beats per minute. Diseases and dysfunctions of the heart can occur with the blood vessels that supply oxygen to the heart, with the conduction system, in the valves, or in the heart muscle itself. The major categories of heart disease are described next.

MAJOR CLASSES OF CARDIAC DISEASE

Four major categories of heart disease are discussed in this chapter: coronary heart disease, arrhythmia, valve disease, and congestive heart failure. Coronary heart disease accounts for the greatest morbidity and mortality each year. These four categories often overlap and interact (i.e., people have more than one type of disease at the same time). In this section, a brief description of the disease category is followed by information on the known causes, after which prevalence data are cited.

Coronary Heart Disease

Coronary heart disease (CHD) is the most common form of heart disease. It is known by several other names, including ischemic heart disease, coronary artery disease, and acute coronary syndrome. No matter what it is called, it is always characterized by atherosclerosis (described subsequently).[1] The majority of people who are hospitalized for CHD are diagnosed with either angina pectoris or myocardial infarction (MI). Angina pectoris refers to chest pain caused by lack of oxygen to the heart. It often occurs on exertion. However, when angina becomes more frequent or intense, or occurs with less physical exertion or at rest, it is called unstable angina, because this implies that there is a change in the aetherosclerotic plaque causing increased ischemia. MI refers to the death of heart muscle cells because of an interruption in blood flow to the heart. The severity of MI can range from mild to severe, depending on the location and extent of the damage.

Causes of Coronary Heart Disease

The primary cause of heart disease is *atherosclerosis*, a progressive disease that begins with fatty streaks in the wall of the coronary arteries that over time increase in thickness and begin to expand into the opening (lumen) of the blood vessel itself. When an artery that supplies the heart muscle becomes partially blocked (occluded), the ischemia (lack of oxygenated blood) can result in angina, often experienced as pressure or burning in the chest that may be accompanied by shortness of breath (dyspnea). If the artery is completely blocked, and especially if the blockage occurs quickly, the heart muscle beyond the obstruction can die from lack of oxygenated blood, causing a heart attack or or MI. Untreated atherosclerosis can reduce or stop blood flow. A partially occluded artery can lie dormant for years, causing no symptoms. But these atherosclerotic plaques can crack or rupture, permitting blood to mix with the cholesterol deposit. Blood platelets treat the plaque rupture as an injury and form a clot that can then partially or completely occlude the artery. Most heart attacks occur through this process (Topol, 2007).

The primary risk factors that contribute to the development of CHD are high cholesterol, cigarette smoking, high blood pressure, and diabetes (American Heart Association [AHA], 2005). All of the risk factors for CHD are discussed in more detail in chapter 2 (this volume).

Prevalence of Coronary Heart Disease

Each year, more than 800,000 people in the United States suffer MI (AHA, 2005). Of those, half a million people have a first MI, and 300,000 have a recurrent MI. On average, a first MI occurs for men at about age 66 and for women at about age 70. Heart disease follows a chronic course, and

---

[1]Although cerebrovascular disease or interruption in blood supply to the brain (stroke) is also characterized by atherosclerosis, this topic is quite broad in its own right. Stroke is not covered in this book primarily because the cognitive and psychological sequelae of stroke are markedly different from those of coronary heart disease.

about 18% of men and 35% of women have another heart attack within 6 years of the initial MI. There are about 175,000 people each year who have no apparent awareness of symptoms but survive "silent" heart attacks that are later evident during medical examination (AHA, 2005). Historically, within 1 year after a diagnosed MI, 25% of men and 38% of women die, but survival continues to improve in the era of modern medicine.

Although cardiac mortality has decreased in the past few decades, the overall incidence of heart disease has not changed. That is, the same number of people develop heart disease each year, but fewer critically ill cardiac patients die from their disease. Today, patients spend far less time in the hospital following a heart attack than in the past, and the odds of a quickly occurring second attack are lower than a decade ago. In 1990, a nonfatal MI would have resulted in a hospital stay averaging about 8 days, but 10 years later the average length of stay for MI was just 4 days. Shorter hospital stays are attributable to shrinking insurance reimbursement, as well as major technological advances in medical treatment for CHD (AHA, 2005).

Arrhythmia

Arrhythmia or disorders in the electrical system of the heart comprise a second major category of heart disease. There are several types of abnormalities that occur with the heart's rhythm system, including a heartbeat that is too slow, too fast, or irregular. These types of arrhythmias are described next.

Atrial Fibrillation

Atrial fibrillation is the most common type of abnormal heart rhythm. When atrial fibrillation occurs, electrical discharges do not come only from the SA node but instead come from other parts of the atria. These electrical discharges cause the atria to fibrillate (quiver), and the ventricles then contract irregularly and rapidly. Atrial fibrillation causes loss of synchrony between the atria and the ventricles. Atrial fibrillation can be transient and convert rapidly back to normal rhythm on its own (paroxysmal atrial fibrillation), or it can continue without reverting (chronic atrial fibrillation; AHA, 2006).

Bradycardia

A heart rhythm that is too slow is called *bradycardia*. People with bradycardia may become dizzy, fatigued, or faint if the heart cannot circulate enough blood because of slow heart rate. There are two common types of bradycardia. If the SA node loses the ability to increase heart rate or initiate the heart beat, the resultant condition is called *sick sinus syndrome*. If the SA node successfully passes the signal but the impulse becomes slowed, irregular, or stopped at the AV node, the resultant condition is termed *heart block*. Heart block is a condition described in terms of the severity. First-degree heart block refers to a condition in which the electrical impulses are slowed as they pass through the conduction system, but all of them successfully reach the ventricles. First-degree heart block rarely causes symptoms. Second-degree heart block occurs when some, but not all, electrical impulses from the atria reach the ventricles, causing slow or irregular heartbeat. Third-degree or complete heart block occurs when all the electrical impulses from the atria are blocked (AHA, 2006).

Tachycardia

Tachycardia refers to a heartbeat that is too fast, causing a person to become dizzy, faint, and develop palpitations, chest pain, or shortness of breath. Tachycardia can be normal, such as during exercise or excitement. Abnormal tachycardia usually occurs when the electrical impulse takes an abnormal pathway, often in an area of the heart that is damaged by disease or previous heart attack. There are two common types of abnormal tachycardia: abnormal tachycardia originating in the atrium (atrial tachycardia) and abnormal tachycardia from the ventricle (ventricular tachycardia). Both atrial and ventricular tachycardia often occur when the electrical impulse enters an abnormal pathway (called a reentry circuit) in the chamber and travels in a circle, making the chamber contract again each time it passes. Ventricular fibrillation, like atrial fibrillation, is a type of tachycardia in which the muscle does not contract but twitches in a disorganized fashion. Ventricular fibrillation occurs when multiple sites in the ventricle fire impulses erratically and the ventricle begins to fibrillate, making it unable to pump blood out. Untreated ventricular fibrillation is lethal and leads to cardiac death within minutes if the electrical rhythm of the heart is not restarted (AHA, 2006).

Sudden cardiac death is also called cardiac arrest and is an unexpected death that occurs almost always as a result of ventricular fibrillation. When the cardiac conduction system is halted and the heart cannot pump blood, death occurs in 4 to 6 minutes (AHA, 2005). Sudden cardiac death is primarily associated with having one or more coronary arteries obstructed by atherosclerotic plaques, especially if this occurs rapidly. Less often, certain drugs such as cocaine and extreme physical exertion can also trigger sudden cardiac death, particularly in people with underlying genetic vulnerability (Grant & Durrani, 2007).

Causes of Arrhythmia

Arrhythmia can be caused by underlying heart disease such as damage from an MI, valve disease, or congenital heart disease. Arrhythmia can also be triggered by thyroid dysfunction, hypertension, certain drugs, overconsumption of caffeine or alcohol, smoking, low potassium, physical exertion, and stress. Wolff–Parkinson–White syndrome, a condition characterized by having an extra conduction pathway for electrical signals, is also a cause of heart arrhythmia.

Prevalence of Arrhythmia

Cardiac arrhythmias are common, and more than 2 million Americans are diagnosed with atrial fibrillation or flutter (AHA, 2005). The average age for men diagnosed with atrial fibrillation is 67 years, compared with 75 years in women. Atrial fibrillation is an independent risk factor for stroke and is responsible for about 15% to 20% of all strokes. Sudden cardiac death accounts for about 335,000 deaths a year in the United States. Put another way, nearly 900 Americans a day die unexpectedly from sudden cardiac death without ever being admitted to the hospital (AHA, 2005).

Valve Disease

Valve disease is a third major category of heart disease. Valves allow blood to flow through each chamber of the heart progressively. Valves have flaps (leaflets) that allow blood to flow in and then to close completely so that blood does not leak backward (regurgitation). The mitral valve has two leaflets and a normal aortic valve has three leaflets, but a common abnormality that requires valve surgery is a bicuspid aortic valve, or an aortic valve with only two leaflets. A valve is diseased when it is too narrow (stenotic) or does not close properly and leaks (insufficient). Valves can become inflamed, stiff, scarred, thickened, shortened, malformed, or be the wrong size. The most common type of valve disease is mitral valve prolapse, a condition that occurs when the valve's leaflets bulge (prolapse) into the atrium as the ventricles contract. Sometimes mitral valve prolapse allows blood to regurgitate into the atrium, but most often mitral valve prolapse is totally benign and has no harmful effects (AHA, 2006).

Causes of Valve Disease

Valve disease can result from rheumatic fever that is caused by bacterial infection, most commonly, untreated strep throat. Other types of bacterial infections that attack the valves result from dental procedures, surgery, intravenous drug use, or severe infection. Congenital abnormalities can cause valve disease. Valve disease can also be caused by prior MI, coronary artery disease, cardiomyopathy, syphilis, hypertension, and connective tissue disease. In rare cases, certain tumors, drugs, and radiation can cause valve disease (AHA, 2006).

Prevalence of Valve Disease

Slightly more than 2% of adults in the United States have mitral valve disease, but aortic valve disorders are the most common valvular cause of hospital discharge. Prevalence of valve disease increases with age and is roughly equal in prevalence between men and women (AHA, 2005).

Congestive Heart Failure

Cardiomyopathy is a fourth major category of heart disease, and the term refers to weakness of the heart muscle. However, this section is titled congestive heart failure because this is the most common presentation of cardiomyopathy. Congestive heart failure or, more properly, just heart failure (HF), is the fastest growing disease category in cardiac medicine (AHA, 2005). Cardiologists tend to use the term *heart failure*, but with patients most clinicians refer to *congestive heart disease*, recognizing that the word *failure* has negative connotations. The term congestive heart disease is not used in this chapter because the acronym CHD is easy to confuse with coronary heart disease. Congestive heart failure refers to a constellation of problems caused by an inability of the heart to pump (systolic heart failure) or to relax (diastolic heart failure) properly. Cardiomyopathy refers to a weakness of heart muscle, whereas HF refers to the process by which fluid backs up into the lungs (congests) because the heart's ability to pump or relax is impaired and fluid accumulates throughout the body. HF is a chronic disease that occurs when one or more chambers of the heart fail to contract properly. As the heart's ability to pump decreases, the heart tries to compensate for its weakness by expanding. This is done by holding on to extra fluid, causing fluid to build up (congest) in tissues throughout the body. The term failure is somewhat misleading in that the pumping action of the heart has not "failed," but rather the heart muscle cannot pump effectively to keep up with the body's demands for oxygen-rich blood supplied to the hands, feet, and organs. To measure the body's efficiency at pumping blood, cardiologists measure *ejection fraction*, or the proportion of blood present at the beginning of a contraction that the left ventricle expels with each beat. Normal ejection fraction is 50% to 70%; the lower the ejection fraction, the weaker the heart's ability to pump (Francis, 2007).

Causes of Congestive Heart Failure

Heart failure has many causes, including previous MI, hypertension, valve disease, arrhythmia, excessive alcohol use, pregnancy, myocarditis (inflammation of the heart muscle from infections or chemicals), obesity, or diabetes. In short, any type of heart disease can eventually progress to HF. As HF worsens, this disease is characterized by high mortality rates and high likelihood of hospital admission. The New York Heart Association uses a classification system for congestive heart failure that ranges from I to IV, with Class IV representing those people who have the most severe HF symptoms and functional limitations (AHA, 2006).

Prevalence of Congestive Heart Failure

People with HF have a very serious illness. One out of five people diagnosed with HF die within 1 year. Half of people with HF die within 5 years. There are 550,000 new cases of HF diagnosed each year, and it is the only heart disease that is increasing in prevalence, according to the AHA (2005). About 2% of people age 40 through 59 have HF, but the prevalence increases dramatically with age, such that over the age of 80, 20% of people are diagnosed with HF.

People with HF must closely monitor their symptoms (e.g., fatigue, urine output, weight) as well as take medication, monitor fluid intake, follow a regimented diet (e.g., avoid sodium), and exercise. When fluid accumulates in the body, it causes shortness of breath and leg swelling. People feel very tired and fatigued when they are symptomatic with HF. Consequences of not sticking to the medical regimen can be severe and even require hospitalization.

SELECTED TREATMENTS FOR CARDIOVASCULAR DISEASE

In this section, certain treatments associated with each of the four major heart disease categories are described. Diagnostic tests are not described, except to say that diagnostic procedures used to diagnose heart disease tend to fall into the category of noninvasive tests (e.g., electrocardiogram, exercise stress test, echocardiogram, magnetic resonance imaging) and nuclear imaging and invasive tests (e.g., cardiac catheterization and angiography). It is helpful to understand the different types of diagnostic procedures, but the breadth of topic and complexity of each type of test render it beyond the scope of this chapter. The interested reader is referred to both the *Textbook of Cardiovascular Medicine: Third Edition* (Topol, 2007) and the AHA's (2006) online *Heart and Stroke Encyclopedia* for additional reading on these topics.

Treatment categories are selective because many aspects of treatment are not discussed in this chapter. These areas are not emphasized because the topics are so broad (e.g., medications to treat heart disease) that it is beyond the scope of the book. However, there are many excellent sources for more in-depth coverage of these topics that are omitted (AHA, 2006; Topol, 2007).

The following sections focus on the most common, invasive treatments for coronary heart disease, arrhythmia, valve disease, and congestive heart failure. Treatments for each of these categories sometimes overlap, for example, open-heart surgery can be used to treat both coronary heart disease and valve disease. It is important to caution the reader that cardiologists always prefer to use preventive and noninvasive treatments over invasive treatments if possible, but these types of behavioral treatment (e.g., diet, exercise) are discussed in other chapters of this book.

Percutaneous Transluminal Coronary Angioplasty

Percutaneous transluminal coronary angioplasty (PTCA) is often referred to simply as angioplasty. About 640,000 people underwent PTCA in 2002 (AHA, 2005). PTCA always follows the diagnostic part of the procedure, the cardiac catheterization or coronary angiogram, when the narrowing of the coronary artery is identified. During PTCA, a balloon catheter is inserted into an artery through the groin and threaded into the coronary artery. Special dye or contrast material highlights obstructions in the vessel that are viewed by the physician on a monitor. A balloon in the catheter is inflated so as to flatten the plaque and improve blood flow. Almost 90% of PTCA procedures also place a stent (an alloyed metal mesh tube) designed to stay in place (similar to a scaffold) to keep the artery open after angioplasty (Anderson et al., 2002). In the 1990s, about 25% to 30% of stents were affected by restenosis (reclosing of the artery after angioplasty) within 6 months (Anderson et al., 2002). More recently, stents coated with time-release medications (drug-eluting stents) that reduce the risk of restenosis by 75% (Roy & Waksman, 2006) have been frequently used. As a result of these technological advances, the rate of coronary stent insertion increased dramatically in the late 1990s, and restenosis following stent placement became an exception rather than the norm. However, a long-term and unanticipated problem began to occur in some patients who received drug-eluting stents. At the site where the stent is placed, blood clot or thrombus formation was more likely to occur. Discussion and evaluation of the risks and benefits of the use of drug-eluting stents is ongoing (Tung, Kaul, Diamond, & Shah, 2006) at the time of this writing.

Patients enter the catheterization laboratory with either a scheduled angiogram to diagnose and treat coronary artery disease or an emergency procedure while the patient is having an MI. In the latter case, patients are diagnosed with MI in some other setting (often the emergency room) and transferred quickly to the catheterization laboratory to have an angioplasty that will open the vessel and mitigate as much damage to the heart muscle as possible.

Open-Heart Surgery

In 2002 there were over 700,000 open-heart surgery operations in the United States (AHA, 2005). The two major categories of open-heart surgery are coronary artery bypass graft operations, sometimes called CABG (pronounced "cabbage") or also called bypass surgery, and valve operations to repair or replace a valve. Although there are newer, less invasive surgical techniques, the majority of patients undergoing open-heart surgery have their sternum broken and recover from this major surgery, with a substantial zipper-type scar running down their chest. A period of postsurgical recovery time is required before normal daily activities can be resumed.

Coronary Artery Bypass Graft Surgery

CABG is the most commonly performed open-heart surgery in the United States, and 515,000 CABG operations were performed on 306,000 patients in 2002 in the United States (AHA, 2005). CABG is used to fix problems with the left main coronary artery, all three coronary arteries, and the left ventricle. CABG is so named because a vein from the leg (saphenous vein), one of the internal mammary arteries, or even an artery from the arm is grafted (attached) to the aorta and to the coronary arteries, beyond the blockage, to create a bypass to allow blood to flow around an obstruction to the heart. CABG surgeries take place either "on pump" or "off pump." On-pump surgery occurs when the heart is stopped, and a cardiopulmonary bypass (CPB) pump, or heart–lung machine, oxygenates blood and reinfuses it into the patient's body. Off-pump surgery occurs when the cardiac surgeon operates on the beating heart (AHA, 2006).

During on-pump CABG surgery, the heart is stopped, and a CPB pump takes over the function of the heart and lungs temporarily. A complication of this procedure is postperfusion syndrome, sometimes called *pump head*. Postperfusion syndrome is characterized by memory problems, confusion, speech problems, and psychological symptoms, but these are typically transient and not evident at 1-year postsurgery (van Dijk et al., 2002).

Valve Repair or Replacement

There are three common valve repairs and replacements: mitral valve repair, mitral valve replacement, and aortic valve replacement. These accounted for about 93,000 open-heart valve surgeries in 2002 (AHA, 2005). Mitral valve repair refers to any of a variety of surgeries to fix rather than replace the malfunctioning valve. Valves that are stenotic can be treated with valvuloplasty in the cardiac catheterization laboratory, whereby a balloon catheter is threaded through the valve and expanded to stretch it open. Regurgitating valves are sometimes repaired with simple sutures (stitches). The decision on whether to replace or repair a faulty mitral valve is based on the etiology and severity of the problem and the relative merits of each treatment approach. If mitral valve replacement is decided on, a prosthetic (artificial) valve is used to repair the mitral valve. Both mechanical valves and biological valves, primarily made from pig aortas or cow pericardium (heart muscle), are used for mitral valve replacements. The aortic valve is almost always replaced rather than repaired, with either a mechanical or biological valve. Biological aortic valves are most often made from pig aortic valves or from cow pericardium but can also be retrieved from human cadavers and sometimes, but not often, the patients' own pulmonary valve (AHA, 2006).

Treatment for Arrhythmia

There are two main types of nonmedication treatments for arrhythmia: implantation of a device or a surgical procedure. The two main categories of device are pacemaker and implantable cardioverter defibrillator.

Pacemaker

A pacemaker is a small, electronic device that is implanted into the body to treat bradycardia. The pacemaker has a pulse generator and one or two leads. The pulse generator contains a battery that supplies electrical energy and circuitry that produces electrical impulses to make the heart beat (pacing). A single-chamber pacemaker has one lead, an insulated wire placed in the right atrium or right ventricle, and is connected to the pulse generator. A dual-chamber pacemaker has two leads, one placed in the right atrium and the other in the right ventricle. The pacemaker functions to sense whether the heart is beating too slowly or pausing too long between beats, and the device sends electrical impulses to stimulate the heart to contract. Impulses from the pacemaker are too mild to be sensed by the patient with the device (AHA, 2006).

Implantable Cardioverter Defibrillator

An implantable cardioverter defibrillator (ICD) is similar to a pacemaker in that it is a small electronic computer device implanted into the body below the collarbone but is used primarily to treat ventricular tachycardia and ventricular fibrillation. Similar to the pacemaker, the ICD also has a pulse generator and one, two, or three leads. A biventricular ICD has three leads placed in the right atrium, right ventricle, and left ventricle. An ICD can deliver mild electrical impulses that may not be felt or may feel like fluttering in the chest. However, when arrhythmias do not respond to mild pacing impulses, the ICD delivers one or more electrical shocks to the heart that may feel like getting hit or knocked in the chest; this is called cardioversion. If the ICD detects a severe and dangerous arrhythmia such as ventricular fibrillation, it will deliver a high-energy shock that may feel like getting kicked in the chest or cause unconsciousness. The ICD stores information about electrical activity of the heart, and this information can be downloaded by the physician over the telephone.

On average, people with ICDs get shocked about twice a year (Godemann et al., 2004b; Sears & Conti, 2003). An ICD "storm" occurs when an ICD fires more than twice in a 24-hour period (AHA, 2006). At least 150,000 people had an ICD implanted in 2006, and more than 500,000 were living with an ICD (AHA, 2005).

Catheter Ablation

During catheter ablation, an electrode catheter is inserted into a vein or artery (most often through the groin) and threaded to the place where the abnormal electrical pathway occurs. Radio-frequency energy is passed through the catheter, causing the tip to heat up and destroy (ablate) the cells causing the arrhythmia and causing a scar that will no longer transmit electrical impulses. People who are at severe risk for sudden cardiac death may be treated with both catheter ablation and ICD (AHA, 2006).

Heart Transplant

Patients with end-stage heart disease sometimes become candidates for heart transplant. About 2,000 heart transplants are performed annually in the United States, and the average survival time is about 10 years (AHA, 2005), but in 2004 there were more than 3,300 patients on a waiting list to receive a heart transplant. The demand for donor hearts far outweighs the supply. In recent years, the development of ventricular assist devices, the improvements in pharmacotherapy, and the advent of the artificial heart have led to the hope that every patient who is in need of heart transplant will one day have the opportunity to be helped through one or more of these treatments. Heart transplant recipients are predominantly male (72.5%) and White (70%), and nearly half (47%) are between age 50 and 64 (United Network for Organ Sharing, 2007).

SUMMARY

Cardiovascular disease is the leading cause of death among men and women across all ethnicities in the United States (AHA, 2005). The prevalence of heart disease escalates dramatically with age. Between the ages of 55 and 64, 21% of men and 9% of women have cardiovascular disease. By the ages of 65 to 74, those proportions increase to 35% and 20% for men and women, respectively, and between the ages of 85 and 94, 74% of men and 65% of women have cardiovascular disease (AHA, 2005). David Waters, retired chief of cardiology at San Francisco General Hospital in California, explained, "We have managed to push coronary disease back into older age ranges, and the average heart attack is milder, and carries a much better prognosis than in years past" (personal communication, February 1, 2007). New technology to treat cardiovascular disease is being developed every day. Despite this, heart disease continues to be the most pressing public health problem facing our country. The contribution of psychological factors to the development and prognosis of heart disease is strikingly evident and the potential for intervention is ripe.

2

RISK FACTORS AND PERCEPTIONS OF RISK FOR CARDIOVASCULAR DISEASE

Modifiable risk factors for heart disease are factors that can be changed. They include high cholesterol, cigarette smoking, hypertension, diabetes, obesity (especially abdominal obesity), and metabolic syndrome. Although psychological factors are also known to incur risk for cardiovascular disease, these are addressed in detail in Part II of this book and are thus not covered in this chapter. Nonmodifiable risk factors for heart disease include older age, male gender, family history, and genetic vulnerability (Topol, 2007). It is important to be aware of both types of risk factors when working with a cardiac population, but behavioral health clinicians typically focus on modifiable risk factors in clinical practice. An overview of each risk factor follows.

CHOLESTEROL

Cholesterol is a fat that the body needs to make cell walls, brain tissue, hormones, and many other substances. Cholesterol and other fats of lipids are transported in the blood with proteins, forming lipoprotein particles. High-density lipoprotein (HDL), the so-called good cholesterol, helps to carry fat and cholesterol away from the artery to the liver. Low-density lipoprotein (LDL), or the bad cholesterol, deposits cholesterol in the arteries. Total cholesterol above 240 milligrams per deciliter (mg/dL) and LDL above 160 mg/dL are considered to be high. Excess LDL cholesterol causes coronary heart disease (CHD) when lipid deposits build up on the walls of the arteries and the resulting plaque begins to obstruct the artery and lies dormant, at risk for rupture (Rader, 2007).

TOBACCO USE/CIGARETTE SMOKING

Cigarette smoking and tobacco smoking using pipes and cigars cause ischemic heart disease because they increase heart rate and blood pressure. The carbon monoxide from cigarette smoke makes blood thicker and more prone to clotting. Smoking damages the endothelial lining of the arteries and decreases oxygen to the heart. Smoking interacts synergistically with other risk factors to incur greater risk for heart disease (Critchley & Capewell, 2003). The topic of cigarette smoking and smoking cessation is important for clinicians working in behavioral cardiology and is covered in detail in chapter 10 of this volume.

HYPERTENSION

Hypertension or high blood pressure is the most common risk factor for heart disease. Blood pressure rises when the heart contracts (systole) and falls when the heart relaxes (diastole). Blood pressure is measured with the top number referring to systolic pressure and the bottom number referring to diastolic pressure. Systolic pressure is recorded as the force of the tension on the walls of the arteries when the heart contracts, and diastolic pressure is recorded as the force of the tension on the walls of the arteries when the heart relaxes between contractions. Normal blood pressure is below 120/70 millimeters of mercury (mm HG); in adults, hypertension is characterized by blood pressure that is higher than 140/90 mm HG. Systolic blood pressure is more closely related to the development of cardiovascular disease than diastolic blood pressure. Hypertension causes CHD because blood vessels with blood flowing through at chronically high rates of pressure are more likely to weaken and rupture and to develop obstructions (Henri & Rudd, 2007).

DIABETES MELLITUS

Diabetes mellitus is a problem of glucose (sugar) metabolism. The pancreas makes the hormone insulin to help glucose enter the body's cells. People who have diabetes do not produce enough insulin, cannot use the insulin efficiently (insulin resistance), or both, and this causes blood glucose to become too high (hyperglycemia). Diabetes has a damaging effect on both big blood vessels (macrovascular disease) and small blood vessels (microvascular disease). People with diabetes are more likely to have atherosclerosis in multiple blood vessels as opposed to a single vessel, more likely to have plaque rupture, and more likely to also have thrombosis in conjunction with these other problems. In addition, people with diabetes often have other risk factors for heart disease (e.g., high cholesterol, obesity, hypertension) that interact with the diabetes to increase risk for heart disease (Aronson & Rayfield, 2007).

OBESITY AND OVERWEIGHT

Excess body fat, particularly abdominal obesity, is associated with greater risk of cardiovascular disease. Being overweight is associated with other cardiac risk factors such as increased blood pressure, high LDL cholesterol and triglyceride levels (triglyceride is the form in which most fat exists in the body), and lowered HDL cholesterol. Obesity is the primary risk factor for the development of adult-onset diabetes. Excess body weight is primarily attributable to both sedentary behavior and poor nutrition. Sedentary lifestyle also makes an independent contribution to increased risk for diabetes, hypertension, and hyperlipidemia.

SEDENTARY BEHAVIOR

Moderate exercise (60% to 75% of age-predicted maximum heart rate) improves functional capacity (Leon et al., 2005). Sedentary lifestyle dramatically increases risk for CHD (Pate et al., 1995). Moderate activity (e.g., walking 6 miles per week) or climbing stairs reduces risk for heart disease (Blair et al., 1995), yet fewer than 20% of adults meet the Healthy People 2000 definition for regular, sustained physical activity of 30 minutes or more of moderate activity per day for at least 5 days a week (Brownson, Jones, Pratt, Blanton, & Heath, 2000). There are numerous programs that are appropriate for adults with orthopedic problems, postangioplasty, exercise-induced ischemia, heart failure, and claudication (Thompson, 2005). The problem, however, is not that safe, effective programs are not available but that people in general are very sedentary. Reasons people give for not exercising include low motivation, no support from family or friends, inconvenience, time constraints, and family or job responsibilities (Mak, Chan, & Yue, 2005; R. Mitchell, Muggli, & Sato, 1999; Sniehotta, Scholz, & Schwarzer, 2006). In addition, poor psychological health and low self-efficacy are associated

TABLE 2.1
Guidelines for Cardiac Risk Factors

Measure	Good	Moderate risk	High risk
Blood pressure (mm Hg)	120/80		
Body mass index (BMI)	18.5–24.9	25–29.9	30+
Total cholesterol (mg/dL)	<200	200–239	240+
LDL cholesterol (mg/dL)	<100	100–129	130+
HDL cholesterol (mg/dL)	60+	50–60	<50 women <40 men
Tryglycerides (mg/dL)	<150	150–199	200+
Glucose (mg/dL)	<100	100–120	120+
C-reactive protein (mg/dL)	<1	1–3	3+
Ejection fraction	50+	<50	

with an inability to adopt an exercise regimen (Dornelas, Swencionis, & Wylie-Rosett, 1994).

METABOLIC SYNDROME

When three or more of the following—large waist circumference >35 inches, high triglyceride levels >150 mg/dL, low HDL levels <50 mg/dL in women and <40 mg/dL in men, high blood pressure >130/85 mmHg, or high fasting glucose level >100 mg/dL—are clustered together, the effect is called *metabolic syndrome*. Metabolic syndrome is a clustering of risk factors associated with increased risk for diabetes and cardiovascular disease (Gami et al., 2007). Table 2.1 lists the guidelines for cardiac risk factors.

OTHER MARKERS OF CARDIOVASCULAR DISEASE

Other markers of cardiovascular disease that can be measured by blood test include the following: C-reactive protein, an indicator of inflammation; homocysteine, an amino acid that can be associated with thickening of the endothelium (arterial lining); fibrinogen, blood protein that is important for clotting; and lipoprotein A, a blood lipid that impairs the ability to dissolve clots (Topol, 2007).

PERCEPTIONS OF RISK FOR CHD

High cholesterol, hypertension, diabetes, smoking, and obesity substantially increase risk for heart disease, but usually people do not think of themselves at being at high risk for CHD because of these factors. In general, people are not very good at correctly estimating their risk for any disease. Risk perceptions are influenced by both thoughts and emotions. In terms of numerical calculations, researchers calculate risk perceptions in either relative (one's own risk compared with another person of same age and gender) or absolute (a quantitative assessment of one's personal likelihood of developing a specific disease) numbers. Relative personal risk assessments are generally thought to be more accurate because the person must consider the risk status of others of the same age and sex, compared with him- or herself (Weinstein, 1982). For example, "Do you think that you have the same, more, or less risk of heart disease as another woman your age?" However, both (relative and absolute) ways of asking about perceptions of risk are important, because each can yield information about educational deficits. For example, a person might accurately state that he or she is at greater risk for a heart attack than another person of the same age and sex but still minimizes his or her overall risk if the person is not aware of the prevalence of heart disease.

One out of two people will die from heart disease, but most people worry little about this. In general, people may have what researchers have termed an *optimistic bias* about their own personal risk. People with an optimistic bias acknowledge some risk and believe the rest of the population does face that risk, but they minimize the relevance of perceived personal risk for themselves (Weinstein, 1998). For example, smokers represent a patient population at elevated risk for heart disease, yet smokers typically underestimate their risk for all diseases, including CHD (Weinstein, 1998). Similarly, people with previous cardiac events also underestimate their risk for heart disease, especially when compared with the estimates provided by their physicians (Bjerrum, Hamm, Toft, Munck, & Kragstrup, 2002). A number of elements influence risk perception, including family history, first-hand experience, and age.

Even though family history is highly correlated with perceptions of personal risk, it is not necessarily correlated with an accurate perception of risk among people with heart disease. Among adult children of people with diagnosed premature CHD, approximately half (47%) still underestimated their relative risk of developing heart disease, compared with other people of the same age (Allen & Blumenthal, 1998), and only 28% correctly identified heredity as a risk for heart disease. However, people perceive themselves as being at higher risk when they have first-hand experience of knowing someone having the disease, the *friend factor* (DiLorenzo et al., 2006; Montgomery, Erblich, DiLorenzo, & Bovbjerg, 2003). The friend factor seemingly operates through a process whereby events that are more salient and familiar (i.e., more easily recalled) are judged as being more likely to occur (Rees et al., 2001). For example, younger people are more likely to overestimate their risk for traffic accidents compared with older people, possibly because of greater exposure to peers who have been in motor vehicle accidents (Tamura &

Kawata, 1997). Similarly, younger people are more likely to underestimate their risk for future diseases (Tamura & Kawata, 1997).

Clinical Example

Jane was a 52-year-old, trim, active legal secretary in good health, except for a 20-year, one-pack-per-day smoking habit. She had been married for nearly a quarter of a century to an affable insurance underwriter about her age. Their children were in their 20s. She lived a highly pressured life working for a prestigious law firm, but she had a strong bond with her boss and supportive relationships with her peers at work. Jane took a kickboxing class twice a week and was active in local politics. On a warm day in the summer, she waited in line with her husband to see a movie matinee. She felt somewhat nauseous and dizzy but attributed this to the unusually warm weather and crowds in the theater. She said nothing to her husband, assuming that these ill feelings would pass. As they sat eating popcorn and watching the coming attractions, she felt distinctly ill with tightness in her neck and jaw. The sensations worsened, and she told her husband but minimized the import, not wanting to cause him to leave the movie early. Jane waited a long time before finally admitting that she needed to go to the hospital. No one was more surprised than she to find that she had had a heart attack. As the physicians questioned her, it became clear that she had ignored prior signs of dizziness, shortness of breath, and neck pain. Her mother had died of heart disease at age 60, and Jane herself was a long-time smoker. Despite all this, she had little sense that she was at risk for heart disease.

Why would a bright, otherwise assertive woman try to wait until the film was over before seeking treatment for a heart attack? One interpretation is that the patient is experiencing a form of self-protective denial, and the topic of cardiac denial is discussed later in this book. However, people generally do not seem to have an accurate handle on risk. They either over- or underestimate risk for disease. Both men and women seem to similarly misperceive personal risk for disease. Wilcox and Stephanik (1999) measured middle-aged women's risk perceptions about CHD and breast, colon, and lung cancers for both men and women. Ironically, women were more accurate in estimating the leading causes of mortality in men than they were in women! About 6 out of 10 women think that they are at greater risk for cancer than heart disease. Only 8% of women correctly identify cardiovascular disease as the leading cause of death in women (Roberts, 2004). This information has led to a wave of public health campaigns dedicated to improving public awareness in this area.

The large public education campaign launched by the National Heart, Lung, and Blood Institute, the American Heart Association, the National Coalition for Women With Heart Disease, and other public health groups has sought media attention to bring greater awareness about the risk for heart disease among women and the importance of physical activity and heart-healthy nutrition. This educational campaign provides a great deal of information that clinicians can use to help in the education of women about their risk for cardiovascular illness. Underlying the educational campaign is the assumption that if people have a heightened awareness of risk, this will translate into behavioral change such that they will begin to take preventive measures against heart disease.

Other public education campaigns (e.g., to wear seatbelts) have been effective in increasing the desired behaviors. The difference, however, is that those campaigns have focused on a single, circumscribed behavior that is easy to dichotomize. Either one wears a seatbelt or one does not. In the case of heart disease, the number of interrelated risk factors and the distal perception of the disease usually lead to a sense of complacency in the general public. From the perspective of the medical professional, general adherence to recommendations from the health care provider leaves much to be desired.

ADHERENCE

Nonadherence to medication and lifestyle change is a major reason for frequent hospitalizations and worsening of cardiac disease (van der Wal et al., 2006). For example, patients with congestive heart failure are typically asked to take medications as prescribed, follow a low-sodium diet, and exercise according to nationally recommended guidelines. This would be a tall order for most people under the best of circumstances. However, people with heart failure are, by definition, chronically ill, often suffer from financial constraints that make it difficult to pay for prescriptions, and may have cognitive impairment as a result of aging, progression of heart failure, or both. Patients may be compliant with some aspects of treatment but not others. For example, a person may have extreme difficulty following a low-sodium diet but be successful at walking regularly and stopping smoking. Therefore, assessing the level of adherence to each particular treatment regimen is critical, rather than giving a patient the general label of "nonadherent."

Adherence has often been studied in the context of cardiac rehabilitation. The primary problem related to cardiac rehabilitation is that it is vastly underused, with fewer than 20% of eligible patients actually attending such a program (Leon et al., 2005). There are many reasons for this. Women, older adults, and racial or ethnic minority patients are less likely to attend cardiac rehabilitation (Cooper, Jackson, Weinman, & Horne, 2002). There are low referral rates for programs, some programs are inaccessible to patients in terms of geographic location, and third-party payers often do not adequately reimburse for services (Cooper et al., 2002; Lane, Carroll, Ring, Beevers, & Lip, 2001b). People who are depressed or poorly motivated are also less likely to attend cardiac rehabilitation and more likely to drop out after they start (Linden, 2000). Because most cardiac rehabilitation programs have the potential to be a strong referral source for behavioral health clinicians, it is useful to have a theoretical framework for understanding how people make the complex decision to stick with or drop out of mainstream treatments such as cardiac rehabilitation.

THE TRANSTHEORETICAL MODEL

A framework for understanding how people change behavior is found in the transtheoretical model (Prochaska & DiClemente, 1983; Prochaska, DiClemente, & Norcross, 1992). The transtheoretical model integrates motivational, cognitive, and behavioral domains to explain the process by which people implement intentional behavioral change, whether the desired outcome is to stop smoking, increase exercise, make dietary change, or some other behavior. The transtheoretical model is a paradigm that can be used to explain how people effect behavior change on their own, and the model suggests that interventions that are matched to the appropriate stage of change will be more effective than behavioral interventions that are applied without regard for the individual's readiness to change.

The transtheoretical model suggests that behavior change involves a progression through five stages over time.

1. *Precontemplation:* A stage in which the individual has no intention of making any behavior change in the foreseeable future, measured as a 6-month period. Individuals in this category may be those who are termed by the provider as being unwilling or resistant to change.
2. *Contemplation:* A stage in which people report that they intend to make a behavior change within the next 6 months. People in the contemplation stage are typically ambivalent in terms of being aware of both the necessity for change and the difficulties in carrying out the change in question.
3. *Preparation:* A stage in which the individual intends to make a change within the immediate future and certainly within the next 30 days. These individuals are those who are on the brink of change and may have sought out methods to help prepare for the change to come, for example, by enrolling in a smoking cessation group or joining a gym.
4. *Action:* A stage in which the person has been actively making a behavior change for less than 6 months. Reaching the action stage requires a specific criterion; for example, cutting back on cigarettes is not enough, complete abstinence is necessary in the action stage. Thus, as must be evident, many

people may cycle between contemplation, preparation, and action as they make an effort to substantively increase their physical activity, change their diet, or stop smoking, enough to reach a desired criterion.

5. *Maintenance:* A stage in which the individual has achieved the behavior change for at least 6 months. People in this category may continue to struggle to prevent relapse or might feel secure in having been successful at making a permanent behavioral or lifestyle change.

If we use dietary sodium as an example, patients who report that they are not considering reducing sodium are at the precontemplation stage. Those who are ambivalent but seriously considering reducing sodium in the next 6 months are at the contemplation stage. Patients who are actively trying to cut back are at the preparation stage. Those who are keeping their sodium intake at the recommended level are at the action stage. Only a minority of people are in the maintenance stage with respect to dietary sodium!

Although the stages of change are hypothesized to occur in sequence, the model has been often depicted as a spiral rather than a linear progression, with expected setbacks and regressions to earlier stages. The developers of the model suggest that most people make multiple attempts at behavioral change before changing for good and that even when attempts at change do not succeed, something is learned each time that will ultimately prove helpful when the individual makes the next attempt. Motivation and confidence (also called self-efficacy) increase at each stage, suggesting that therapists should tailor their approach according to the patient's readiness to change (DiClemente et al., 1991; Prochaska & DiClemente, 1984). For example, precontemplators who are not thinking about making a change will benefit more from an approach that establishes rapport and plants a seed rather than frank discussion of actual behavioral change strategies. An individual who is contemplating change may benefit most from a motivational approach that addresses his or her ambivalence about change. A person in the preparation stage can gain far more from discussion of behavioral interventions (e.g., joining a smoking cessation program) than will a person who is in the precontemplation or contemplation stage. An individual who is actively making behavior change can be helped through support and techniques to achieve the desired criterion (e.g., keeping a food diary or exercising with a partner). Finally, the person in the maintenance stage may need coaching to prevent relapse, particularly during times of stress.

One of the more poignant public examples of vulnerability to relapse under stress, even after a long period of maintenance, came from ABC news anchor Peter Jennings, who had stopped smoking in the 1980s. After he received a diagnosis of lung cancer in April 2005, Jennings reported that he had relapsed to smoking after the terrorist attacks on the United States on

September 11, 2001. When asked to describe Jennings's finest hour, Michael Clemente, former senior writer and producer for *World News Tonight With Peter Jennings*, said, "I guess 9/11 because he was involved in about four days straight full coverage." Clemente added later in the interview, "I helped convince him to go to a hypnotist in the mid-1980s so he could quit and he did, until 9/11 happened and he slowly drifted back into it." Jennings died in August 2005 of lung cancer (Clemente, 2005).

Many people who work in the behavioral sciences are familiar with the stages of change, but the transtheoretical model also identifies *processes of change*, or mechanisms that people use to change behavior. The processes of change underscore the importance of emotional arousal, alteration in the environment, supportive relationships, cognitions, and behavioral reinforcement as some of the dimensions that are critical in helping people to be successful in intentional behavioral change. The transtheoretical model is introduced in this chapter because it is relevant to all of the modifiable risk factors for cardiovascular disease discussed in the chapter. The transtheoretical model is also easily incorporated into many psychotherapeutic approaches and thus is helpful in matching a therapeutic intervention to a patient's readiness to change.

3

EMOTIONS AND THE HEART

How is it that human beings seem to universally agree that emotions are experienced by the heart? Can people die of a broken heart? Phrases such as "absence makes the heart grow fonder" (love), "heart in my throat" (fear), "to my heart's content" (joy), "a bitter heart" (anger), "broken heart" (grief), and "heart of stone" (devoid of feeling) make the point that people have long recognized that emotions seem to be felt by the heart. Human behaviors also seem to indicate that the heart is somehow linked to the strongest intensity of emotion, as evidenced by placing the hand over the heart while pledging allegiance or singing the national anthem. Despite the abundance of these phrases in colloquial language and references linking emotion to the heart from some of the earliest published literature, it is only in more recent decades that scientists from a variety of disciplines have made more progress in understanding the mind–body connection. Before examining the relationship between affect and the cardiovascular system, this chapter first discusses how emotions are processed in the brain.

The nascent field of affective science (Ekman & Davidson, 1994) has the potential to greatly influence the direction of research in the field of behavioral cardiology. The understanding of emotion took a leap forward with the publication of an article by Antonio Damasio (2001) called "Fundamental Feelings" in the journal *Nature*. In this article, Damasio advanced the understanding of the difference between emotion and feeling. *Affect* is an umbrella term that has been used synonymously with both emotion and feeling. However, emotions have been differentiated from feelings. According to a growing body of research by Damasio and others, emotions are automatic responses of the body to a stimulus, for example, quickening of the heart in anger or the flush of the skin in shame. Feelings are the "mental representations of the physiological changes that characterize emotions" (Damasio, 2001, p. 781). As automatic bodily reactions, emotions are unconscious, whereas feelings are the conscious perceptions of emotions. Human beings are evolutionarily determined to respond to certain stimuli with a particular emotional response (e.g., physiological arousal indicating fear in response to threatening stimulus). Although I use the terms *emotion, feeling,* and *affect* interchangeably in this book, it is with the understanding that emotional responses are manifested in bodily response, often without conscious awareness. Emotional experience reflects multiple systems of the body responding together. As the neuroscience of emotion has evolved, it has become increasingly evident that emotions are not "in the head" and that affects, cognitions, and bodily responses take place through interrelated and connected neural circuits (R. J. Davidson, 2003c). Most clinicians are aware that emotions generate response from the sympathetic nervous system.

CENTRAL NERVOUS SYSTEM

The central nervous system controls a number of automatic processes, including breathing, heart beat, digestion, and so on. It communicates through either hormonal or electrical impulses. The autonomic nervous system is ideally balanced between the functions of the sympathetic nervous system, which generates the stress response, and the parasympathetic nervous system, which generates the relaxation response.

Emotional arousal has long been associated with increased sympathetic activity, which is often referred to as the *fight-or-flight* response first described by Walter Cannon (1929). In response to a trigger, this physiological response pattern occurs when blood pressure, heart rate, glucose levels, adrenaline, oxygen circulation to vital organs, and blood clotting increase through activation of the hypothalamus and hypothalamic-pituitary-adrenal (HPA) axis. Activation of the HPA axis leads to the release of stress hormones such as cortisol and epinephrine (adrenaline) as well as the release of neurotransmitters such as dopamine, which are associated with depression. Hans Selye (1956) described the general adaptation syndrome model, a theory that describes how stress negatively affects the body. In short, this model argues that when levels of stress hormones such as cortisol are chronically high, the net effect can increase blood pressure, triglyceride, and low density lipoprotein, or LDL, cholesterol levels.

Parasympathetic innervation of the heart is mediated by the vagus nerve, the cranial nerve that starts in the brainstem and extends down through the chest and abdomen. The right vagus stimulates the sinoatrial node. When the vagus nerve is activated, heart rate and blood pressure can be reduced. Chronic sympathetic arousal is associated with impaired vagal control, which later research has shown incurs increased risk for cardiac events (Carney et al., 1988; Rozanski, Krantz, & Bairey, 1991). In sum, substantial evidence exists that negative affect appears to put the sympathetic nervous system in a permanent state of red alert, which can wear down the cardiovascular system. However, as neuroscience has developed greater understanding of emotional states and brain response, a more nuanced understanding of individual variation in emotional arousal has developed.

EMOTIONS AND THE BRAIN

Although both halves of the cerebral cortex process emotions and motivation, the right side is more active in response to sadness, whereas the left side is more active in response to happiness (R. J. Davidson, 2004b). In addition, the right side of the cerebral cortex is more involved in what researchers have termed *withdraw* motivation, whereas the left side is more active during *approach* motivation (Harmon-Jones, 2003; Selye, 1956). The carrot and the stick is a metaphor for approach–avoid motivation. Approach motivation refers to the direction of behavior toward positive stimuli (objects, events, possibilities), whereas avoidance motivation is the direction of behavior away from negative stimuli (objects, events, possibilities; Elliot, 2006).

There is a vast literature showing that there are specific regions of the brain that distinguish between emotions and regions that modulate intensity of emotional response (R. J. Davidson & Irwin, 1999). A few selected examples are provided to illustrate this point. In a laboratory study, the emotions of happiness, sadness, and disgust were elicited from participants by film and recall. Recalled sadness was associated with increased activation in the anterior insula, whereas happiness was distinguished from sadness by greater activity in the vicinity of the ventral medial frontal cortex (Lane, Reiman, Ahern, Schwartz, & Davidson, 1997). Laboratory studies of college students who listened to music that increased positive affect showed greater left-sided activation of the prefrontal cortex (W. S. Kim, Yoon, Kim, Jho, & Lee, 2003). In an article called "Making a Life Worth Living: Neural Correlates of Well-Being," greater levels of *eudaimonic* well-being (defined as autonomy, mastery, personal growth, positive relationships with others, purpose in life, self-acceptance) and *hedonic* well-being (defined as the frequent experience of positive affect, life satisfaction, infrequent negative emotions, and satisfaction with important domains such as work or family) were associated with greater left than right superior frontal activation of the prefrontal cortex (Urry et al., 2004).

If greater levels of left-sided activation are associated with higher levels of psychological well-being, then it follows that attachment might be reflected by differential patterns of responses in specific regions of the brain as well. Babies who cry when their mothers leave show greater levels of left prefrontal activation compared with babies who do not cry after maternal separation (R. J. Davidson & Fox, 1989). Among adults, similar findings emerge. In a study with 20 female subjects, researchers asked participants to think about—or stop thinking about—positive and negative relationship scenarios. During negative scenarios (e.g., conflict, breakup, death of partner), level of attachment anxiety was positively correlated with activation in the anterior temporal pole, which is more active when sadness is experienced. Attachment anxiety was inversely correlated with activation in a region associated with emotion regulation (orbitofrontal cortex). This study provides neurobiological evidence that people with an anxious attachment style react more strongly to thoughts of loss and have more difficulty regulating their negative emotions compared with those with less anxious attachment styles (Gillath, Bunge, Shaver, Wendelken, & Mikulincer, 2005). Overall, evidence is emerging that there are differential neural activation patterns in response to healthy attachment compared with poor attachments (Noriuchi, Kikuchi, & Senoo, 2007).

All emotions have evolutionary value. Emotions play a key role in motivating people and helping to discern which environmental features are salient and which to ignore. Positive emotions help guide people in determining what they should do (approach motivation), whereas negative emotions help the individual gauge what *not* to do (avoidance motivation; Klein, 2002). However, even the terminology of *positive* and *negative* emotion may be a bit misleading. In a related line of research from the psychotherapy literature, theorist Leigh McCullough described anger as an activating (approach) emotion that energizes and stimulates greater levels of activity as opposed to an inhibiting (avoidance) emotion such as fear (McCullough et al., 2003). Although anger is often thought to be a negative affect, it is associated with greatly increased motivation and greater levels of left-sided prefrontal activation (Harmon-Jones, 2003). Why should the relationship between emotional states and differential activation of brain regions matter to psychotherapists? The lessons from neuropsychology are particularly encouraging in this regard. Strong arguments have been made that the brain can be trained to experience positive emotions more frequently and for longer duration (Klein, 2002). In other words, people can learn to become happier. This line of neurobiology research provides support to those psychotherapists who propose that emotional activation is a primary catalyst of psychological change (Greenberg & Pascual-Leone, 2006; Johnson & Greenman, 2006; Magnavita, 2006; McCullough et al., 2003).

AFFECTIVE STYLE AND BRAIN PLASTICITY

Clinicians often observe that clients vary widely in their sensitivity to emotional stimuli. A substantial part of this individual variance in affective style is reflected in differential neurobiological response to emotional stimuli. The time that it takes for the brain to respond to affective cues, the magnitude and duration of the response, and the time it takes to recover from emotional arousal are largely attributable to individual differences in neurobiology (R. J. Davidson, 2003c). Neuropsychologist Richard Davidson, from the University of Wisconsin–Madison, has reviewed many years of research from his and other laboratories and examined the results of neuroimaging and psychophysiological measures and studies of individuals of different ages ranging from early childhood to old age. The majority of studies reflect that a resilient affective style is associated with high levels of left prefrontal activation, ability to modulate activity in the amygdala, and quick recovery from negative emotions and stressful events. A resilient affective style is also associated with lower levels of stress hormones such as cortisol and better immune response (R. J. Davidson, 2003b, 2004a).

Perhaps the most exciting aspect of work in this area is the implication that neural circuitry can be shaped by experiences that might potentially promote a more resilient, positive affective style (R. J. Davidson, 2003a). Preliminary research indicates both that people can be trained to experience more positive feelings and that this experience can be measured in terms of activation of the left prefrontal cortex, as well as in terms of markers of immune response. For example, one of Davidson's studies was designed such that 25 participants were randomly assigned to a mindfulness meditation group or to a wait-list control condition. Participants who learned to meditate had significant increases in left-sided anterior activation of the brain (the region associated with positive emotion) and also had greater increases in immune response, as measured by antibody titers to influenza vaccine (R. J. Davidson et al., 2003). This line of research gives psychotherapists strong reasons to consider how one might work with emotions more effectively in therapy. However, what is the evidence that emotions are specifically linked to cardiovascular response?

EMOTIONS AND CARDIOVASCULAR ACTIVATION

The sympathetic and parasympathetic branches of the autonomic nervous system connect the neural pathways between the brain and the heart to mediate cardiovascular response. Cardiovascular response is measured in terms of multiple parameters, including heart rate (number of beats per minute), systolic and diastolic blood pressure, contractility of the myocardium (calculation of the maximum diastole to the maximum systole), stroke volume

(volume of blood pumped per beat), and cardiac output (stroke volume multiplied by heart rate). In turn, these measures reflect multiple physiological indices, including respiration level, vagal activation, sympathetic activation, physical activity levels, and circadian (day–night) rhythm. When heart rate increases, total cardiac output increases.

Emotions affect the heart with distinct patterns of physiological response (Rainville, Bechara, Naqvi, & Damasio, 2006). Anger produces greater increases in diastolic pressure and heart rate and slower recovery of systolic pressure following exercise. Sadness produces systolic pressure and heart rate changes and is the one emotional state that interferes with the cardiovascular adjustments normally associated with exercise (Schwartz, Weinberger, & Singer, 1981). Anger, compared with joy, fear, and sadness, shows the largest effect on the cardiovascular system. Sadness produces decreases in cardiac output (Sinha, Lovallo, & Parsons, 1992) as does fear, whereas anger produces increases in cardiac output (Montoya, Campos, & Schandry, 2005).

When people with social phobia are asked to give a public speech, their anxiety is evident through right-sided cortical activation as well as increased heart rate (R. J. Davidson, Marshall, Tomarken, & Henriques, 2000). Two-year-olds given challenging tasks that are designed to elicit negative emotions show increased heart rate and other markers of cardiovascular response (K. A. Buss, Goldsmith, & Davidson, 2005). Depression can trigger increased heart rate and reduce heart rate variability in cardiac patients (Carney et al., 2003, 2007). Frasure-Smith and colleagues found that depressed post–myocardial infarction (MI) patients with more than 10 premature ventricular contractions (PVCs) per hour were 60% more likely to die within 18 months after MI than depressed patients with fewer PVCs (Frasure-Smith, Lesperance, & Talajic, 1995a). Serious arrhythmias can be triggered more easily in people who are depressed (Musselman, Evans, & Nemeroff, 1998; Nemeroff, Musselman, & Evans, 1998). A large study of 2,627 postmenopausal women enrolled in the Women's Health Initiative observational study confirmed that the association with depression and heart rate variability also holds true for healthy women without cardiac disease. Women with depressive symptoms showed significant reductions in heart rate variability and higher heart rates compared with nondepressed participants (C. K. Kim et al., 2005). Using functional magnetic resonance imaging to scan both the heart and the brain at the same time, University of Wisconsin researcher Kim Dalton and colleagues showed that high levels of anxiety were associated with both greater activation in brain regions associated with negative emotion and increased cardiac contractility (Dalton, Kalin, Grist, & Davidson, 2005).

Feelings of love, warmth, and affection are also manifested in the body through endocrine changes (increases in oxytocin) and cardiovascular response. Most of the research in this field has focused on the detrimental effects of social isolation as a risk factor for morbidity and mortality. Even when disease severity, demographic factors, and psychological distress are controlled, people with heart disease who are more socially isolated have far greater risk of dying from cardiovascular disease or any other cause than those with a stronger network of support (Brummett et al., 2001). However, this begs the question "do warm and affectionate ties actually improve heart health"? Preliminary research in this area suggests that the study of attachment and positive emotion will be a fruitful area of focus for future behavioral cardiology researchers. In a study of 183 cohabitating couples, those who were randomized to receive a warm hug prior to a public speaking task had lower blood pressure and heart rate compared with those who had no contact (Grewen, Anderson, Girdler, & Light, 2003). Warm contact presumably elicits feelings of affection and love and lowers blood pressure and heart rate (Light, Grewen, & Amico, 2005). Many years of animal research on rats, primates, prairie voles, and other mammals have shown that caretaking and attachment behaviors are reliably associated with favorable neurobiological effects on the cardiovascular system (Insel & Young, 2001). Although pleasurable feelings such as happiness, joy, love, and affection have been less studied (perhaps because positive emotions are more difficult to reliably produce in laboratory settings), the existing research offers support that positive emotions have their own distinctive patterns of response manifested in the brain, heart, and rest of the body.

EMOTIONS AND IMMUNITY

There is a large body of research demonstrating that high stress levels are associated with depressed immune response (McClelland, Floor, Davidson, & Saron, 1980) and, conversely, that efforts to reduce distress are associated with favorable immune response (Selye, 1974). Neurologist Robert Sapolsky has written extensively about how the stress response has great evolutionary value in the wild but in humans creates a host of disease-producing bodily responses when it cannot be turned off (Sapolsky, 2004). The link between negative emotions, higher levels of right-sided cortical activation, and depressed immune response in the body has also been studied. People with greater levels of right prefrontal activation have lower levels of immune functioning (R. J. Davidson, Coe, Dolski, & Donzella, 1999). People who are depressed show signs of exaggerated platelet reactivity (Musselman et al., 1996) and higher levels of interleukin 6, a protein in the blood. Inflammation is one marker of immune response and is the body's way of responding to injury to promote healing.

Negative mood is thought to affect the heart through the immune system's proinflammatory mechanisms. Negative emotions affect the way that various markers of inflammation respond in the body in terms of adhesiveness (stickiness) and aggregation (tendency to clot together; Maes, 1999).

Overall, inflammatory responses promote progression of heart disease by increasing the tendency to build up plaque within coronary arteries, by increasing the stickiness of the platelets that form in blood vessels, and through overreaction of platelets in response to rupture of atherosclerotic lesions. If future research indicates that the use of psychotherapeutic techniques to treat negative emotions is shown to produce anti-inflammatory responses, this may be an important key to slowing down atherogenesis (Gidron, Kupper, Kwaijtaal, Winter, & Denollet, 2007).

EMOTIONS AND GENETICS

Genetic vulnerability accounts for individual variation in emotional regulation as well as increased risk for heart disease. One gene involved in transport of serotonin, a neurotransmitter for mood regulation, is implicated as a potential mediator of heart disease through psychological mechanisms. Serotonin is a neurotransmitter with multiple sites of action (e.g., cortex, amygdala, hippocampus) with effects on mood, anxiety, sensory processing, cognition, and sleep. A low-activity promoter polymorphism (5-HTTLPR) of the serotonin transporter gene (SLC6A4) is associated with greater vulnerability to developing depression, greater likelihood of persistent negative affect, and poorer response to selective serotonin reuptake inhibitor antidepressant medications.

The 5-HTTLPR polymorphism is associated with a heightened response in the brain's amygdala from environmental cues (Hariri et al., 2005). 5-HTTLPR has been examined in a Japanese sample of 2,509 cardiac patients, and results showed that depressive symptoms were more common in carriers of the low-activity transporter polymorphism compared with noncarriers (48.3% vs. 35%). Long-term (2-year) recurrent cardiac events were also more common in carriers than noncarriers (31.3% vs. 22.3%), but the effect was rendered nonsignificant when depression was statistically controlled, suggesting that depression mediated the relationship between the genetic vulnerability and cardiac outcome (Nakatani et al., 2005). Many genetic factors are likely to underlie the susceptibility to risk factors for cardiovascular disease, and this example focuses on just one candidate gene. However, such research demonstrates the complex interplay of genetic factors with susceptibility and risk.

CLINICAL IMPLICATIONS OF EMOTION RESEARCH

As must be evident from the discussion in this chapter, there is no single neurobiological pathway connecting emotions and heart disease. Redford Williams and his colleagues have suggested that psychological risk factors tend to cluster together and interact in both additive and synergistic ways to influence risk for heart disease (Williams, Barefoot, & Schneiderman, 2003). Genetic vulnerability combined with environmental factors also plays a critical role in an individual's cardiovascular susceptibility to the effects of negative emotions. The changes in neural circuitry that occur as a result of positive emotions and healthy attachments are only beginning to be understood by researchers (Insel & Young, 2001).

Klein (2002) provided an extensive review of the neuropsychological research on positive emotions and made a strong case that the brain can be trained to react less to negative emotional cues, to experience negative emotions less frequently and for shorter duration, to experience positive feelings more frequently, and to savor pleasurable feelings for a longer period of time. Quick awareness of negative emotion allows a person to become more adept at consciously pushing the emotion out of his or her mind. Just as emotions are manifested in bodily response, so too can the body produce feelings. For example, physical activity is consistently shown to produce favorable improvements in mood through increased endorphin levels. In general, psychotherapists who work with cardiac patients can be informed by neurobiological research on emotions through the following:

- Greater efforts to sensitize cardiac patients about their own emotional states.
- Techniques to elicit positive emotions during interventions addressing the importance of attachment and social ties for good cardiovascular functioning.
- Recognition that mood is manifested in bodily response and the body influences mood. People with good nutritional habits who practice some form of invigorating physical activity tend to be in better moods.

Each chapter that follows is devoted to the topics of depression, anxiety, hostility, interpersonal relationships, coping with chronic disease, and existential issues, respectively, and covers psychotherapeutic approaches to working with each focus. This chapter has served to introduce this subject matter by providing background studies that have examined the physiological link between emotions and the body.

Psychological and behavioral treatments must be developed and implemented in the absence of a complete understanding of the impact of emotions on heart health. In the years to come, the field of behavioral cardiology will no doubt arrive at a more nuanced understanding of how these physiological states that are stimulated by emotions interact with each other to influence the development and course of cardiovascular disease.

II

PSYCHOSOCIAL FACTORS AND CARDIOVASCULAR DISEASE

4

DEPRESSION

Of all the emotion-related factors that have been studied with respect to heart disease, depression has been shown most consistently to be linked with the development and prognosis of cardiovascular disease. For many people, it is intuitive that feelings of depression might follow a heart disease diagnosis, but, in fact, the literature shows a bidirectional relationship, with depression also increasing risk for heart disease. The information on depression and cardiovascular illness in this chapter is based on a rich literature base that continues to grow exponentially.

In contrast to some psychiatric diagnoses, there is relatively good agreement on the symptoms of depression, which include the following: prolonged sadness and/or loss of interest in pleasure most of the day, nearly everyday; significant weight loss or gain when not dieting; insomnia or hypersomnia; psychomotor agitation or retardation; fatigue or loss of energy; feelings of worthlessness or excessive guilt; diminished ability to think, concentrate, or make decisions; and recurrent thoughts of death, suicidal ideation, or suicide attempt. However, it is important to note that the scientific literature has often focused on symptoms of depression, not depressive disorders that meet diagnostic criteria. The bulk of the behavioral cardiology research showing a strong relationship between depression and cardiovascular disease has used self-report questionnaires to assess the level of depressive symptoms. The symptoms of depression in cardiac populations are sometimes less specific and more mild than in noncardiac populations (Lesperance & Frasure-Smith, 2000).

PREVALENCE OF DEPRESSION IN PEOPLE WITH HEART DISEASE

To the extent that a diagnosis of heart disease is associated with a transient increase in depressive symptoms and loss of functional coping abilities, it is likely that a high proportion of cardiac patients might meet criteria for adjustment disorder with depressed mood after an acute coronary event or surgical procedure. About one out of five patients with myocardial infarction (MI) has diagnosable major depression, and more than a quarter meet criteria for minor depression (Carney et al., 1987). Similarly, about one out of five patients with ventricular tachycardia meets diagnostic criteria for major or minor depression (Carney, Freedland, Rich, Smith, & Jaffe, 1993). Depression rates in patients hospitalized for heart failure are similar to those of patients following MI, but 40% of the class of most severely ill patients with heart failure meet criteria for major or minor depression (Freedland et al., 2003). Among patients undergoing coronary artery bypass graft operations (CABG), more than one out of four has elevated depressive symptoms prior to, immediately following, and 3 months after surgery (Rymaszewska, Kiejna, & Hadrys, 2003). A study of 100 stable outpatients with coronary heart disease (CHD) showed that prevalence of past major depressive episode was 29%, recurrent major depressive disorder with current major depressive episode was 31%, and current dysthymic disorder was 15% (Bankier, Januzzi, & Littman, 2004).

DEPRESSION AS A PREDICTOR OF
MORBIDITY AND MORTALITY

Studies from the Montreal Heart Institute showed that depression following MI was an independent risk factor for mortality at 6 and 18 months postdischarge, equal in effect to that of left ventricular dysfunction and history of previous MI (Frasure-Smith, Lesperance, & Talajic, 1995a). More recent studies from their group indicate that depression also predicts long-term (5-year) cardiac mortality (Lesperance, Frasure-Smith, Talajic, & Bourassa, 2002). Even when depression occurs up to 1 year after the initial cardiac event, it still holds prognostic significance, although as treatment for cardiac care has improved, the strength of the relationship between depression and cardiac outcome has attenuated. A meta-analysis of 22 studies with 6,367 MI patients conducted by van Melle et al. (2004) concluded that depression following MI is associated with a 2- to 2.5-fold increased risk of impaired cardiovascular outcome but that this effect was most pronounced in studies that were conducted on patients treated before 1992.

Similarly, depression predicts morbidity and mortality in people with other types of heart disease. More severe depressive symptoms are associated with greater likelihood of shock among patients with implantable cardioverter defibrillators (Whang et al., 2005), are predictive of mortality in people with heart failure (Jiang et al., 2004), and are associated with higher short- and long-term mortality rates among patients who have undergone CABG surgery (Burg, Benedetto, Rosenberg, & Soufer, 2003; Burg, Benedetto, & Soufer, 2003).

PATHWAYS BY WHICH DEPRESSION MAY AFFECT MORBIDITY AND MORTALITY

Depression in patients with CHD is associated with autonomic nervous system dysfunction, including elevated heart rate, low heart rate variability, exaggerated heart rate responses to physical stressors, high variability in ventricular repolarization (Carney, Freedland, & Veith, 2005), and differences in markers of inflammation and coagulation (Carney et al., 2007). Additionally, depression is linked with morbidity and mortality through behavioral pathways in that depressed individuals are less likely to take good care of their health, as evidenced by being less likely to attend cardiac rehabilitation programs (Glazer, Emery, Frid, & Banyasz, 2002), and are at higher risk for tobacco use (Freedland, Carney, & Skala, 2005), problem drinking (Kendler, Heath, Neale, Kessler, & Eaves, 1993), and drug use (Kessler, Zhao, Blazer, & Swartz, 1997). Of the more than 900 participants evaluated in the Heart and Soul Study, 22% had current depression as measured by the Diagnostic Interview Schedule (Gehi, Haas, Pipkin, & Whooley, 2005). The depressed patients in the Heart and Soul Study were more likely to forget to take medications, to skip medications, and not to take medications as prescribed compared with nondepressed patients.

PREEXISTING VERSUS REACTIVE DEPRESSION

For half of depressed post-MI patients, the depression predates the cardiac event (Lesperance, Frasure-Smith, & Talajic, 1996). The time of onset of the depressive symptoms provides information that guides the course of therapy. People with longstanding, preexisting depression require different psychotherapeutic techniques than people with first episodes of depression. Depression that precedes a cardiac event is explored to determine the extent of depressive history, previous treatments, and potentially related stressors, such as marital discord or work-related problems. These same topics are also explored for people with first episodes of depression, but the physical symptoms, reactions to medications, effect of the cardiac event, and hospitalization (if applicable) are considered as potential triggers. A high proportion of patients have a transient increase in depressive symptoms (Carney et al., 2004), possibly as a result of the effect of being diagnosed with heart disease and temporary loss of functional coping abilities, but there is little research that has yet differentiated the characteristics of patients whose depression remits from those whose depression persists long term. In the absence of such guidance, traditional markers of chronic depression in noncardiac patients (e.g., prior history of depression, other comorbid psychiatric illness, suicidality) should be considered when trying to identify whether the depressive symptoms are likely to remit with the passage of time.

ASSESSMENT OF DEPRESSION

There are many measures of depression. This section focuses on several questionnaires that have often been used in studies with cardiac patients. A consensus statement by a working group of researchers assembled by the National Heart, Lung, and Blood Institute generally endorsed the Beck Depression Inventory (BDI) and the 17-item Hamilton Rating Scale for Depression for the assessment of depression severity (K. W. Davidson et al., 2006). The panel focused on developing a consensus statement regarding the assessment of depression in randomized controlled trials and for epidemiological studies rather than during the routine delivery of clinical care. In practice, most therapists would be likely to include a self-report measure of depression to accompany their clinical interview but would probably not rely on a structured interview such as the Hamilton Rating Scale for Depression. Thus, this section covers two questionnaires that have been commonly used with cardiac populations and one that was specifically designed for use with this patient population.

Beck Depression Inventory

Many therapists use the BDI to assess depression in cardiac patients (Beck & Steer, 1984; Furlanetto, Mendlowicz, & Romildo, 2005). The revised version of this self-report measure (BDI–II) has 21 items that correspond to depressive symptoms consistent with the *Diagnostic and Statistical Manual of Mental Disorders, Fourth Edition, Text Revision* (DSM–IV–TR; American Psychiatric Association, 2000). The questionnaire takes about 5 to 10 minutes to complete and assesses for symptoms that have occurred in the past 2 weeks. It is appropriate for adults with at least a sixth-grade reading level and is sensitive to change over relatively brief periods of time. The BDI has face validity; the disadvantage of this is that patients who are intent on minimizing or overreporting their symptoms can easily do so. Thus, the BDI alone is not sufficient to make a clinical diagnosis of depression. An advantage of the BDI is that it is more sensitive to lower levels of depression. The BDI–II is a revision of the original BDI. Most of the validation studies with cardiac patients used the original BDI. Scores on this measure have been found predictive of mortality and reinfarction in patients after acute coronary syndrome and CABG (Burg, Benedetto, & Soufer, 2003).

The BDI includes items about physical health that could be caused by any number of medical reasons. Disentangling the somatic symptoms of depression can be extremely difficult. Patients who are depressed often present with vague complaints of insomnia, fatigue, headache, memory problems, and bodily discomfort. It is not uncommon that many medical patients seek treatment from their cardiologist for sleep problems, fatigue, and lack of appetite. Some researchers have tried summing the first 14 items of the BDI to create a cognitive–affective subscale and to sum the somatic items (15–21) separately to gauge the relative contribution of physical distress to the diagnosis of depression (Zemore & Eames, 1979). However, there is also a Beck Depression Inventory for Primary Care measure that, when a cutoff of 4 is used (Steer, Cavalieri, Leonard, & Beck, 1999), has been shown to yield 97% sensitivity and 99% specificity rates, respectively, for identifying primary care patients with and without major depression.

Cardiac Depression Scale

The Cardiac Depression Scale (CDS; Hare & Davis, 1996) is a 26-item self-report measure that was developed as an index of quality of life specifically for cardiac patients. The questionnaire takes about 5 minutes to complete. Birks, Roebuck, and Thompson (2004) assessed depressive symptoms using the CDS among a British cardiac population and found that scores on the CDS correlated with scores on the BDI–II and the Hospital Anxiety and Depression Scale. There are a limited number of studies that report using the CDS (Di Benedetto, Lindner, Hare, & Kent, 2006; Wise, Harris, & Carter, 2006). The advantage of the CDS is that it has face validity and is specifically designed for cardiac patients. The disadvantages are that there have been relatively few validity studies of this measure, there is no consensus in the literature that "cardiac" depression differs substantially from depression in noncardiac populations, and there is no evidence about what a meaningful clinical cutoff would be for depression. Astin, Jones, and Thompson (2005) used the CDS in 140 patients undergoing first-time elective percutanaeous transluminal coronary angioplasty and used cutoff scores of 104 for men and 113 for women, but there is nothing to support that these scores represent clinically meaningful cut points. If this questionnaire is incorporated into clinical practice, it should be used in conjunction with other measures. Nonetheless, this questionnaire is helpful as a measure of adjustment to heart disease, and in contrast to many other depression measures, patients often find it very relevant to their current situation.

Brief Symptom Inventory

The Brief Symptom Inventory (BSI) is a 53-item self-report measure of psychiatric symptom distress that takes about 8 to 10 minutes to complete (Derogatis & Melisaratos, 1983). This questionnaire is the brief version of the 90-item, revised Symptom Check List (SCL–90–R). The BSI measures nine symptom dimensions, including depression, and has three global scores for symptomatic distress. The questionnaire measures symptomatic distress in the past 7 days, including the current day. The disadvantage of the BSI is that the subscale items correlate highly with each other, making it difficult to pinpoint diagnosis with any degree of precision. The advantage of this measure is that it serves as a quick screen for more severe psychopathology. Use of the BSI in cardiac populations has been limited, although there has been some support for the BSI as method of quick assessment for psychiatric pathology in cardiac subgroups (De Jong, Moser, An, & Chung, 2004; O'Farrell, Murray, & Hotz, 2000).

In summary, the assessment and diagnosis of depression in the cardiac population by practitioners generally relies on clinical interview and might include one or more paper-and-pencil measures. Patients with symptoms of depression may meet criteria for major depression, dysthymia, adjustment disorder, or bereavement. The most difficult aspect of diagnosing depression in this population is judging whether physical symptoms of depression (e.g., low energy, sleep problems, appetite problems) are a result of depression, medical illness, medication regimen, or multiple factors.

PSYCHOTHERAPEUTIC TECHNIQUES FOR DECREASING DEPRESSIVE SYMPTOMS

Psychotherapy treatments for depression that are most often recommended for cardiac patients include cognitive behavioral and interpersonal therapies. Marital therapy (for patients with marital discord) has also been shown to be effective in treating depression in the general adult population and is a good choice when depressed mood is attributable to poor marital quality. Some variant of psychodynamic therapy is practiced by at least 30% of clinicians registered in a large database of more than 13,000 psychologists in the United States (National Register of Health Service Providers in Psychology, 2007), and so it is important that this therapy modality also be adaptable for the treatment of this patient population. Although each therapy modality differs in terms of emphasis and technique, any of these orientations can be adapted to address the various presenting problems that propel people into therapy.

Clinical Example

Estelle and James were an African American couple in their 70s who were referred for therapy by the cardiac rehabilitation program. James had suffered an MI 6 months ago and had been treated with angioplasty and three stents. Estelle was devoted to his recovery and attended each rehabilitation class on exercise, stress, nutrition, and the like. She sought out therapy after seeing a brochure. In the initial evaluation, the therapist was a little puzzled about the reason for their visit. Estelle was the first to attempt to explain why they sought treatment, but her voice broke before finishing the first sentence. "Our son, Rick was killed in a motorcycle accident." James's voice was flat, but he picked up where Estelle left off, grimly describing the tragedy of their loss. Rick, their athletic, outgoing son, had died at age 36. They had one daughter, who lived nearby with their two granddaughters. Although they had outwardly managed to continue to function, James had become numb with grief and Estelle had sunk deep into a depression. Rick's death preceded James's heart attack. Ultimately, it was the heart attack that allowed this couple to seek therapy. They came for 12 therapy appointments over 6 months, and the focus of therapy was on their grief. Estelle coped by looking at photographs and scrapbooks of her son and by immersing herself in taking care of her granddaughters and of James. She worried that James's heart attack was a signal that she would soon lose him as well. For his part, James was unable to talk about his son and was unreceptive to being "coddled." Each partner had difficulty initially in understanding the response of the other. Therapy offered them a place to grieve together and to come to a shared respect for each other's coping mechanisms.

Every therapy modality addresses issues of loss, but interpersonal therapy offers a model that is explicitly designed for grief and loss issues.

Interpersonal Therapy

Interpersonal therapy (IPT) is a 12- to 16-week individual psychotherapy treatment designed to treat unipolar major depression (Klerman, Weissman, & Rounsaville, 1984). The goals of IPT include the reduction of depressive symptoms and conflict in interpersonal relationships. Interpersonal conflicts that may have precipitated the current depressive episode are a major area of emphasis when working within an IPT model. Presenting problems with interpersonal conflict fall into four general categories: (a) grief related to loss of a loved one (e.g., "My son died in a car accident last year and I haven't ever cried about it"); (b) problems navigating life transitions (e.g., "I retired after my bypass surgery last year and I don't feel any purpose to getting up each day"); (c) relational conflicts with an important other person (e.g., "I hate my boss but I have to deal with him every day"); and (d) isolation resulting from deficits in the support network (e.g., "I live alone and have only myself to rely on"). The IPT model assumes that depression is a biologically based medical illness. Viewing depression as stemming solely from physiological vulnerability can decrease feelings of shame or stigma, making the treatment more appealing and understandable to many depressed cardiac patients.

There is one large-scale clinical trial of IPT for cardiac depression completed in Canada (Lesperance et al., 2007). The pilot study for the Canadian Cardiac Randomized Evaluation of Antidepressant and Psychotherapy Efficacy (CREATE) trial (Koszycki, Lafontaine, Frasure-Smith, Swenson, & Lesperance, 2004) showed that more than half of the patients treated using this model experienced a reduction in symptoms of depression. Seventeen patients with coronary artery disease who met criteria for major depression were enrolled, all received 12 weekly sessions of IPT, and 10 of the 17 patients also received antidepressant medication. At the end of treatment, 53% of the sample met criteria for clinically significant reduction of depressive symptoms, defined as scores of less than or equal to 7 and 14 on the Hamilton Rating Scale for Depression and BDI–II, respectively. IPT was considered a promising treatment because there is a large literature establishing the efficacy of IPT as a treatment for depression in general and for primary care patients in particular (Barkham & Hardy, 2001; Schulberg, Pilkonis, & Houck, 1998; Schulberg et al., 2007). Thus, it was thought that therapists with an IPT orientation would find this modality particularly easy to adapt to the treatment of depressed cardiac patients. In turn, people with heart disease are particularly receptive to a relatively brief psychotherapy treatment model that removes some of the stigma traditionally associated with mental illness by emphasizing depression as a biologically based disease process.

The larger randomized CREATE trial tested 12 sessions of IPT plus clinical management against clinical management alone, with and without citalopram (Celexa) in each arm of treatment. There were 284 patients in the study, and citalopram was found to be superior to placebo in reducing depressive symptoms over 12 weeks. However, there was no evidence that IPT improved outcomes over clinical management. This raised questions as to the specific components of the "clinical management" comparison.

Clinical management was developed in the National Institute of Mental Health Treatment of Depression Collaborative Research Program (Elkin et al., 1989) and is a brief (approximately 20-minute) education and support session that assesses depressive symptoms, provides information about depression and support, and promotes compliance with taking medication and keeping study appointments. Clinicians who were providing clinical management sessions avoided interpreting behaviors, exploration of affect, or relational issues. However, and this is important, the IPT study therapists delivered both the clinical management sessions and the IPT. Participants who were randomized to the clinical management arm had a 20-minute session, and those randomized to clinical management plus IPT had 20 minutes of clinical management followed immediately by an average of 48 minutes of IPT. Adherence was good. All ($N = 284$) of the study subjects in the CREATE trial came to at least one clinical management or IPT plus clinical management session, and 86% of the sample completed 12 sessions. However, the CREATE trial illustrated how difficult it is to design an ideal placebo for psychotherapy. Having the same therapists deliver both clinical management and IPT avoided individual therapist effects and also dealt with the possibility that patients might inflate their scores to please their clinician. A problem with this design is that the control condition does not translate well into clinical practice. Clinical management as delivered by trained psychotherapists is not available in real-life medicine.

Where does this leave the therapists? Is it true, as the authors concluded, that IPT is no more effective for treating depression than a 20-minute clinical management session? Or perhaps, did this carefully designed study create some considerable artifice in the control condition? This study certainly underscores that the nonspecific factors that account for most of the variance in psychotherapy outcome seem to have accounted for the benefit of face-to-face interaction. This study also demonstrates that 20 minutes of face-to-face clinical intervention for 12 weeks is sufficient to improve symptoms of depression. Limited contact with a skilled therapist is evocative, often creating a greater level of intensity and deepening the process more than might otherwise occur. Perhaps the 20 minutes of clinical management, coupled with the additional average of 48 minutes of IPT, actually diluted the effect of the intervention. There is little research on the optimal amount of time for psychotherapy sessions, and the traditional 50-minute sessions is an artifact of historical precedent and reimbursement issues. Could clinical management work in real life? To know if clinical management will be effective in practice, one would need to test it using the nurses or physicians assistants who are actually available in such settings to perform the intervention. Given the lack of long-term data from the CREATE trial, the good outcomes shown by IPT in primary care practices, the relative availability of IPT-trained therapists, and the comparative scarcity of well-trained therapists who are available and can get reimbursed for clinical management, it seems that IPT remains a viable treatment for depression with cardiac patients.

Cognitive Behavioral Therapy

Cognitive behavioral therapy (CBT; Beck, Rush, Shaw, & Emery, 1979) was the first psychotherapy treatment that underwent a large-scale clinical trial (described in the following section), demonstrating its effectiveness in cardiac patients. There is a plethora of empirical evidence showing that CBT is an effective treatment for depression in general and specifically for medical patients (L. A. Robinson, Berman, & Neimeyer, 1990). CBT assumes that recurrent negative or self-critical thoughts lead to depressive feelings and that how people think (cognition) affects what they do (behavior). A primary goal of CBT involves altering thoughts, beliefs, attitudes, and mental images, as well as honing the ability to selectively focus attention. The other major goal of CBT is to adopt behaviors that are congruent with rational thoughts by increasing the amount of time spent in pleasurable activities, decreasing social isolation, and problem solving. For example, cognitions that are the focus of treatment may include catastrophic thinking (e.g., "I had a heart attack and I'll die before I'm 50, just like my father did") or misattribution, (e.g., "My wife is nagging me all the time, and she is the reason for my chest pain"). There have been many compilations of the most salient cognitive distortions. Exhibit 4.1 is not comprehensive but includes those often seen in a cardiac population.

The three basic therapeutic strategies used by CBT therapists are behavioral activation, alteration of automatic thoughts, and active problem solving. These are generally well received by cardiac patients because the treatment is short, the goals are easy to understand, and the approach is collaborative.

The Enhancing Recovery in Coronary Heart Disease (ENRICHD) trial, funded by the National Heart, Lung, and Blood Institute, was the first large, randomized controlled trial of a psychotherapeutic treatment for depressed cardiac patients (Berkman et al., 2003). ENRICHD was designed to determine whether individual and group psychotherapy for acute MI patients was effective at treating depression or low social support and to determine whether this therapeutic approach affected cardiac outcomes. ENRICHD enrolled 2,481 patients within 1 month following MI. Standard, face-to-face CBT as developed by Aaron Beck (Beck et al., 1979) was provided to participants in the experimental condition, and when possible, group therapy was also added to the treatment regimen. CBT lasted 6 months, with a median of 11 individual therapy sessions attended. In many instances, the initial sessions of therapy were conducted in the patients' homes so that medically compromised participants could receive treatment within the time frame specified by the study protocol. Participants scoring very high initially on the Hamilton Rating Scale for Depression or whose depression was not reduced by 60% after 5 weeks also received Zoloft (generic name sertraline hydrochloride) selective serotonin reuptake inhibitor (SSRI) antidepressant medication donated by Pfizer. Approximately 3 out of 4 participants were still alive 29 months after initiation of the study, and there was no difference between the experimental and control groups in terms of effect on cardiac mortality or morbidity. CBT was shown to be an effective treatment for depression and low social support following MI, but the magnitude of the effect was not as

EXHIBIT 4.1
Examples of Cognitive Distortions

- *All-or-nothing thinking:* The tendency toward rigid conceptualizations of problems as having black-or-white solutions. Example: "If I don't attend each cardiac rehabilitation class, I might as well not exercise at all."
- *Overgeneralization:* Applying a good rule without discrimination or effort to place the principle in context. Example: "I must open and read all of my hospital bills as soon as possible or I might miss something important."
- *Disqualifying the positive:* Inability to realistically perceive good aspects of oneself or a situation. Example: "I have been really lucky to lose this weight."
- *Jumping to conclusions:* Drawing an interpretation without rational evaluation of all potential explanations or contributing factors. Example: "My wife isn't paying attention to me, now that I left the hospital. It is probably because she thinks I am a burden."
- *Catastrophic thinking:* Negative, exaggerated predictions about an improbable and horrific consequence. Example: "Getting shocked by my ICD (implantable cardioverter defibrillator) must mean that I'm getting sicker and my time is up."
- *Minimization:* The tendency to ignore or remain emotionally detached from important issues, especially emotional or physical needs. Example: "Although I have had open heart surgery, I feel normal now. I should be able to go right back to work."

great as the investigators might have hoped. At 6 months, depressed patients in the CBT treatment condition had a 57% reduction in depression versus a 47% reduction in the usual-care group. Patients with low social support who received the CBT treatment had a 27% improvement compared with an 18% improvement in usual medical care.

The usual-care arm of the ENRICHD study had a better-than-expected improvement in depression in the 6 months following the initial heart attack. The research community speculated that there were many possible explanations. The study was difficult to conduct. Because of changes in managed care, length of stay in the hospital decreased substantially during the recruitment period, forcing research staff to recruit participants through a laborious combination of study visits conducted during the hospitalization and in the participants' home. The study underscored that the trajectory of depression in cardiac patients has innumerable permutations. Some depressive reactions following a cardiac event are reactive, not prognostically significant, and may even spontaneously remit. For other patients, depression precedes the MI. In still other instances, history of prior depression incurs an increased vulnerability to depression after the trigger of a cardiac event. A subgroup of 1,165 ENRICHD participants enrolled in the treatment arm whose depression did not improve had higher late ($\geq$6 months post-MI) cardiac mortality rates compared with intervention patients whose depression responded to treatment (Carney et al., 2004), indicating that treatment refractory depression may be particularly lethal for cardiac patients. Although the ENRICHD study did not show that treatment for depression affects cardiac morbidity or mortality, it did advance the knowledge in the field of behavioral cardiology and confirmed that CBT is effective for the treatment of depression following heart attack.

Marital Therapy

Marriage, marital quality, and living alone have all been linked with depression in cardiac patients (Bramwell, 1990; Case, Moss, Case, McDermott, & Eberly, 1992; Waltz, 1986). A good relationship with a spouse or partner might provide the support necessary to adhere to treatment recommendations and provide some buffering against the stress of a cardiac event (Brecht, Dracup, Moser, & Riegel, 1994). Conversely, a marriage marked by conflict and anger may result in sympathetic arousal, impairments in immune function, and a depressive response (Orth-Gomer et al., 2000). Multiple laboratory experiments have documented the ill effects of marital conflict on hormone levels, immune system markers, cardiovascular reactivity, and depression (Carels, Szczepanski, Blumenthal, & Sherwood, 1998; Dopp, Miller, Myers, & Fahey, 2000; Newton & Sanford, 2003). In these types of research studies, partners are brought together in a research setting and asked to discuss a topic known to be a source of disagreement or frequent argument. Verbal and physical behaviors (e.g., lack of eye contact, refusing to talk, raising the voice, emotional withdrawal, complaining, criticizing, sarcasm) are observed and rated. Physiological parameters (e.g., cortisol levels, blood pressure, heart rate) are also measured. Although the research on marital therapy for depressed cardiac patients is quite limited, there is little question that poor marital quality is related to depression and, if it is present, must be addressed in the treatment plan.

The Relationship Support Program is an example of marital therapy that has been adapted to the treatment of cardiac patients (Rankin-Esquer, Deeter, & Taylor, 2000). This program is designed to complement medical interventions and to help couples examine how relational issues are affected by the cardiac event. A review of eight studies on marital therapy for depression (Barbato & D'Avanzo, 2006) provided support that marital therapy is as effective for the treatment of depression as individual therapy, and this choice should be determined by patient preference.

Psychodynamic Psychotherapy

Under the umbrella term psychodynamic psychotherapy, there are a number of models for intervention that have been shown to be effective in treating depression in the general population. Psychodynamic psychotherapy focuses on early or recent past experiences with important other people in a person's life. This therapeutic model assumes that maladaptive patterns are doomed to repeat themselves until a person gains insight into the pattern and resolves to change it. Therapy may be focused on a precipitating event or on a central conflict. A goal of therapy may be to change maladaptive personality traits. Psychodynamic therapy typically makes use of both interpretations and transference interpretations. One of the difficulties in reviewing the literature is that psychodynamic psychotherapy models vary widely, are not easily described in treatment manuals, and thus have not traditionally lent themselves to empirical study. Nonetheless, a large proportion of practicing therapists describe themselves as either using a psychodynamic orientation or incorporating some principles from this therapy modality. Traditionally, psychodynamic therapy was often provided in an open-ended fashion and might even go on for years. In the 1980s, it became more common to practice time-limited psychodynamic psychotherapy, with the number of therapy sessions limited to 12 to 40 sessions. Clinically, an explicit focus on time can be useful in conducting psychotherapy for cardiac patients because it capitalizes on the natural reminder of mortality precipitated by a heart attack or hospitalization.

A meta-analysis by Crits-Christoph (1992) of 11 studies of time-limited psychodynamic psychotherapy showed that this model, delivered with use of a treatment manual, demonstrated large effects compared with waiting list control conditions and was equivalent to other psychotherapies and medication. More recent studies have provided support that time-limited psychodynamic therapy is roughly equivalent in terms of effects to cognitive therapy and supportive therapy for the treatment of depression and anxiety (Svartberg, Seltzer, & Stiles, 1998; Svartberg, Stiles, & Seltzer, 2004). At the time of this writing, only one randomized trial of psychodynamically oriented treatment in a primary care practice setting was found, and that study demonstrated limited evidence of improved outcomes as a result of counseling. However, the authors cautioned that the eligibility criteria allowed more mildly depressed patients into the study, and restricting the inclusion criteria to more severely depressed patients might have yielded more conclusive results (Simpson, Corney, Fitzgerald, & Beecham, 2003).

Clinical Example

> Ryan was a 53-year-old White male who presented for treatment following a first heart attack. He was referred by one of the nurses who noted that he had an elevated depression score when screened in the cardiac rehabilitation program. He described himself as being unable to express himself emotionally with anyone. His second wife was supportive but unable to understand why it seemed not only difficult but also painful for him to have any emotional intimacy. He said that he feared his inability to express emotion might be linked to his heart disease, and even if not, he worried that it was negatively affecting his second marriage. In psychotherapy sessions, Ryan indicated a wish to feel closer to the therapist as well as a great deal of anxiety about that wish. Ryan described his

relationship with his mother as being fraught with angst. He described her as being irrepressibly overbearing both during his childhood and as an adult. As an introverted child, he felt that she had pushed him considerably beyond his comfort zone in a misguided effort to help him overcome his shyness. In adulthood, he looked forward to her visits with all the enthusiasm of a man anticipating an Internal Revenue Service audit. In therapy, Ryan was able to see how his main coping strategies of intellectualization and emotional detachment served to keep people at a distance and kept himself cut off from his emotions. Therapy terminated after there was evidence that he had improved his ability both to identify what he was feeling and to express those feelings in therapy as well as in relationships with other important current figures such as his wife and mother.

Psychodynamic psychotherapy was appropriate for Ryan and was successful in helping him see the recurrent pattern of avoidance of emotional intimacy with his wife and with the therapist that stemmed from his relationship with his mother. Other therapeutic approaches might also have worked well for Ryan. Although there are many differences in language and techniques between therapies, the acquisition of adaptive skills is common to all therapies (Badgio, Halperin, & Barber, 1999). Put in another way, using different strategies and techniques, it is possible to arrive at the same end point (resolution of depressive symptoms) using multiple therapy modalities. In the next section, rumination is discussed from these three theoretical orientations.

RUMINATION

People who are depressed often tend to ruminate or to become introspective and inwardly focused on situations that cause distress (Kubzansky, Davidson, & Rozanski, 2005). People who ruminate more are more likely to become depressed (Nolen-Hoeksema, 2000). Ruminating has been hypothesized as one possible pathway linking depression to heart disease in that people who ruminate tend to have protracted periods of increased heart rate and high blood pressure. Multiple laboratory experiments have demonstrated that when rumination is induced, people are more likely to feel angry in response to environmental stressors, to have difficulty in concentrating, and to have elevated blood pressure even after the original stimulus is removed (Bushman, Bonacci, Pedersen, Vasquez, & Miller, 2005; Gerin, Davidson, Christenfeld, Goyal, & Schwartz, 2006). From a cognitive behavioral perspective, it is important to interrupt the cognitive process of ruminating through distraction, thought stopping, cognitive reappraisal, or behavioral activation (Ray et al., 2005). Viewed through an interpersonal lens, engagement with another person can refocus attention outside the self and resolve relational difficulties that might exacerbate the ruminative process. By using a psychodynamic framework, rumination can be viewed as a defensive process stemming from an underlying conflict. The introspective qualities associated with rumination are not pathological in isolation. In fact, there is evidence that rumination accounts for the long-observed link between creativity and depression, or the tendency of artists to be more prone to low mood (Verhaeghen, Joorman, & Khan, 2005). It is the negative affect often induced by the ruminative process, rather than the rumination itself, that is detrimental to emotional health.

SUMMARY

Depression following heart attack can present a new opportunity for cardiac patients' emotional growth, as relationships and values are reexamined in light of limited time. Therapists can incorporate reference to the MI or angioplasty as a catalyst that forces psychological maturation with statements such as, "The heart attack seems to have brought home the importance of making substantial change in your life right now, rather than waiting."

The number of published results from large-scale trials of psychotherapy to treat depression in cardiac patients is limited, with only two available at the time of this writing. It is probably safe to assume that talk therapies that are effective for the treatment of depression in general will also be effective for the treatment of depression in a cardiac population. Adapting therapy for the treatment of the depressed cardiac patient involves giving special attention to the areas that are known to have an impact on heart health: social isolation, negative affect, adjustment to a new diagnosis of heart disease, lifestyle change, and adherence to the medical regimen. Because depression follows a chronic course and is associated with increased risk for suicide (Kessler et al., 1997), recognizing and treating depression in this population are priorities for cardiac care. Anxiety, the frequent sidekick of depression, is the psychological focus of the following chapter.

5

ANXIETY

Anxiety has been described in terms of both negative emotions (nervousness and worry) and physiological characteristics (increased blood pressure, rapid heart rate, sweating, dry mouth, nausea, vertigo, breathing problems, restlessness, tremors, and feelings of weakness). As is the case for depression, operational definitions of anxiety vary widely across research studies. It is difficult to make conclusive statements about the relationship between anxiety and cardiac disease because researchers typically focus on only one or two manifestations of the construct. Anxiety has been conceptualized as a stable personality trait (trait anxiety), a symptom elicited through provocation (state anxiety), and a psychiatric disorder. The primary categories of anxiety disorders that have been studied in cardiac populations are generalized anxiety disorder, panic disorder, and posttraumatic stress disorder (Dew et al., 2001; Fleet, Dupuis, Marchand, Burelle, & Beitman, 1994; Kubzansky, Koenen, Spiro, Vokonas, & Sparrow, 2007; Wittchen et al., 2002). Although multiple manifestations of anxiety often coexist within the same individual, this is not typically captured in empirical research. Similarly, it can be difficult to generate operational definitions because the term *stress* is used often to describe such a wide spectrum of problems. In this chapter, anxiety refers to symptom distress, whereas stress refers to the perception of hardship posed by adverse conditions.

PREVALENCE OF ANXIETY IN PEOPLE WITH HEART DISEASE

The prevalence of anxiety in hospitalized cardiac patients is high, with about half of patients reporting significant anxiety in the hospital (Moser & Dracup, 1996). About 16% of men and 24% of women undergoing cardiac catheterization have state anxiety scores comparable with psychiatric patients. It is not surprising that people are wracked with nerves in the hospital. Psychologist Ron Levant was hospitalized six times over 2 years while being treated for atrial fibrillation. Levant explained, "In the hospital, medical practitioners take over your life. You can't count on clinicians in the hospital to take care of your emotional needs. In fact, you can count on the fact that they will not" (personal communication, February 28, 2007). The act of waiting for a medical procedure, surgery, or diagnosis is also scary. Although most studies have found that anxiety decreases following a cardiac catheterization procedure, a substantial proportion of people, particularly women, still have persistent anxiety 6 months afterward (Astin, Jones, & Thompson, 2005).

Before coronary artery bypass graft operations (CABG), 28% to 55% of people have elevated symptoms of anxiety, and about one third of people still have clinically relevant symptoms of anxiety at 3 months postsurgery (Rymaszewska, Kiejna, & Hadrys, 2003). Among patients with heart failure, 18% meet criteria for an anxiety disorder (Haworth et al., 2005). Following myocardial infarction (MI), more than one third (36%) of women and 19% of men screen positive for anxiety (Frasure-Smith, Lesperance, Juneau, Talajic, & Bourassa, 1999). In implantable cardioverter defibrillator (ICD) recipients, 13% to 38% of patients have diagnosable anxiety (S. F. Sears, Todaro, Lewis, Sotile, & Conti, 1999). There are also high rates of panic disorder among people who present to the emergency room with chest pain; this is discussed later in the chapter.

ANXIETY AS A PREDICTOR OF CARDIAC MORBIDITY AND MORTALITY

There is little evidence of anxiety as a predictor of mortality. In general, anxiety is not nearly as robust a predictor of cardiac morbidity as is depression. There are some studies showing that anxiety does predict cardiac events following MI (Frasure-Smith, Lesperance, & Talajic, 1995b; Pfiffner & Hoffmann, 2004; Strik, Denollet, Lousberg, & Honig, 2003), whereas others have failed to show a relationship (Lane, Carroll, Ring, Beevers, & Lip, 2001a). Symptoms of anxiety have also been linked to complications following MI (Moser & Dracup, 1996), and one study has shown that over the long term, worry is predictive of nonfatal MI (Kubzansky et al., 1997). Anxiety has not been linked to morbidity in patients with heart failure (Jiang et al., 2004), and no studies have shown that anxiety predicts morbidity in patients with ICD. One difficulty in this line of research is that symptoms of anxiety are highly correlated with other psychological factors, especially depression (Ketterer et al., 2002), and whereas depression is a strong predictor of cardiac morbidity and mortality in people with established heart disease, anxiety by contrast is more strongly linked with onset of heart disease (Kubzansky & Kawachi, 2000).

DOES STRESS PLAY A ROLE IN THE PATHOGENESIS OF CARDIAC EVENTS?

There is evidence that stressful life events play a role in first-occurrence, nonfatal cardiac events such as a first-time heart attack. A study of 97 Italian cardiac patients matched with 97 community control subjects showed that, independent of mood disorders, cardiac patients reported greater numbers of stressful life events compared with control subjects (Rafanelli et al., 2005). A very large study, the INTERHEART trial, was conducted in multiple sites across the world and compared 11,119 first-time MI patients with 13,648 matched control subjects. INTERHEART also showed that stressful life events in the year preceding the index MI were more common in cardiac patients compared with the control group, a finding that is compelling because of the size of the sample (Rosengren et al., 2004). When queried, patients who survive MI tend to attribute their heart attack to "stress" more often than any other cause, such as smoking, family factors, high fat diet, and work (Gudmundsdottir, Johnston, Johnston, & Foulkes, 2001). Cardiac patients who are more anxious are also more likely to believe that their negative emotions caused their heart disease (Day, Freedland, & Carney, 2005). These findings raise the question, how do anxiety and stress affect cardiac function?

HOW DO ANXIETY AND STRESS HARM THE HEART?

There is substantial evidence that acute and chronic anxiety and stress do have an impact on the heart (Buchholz & Rudan, 2007). Imagine that a friend told you of a loved one's death. An observational study cited in the New England Journal of Medicine in 2005 reported that sudden emotional stress (e.g., tragic news such as a close relative's death) can precipitate severe but reversible left ventricular dysfunction in patients without prior cardiac disease, a condition that has been called Tako-Tsubo syndrome (Buchholz & Rudan, 2007). This phenomenon has also been observed after natural disasters such as earthquakes (Kurita, Takase, & Ishizuka, 2001). After the World Trade Center attack, U.S. researchers found that defibrillator shocks increased by 68% in the relatively distant locale of Florida (Shedd et al., 2004). Patients often complain of the "Sunday night blues" in anticipation of the workweek. Indeed, sudden cardiac death occurs most often on Monday morning (Witte, Grobbee, Bots, & Hoes, 2005), and among people with ICDs, ventricular tachycardia occurs more frequently on the first day of the workweek.

Stress has been hypothesized to affect the heart through the autonomic nervous system. Recall the discussion in chapter 3 of this volume, in which acute stress causes the sympathetic nervous system to generate the fight-or-flight response, characterized by elevations in blood pressure, heart rate, glucose, cortisol, adrenaline, and oxygen circulation to vital organs. Anxiety also may trigger inflammatory responses that increase the stickiness of the platelets that form in blood vessels and lead to an overreaction of platelets in response to rupture of atherosclerotic lesions (Maes, 1999). Anxiety and acute stress have also been proposed to affect the heart through coronary artery vasospasm, calcium overload, and disrupted fatty acid metabolism (Buchholz & Rudan, 2007). In summary, most people react to stressful life events with anxiety and some people are predisposed to respond to stress with heightened cardiac reactivity.

EXAMINING THE RELATIONSHIP BETWEEN STRESS AND ANXIETY IN ICD PATIENTS

The population of patients with ICD offers unique opportunities to understand the interrelationship between stress and anxiety. "This is the first generation of people to have survived cardiac arrest. Not along ago, these patients would have died prematurely from sudden cardiac death," stated Sam Sears, a psychologist whose research focuses on patients with ICD (personal communication, March 2, 2007). Sears noted,

> An ICD is a life-saving device but is also adverse because it delivers shock. An ICD is invasive because the device is implanted in the body. A person with an ICD must rely on medical technology and requires a great deal of faith in the medical provider as well as the device itself. . . . The challenge for patients is that they need to learn to find security from this device. The primary benefit of ICD is the perceived security, similar to the feeling people have toward a security alarm on their home. (personal communication, March 2, 2007)

Just as some people worry more about a break-in to the home, people who are more prone to anxiety and negative affect fare more poorly in terms of their adjustment to ICD.

Approximately 30% to 50% of people experience distress following ICD implantation (Sears et al., 2000). The incidence of anxiety disorders among ICD patients who have been shocked is 21%, more than three times the incidence in people who have had no ICD discharge (Godemann et al., 2004a). Godemann et al. also found that the majority (62%) of people who have two or more ICD discharges a year meet criteria for panic disorder and agoraphobia. Table 5.1 examines the characteristics of a sample of 48 patients with ICD who had anxiety disorder compared with those who did not. ICD patients with anxiety disorders were more likely to be younger, to have been shocked more often, to feel fearful, to be attentive to bodily cues, and to report that they "constantly" anticipate the next triggering of the device.

The variability in quality of life is not accounted for by shock alone. Together, history of depression, trait anxiety, optimism, social support, and ICD shocks account for about half the variance (42%–65%) in quality of life. These variables are as strong in their predictive ability to determine quality of life as demographic and medical variables such as age, ejection fraction, and ICD shocks (Sears, Lewis, Kuhl, & Conti, 2005).

Clinical Example

Tito was a muscular Latino male in his early 40s who was urged by his wife to seek counseling for his acute worry about his heart health. Five months ago, a virus had attacked his heart, causing him to be hospitalized for 4 weeks, with 4 days in intensive care. He was diagnosed with congestive heart failure and was vulnerable to ventricular tachycardia. He was scheduled to have an ICD implanted in the next week or so but was extremely nervous. "I lie awake at night, and I can feel my heart beat. I can tell sometimes when it is not right. My wife can feel it too. It scares the heck out of me." Tito's father was a smoker who had died at age 58 of sudden cardiac arrest. Referring to his father, Tito said sadly, "He survived the heart attack but he was too macho to get the pacemaker. Two weeks later, he died in bed. Now they are going to put the ICD in me but I wonder if I'm still going to die before my time, like my Pop."

This is an example of the type of cardiac patient who suffers a great deal but would be unlikely on his own to seek out mental health treatment. Therapy for Tito consisted of three 1-hour sessions the month prior to ICD implantation and four follow-up sessions over the subsequent 2 months. Tito needed help with articulating his fears and taking stock of the radical, unexpected change in his heart health. Although he had not been prone to anxiety before his hospitalization, the onslaught of so many health problems generated fear in this intensely proud man. Additionally, the diagnosis of the same condition that had caused his father's premature death generated considerable fear that he would suffer the same fate. Not only did the ICD prevent arrhythmia, but the biventricular pacing function also improved his ejection fraction (contractile force), which helped him to feel more energized. (Biventricular pacing is also called cardiac resynchronization therapy, and it refers to the fact that a biventricular ICD makes both the left and right ventricle

TABLE 5.1
Shock Experience and Assessment of 48 ICD Patients

	Without anxiety disorder (N = 38)	With anxiety disorder (N = 10)	t	P
Age, y	61.6 ± 10.0[a]	55.2 ± 7.4	2.01	.048*
Years with ICD	3.7 ± 1.9	3.7 ± 1.8	-0.22	.827
No. of ICD shocks	8.9 ± 19.1	30.4 ± 29.8	-2.37	.037*
ICD shocks per year	1.1 ± 1.1	2.0 ± 1.4	-2.44	.019*
No. of defibrillation episodes	4.0 ± 6.0	7.5 ± 5.5	-2.42	.018*
Triggering was painful	2.7 ± 1.5	3.4 ± 1.9	-1.11	.137
Triggering saved my life	4.0 ± 1.4	3.5 ± 2.0	0.76	.465
I can perceive dangerous pulse irregularities	2.7 ± 1.4	3.8 ± 1.2	-2.39	.021
I presented to a physician immediately after the triggering	3.0 ± 1.9	3.1 ± 2.0	-0.07	.946
The triggering frightened me	2.8 ± 1.5	4.4 ± 1.3	-2.84	.007*
The triggering gave me a feeling of security	3.5 ± 1.5	2.9 ± 1.9	1.04	.303
I constantly expect the next triggering	1.7 ± 1.1	3.8 ± 1.4	-5.51	.000*
I feel downcast after the triggering	2.7 ± 1.4	3.7 ± 1.6	-1.8	.78
I pay attention to bodily changes to avoid being surprised by the next triggering	2.9 ± 1.5	4.3 ± 1.3	-2.7	.010*
The triggering does not influence my lifestyle	2.1 ± 1.0	4.0 ± 1.2	-4.78	.000*

Note. ICD = implantable cardioverter defibrillator. y = years. From "Classic Conditioning and Dysfunctional Cognitions in Patients With Panic Disorder and Agoraphobia Treated With an Implantable Cardioverter/Defibrillator," by F. Godemann et al., 2001, *Psychosomatic Medicine*, 63, p. 234. Copyright 2001 by Lippincott Williams & Wilkins. Reprinted with permission. [a]Values are mean ± SD. *Significant difference.

of the heart beat together, in synchrony, which makes the heart pump more effectively.) Although Tito's physician gave him a prescription for Ativan, he proudly reported that he never filled it. As his health returned, his anxiety diminished and he became less sensitized to hearing his heartbeat. He terminated therapy after his adjustment issues and anxiety symptoms related to the ICD implantation had resolved.

Implantation of an ICD device presents its own unique kind of stress. People with an ICD wonder, "How will I know it is working? How can I be sure the battery won't fail?" It is unnerving to contemplate, let alone experience, having one's heart jolted back into rhythm. The ICD can force a person to make significant lifestyle changes. In particular, handheld impact devices such as power tools and chainsaws are more likely to cause the ICD to misfire. Professionals who need to change occupations may need help when they must adjust to having a life-threatening cardiac disease as well as dealing with the threat to their livelihood, adjustments that have been termed *patient acceptance* (J. L. Burns, Serber, Keim, & Sears, 2005).

CHEST PAIN

Chest pain is so common that it accounts for about 8% to 10% of all emergency room visits annually. However, more than one out of four people who come to the hospital with chest pain have no underlying cardiac cause and are diagnosed with noncardiac chest pain (Eslick, 2004). There are many potential causes of noncardiac chest pain, including gastroesophegeal reflux disorder, esophageal spasm, psychiatric disease, and musculoskeletal pain (Eslick, 2004). Anxiety is ubiquitous among emergency room patients and is the primary cause of about 20% of chest pain cases (Katon, Von Korff, & Lin, 1992; Yingling, Wulsin, Arnold, & Rouan, 1993). In particular, anxiety is often manifested in the form of a panic attack.

Panic Attack

People who are having a panic attack often interpret their symptoms as being heart related. Panic attacks are characterized by intense fear, with rapid development of symptoms within 10 minutes. People having panic attacks can have symptoms such as palpitations or racing heart, sweating, trembling, shortness of breath, feeling of choking, chest pain, nausea, dizzy or lightheaded, derealization or depersonalization, fear of losing control or going crazy, fear of dying, numbness or tingling, and chills or hot flushes.

In the general population, less than 4% of people have panic disorder, whereas it is diagnosed in 15% to 20% of emergency room patients with chest pain (Rozanski, Blumenthal, Davidson, Saab, & Kubzansky, 2005). Patients with chest pain who do not meet diagnostic criteria for panic often still have subsyndromal panic disorder that interferes with their functioning, treatment adherence, and quality of life. Cardiac patients who develop symptoms of anxiety are in a difficult bind. To ignore chest pain is dangerous, yet it is difficult and sometimes impossible to discern the difference between chest pain caused by anxiety and that caused by ischemic heart disease. Highly anxious patients with established cardiovascular disease can feel very embarrassed by the experience of going to the emergency room with chest pain, only to be told that "it is not your heart." Treatment for such patients involves efforts to attenuate the feelings of shame. Such an approach usually concentrates on educating the patient that some people have a high degree of sensitivity to their bodily cues and are very attentive to even small perturbations in bodily sensations. Both cognitive behavioral and relaxation therapies, discussed later in this chapter, can be effective in reducing anxiety and helping patients to interpret their bodily sensations more accurately.

Cardiac Syndrome X

The primary symptom that characterizes cardiac syndrome X is also chest pain, but this syndrome is puzzling because, by definition, patients present with angina pectoris and have a positive exercise electrocardiogram for myocardial ischemia but show no evidence of atherosclerosis on angiogram (Asbury & Collins, 2005). Cardiac syndrome X is hypothesized to be associated with microvascular dysfunction in the endothelium that lines the coronary arteries and has also been linked to insulin resistance (Botker et al., 1997; Hurst, Olson, Olson, & Appleton, 2006).

In summary, some types of chest pain are noncardiac in nature and attributable solely to psychological factors. But many types of chest pain are caused by medical problems such as coronary heart disease, cardiac syndrome X, or some other noncardiac medical problem such as gastroesophageal reflux disorder. Cardiac syndrome X is not well understood but underscores the importance of not rushing to assume that chest pain is, or is not, cardiac in nature.

CARDIAC DENIAL

Ironically, the overt absence of anxiety in cardiac patients can also be problematic. The term *cardiac denial* has been coined to refer to the tendency to fail to recognize cardiac symptoms (chest pain, shortness of breath) as being attributable to heart problems.

Clinical Example

Joe was a 46-year-old White male with a family history of heart disease, diffuse back pain from a car accident, and poorly controlled diabetes. He was initially referred for smoking cessation and seen for about 6 months, coming to therapy weekly for 2 months then tapering down. He terminated therapy with many gains, including smoking cessation, but still seemed to have little appreciation of his fragile physical health. Joe had chronic heart problems but did not view himself as a person in poor health. He saw his endocrinologist regularly but still suffered from uncontrolled diabetes with many episodes of hypoglycemia and loss of consciousness. Unbeknownst to any of his health care providers, Joe began to experience chest pain intermittently but dismissed it as one of his many aches and pains. Although his wife was concerned and urged him to talk with his doctor about the chest pain, he shrugged off her advice. According to his wife, Joe seemed to believe it was just one of many medical problems competing for his time and attention. He was fatalistic and often stated, "When it is my time, it is my time. There isn't much I can do about it." On a sunny autumn day, Joe collapsed while his family looked helplessly on. He died from sudden cardiac death, much the same way that 500,000 Americans die each year. His wife called the therapist a month after he had died, to try to make some sense out of his premature passing. With only 4 minutes to shock the heart back into a normal rhythm, there was not enough time for the ambulance to reach him. Joe's case illustrates a common way that cardiac denial operates in that he did have some physical warning signs ahead of time but minimized the personal relevance and had a relatively fatalistic outlook on life.

Cardiac denial is powerful. Whether it is construed as a cognitive distortion or as an unconscious effort to reduce anxiety by ignoring danger signals, there is no question that cardiac denial exists and is more common among people who believe that their health is largely a result of chance factors outside their own personal control (external locus of control). Some studies of patients who were interviewed after MI have showed that the most compelling factor involved in prompting a person to seek medical attention is the belief that the symptoms are indeed heart related (Carney, Fitzsimons, & Dempster, 2002). Conversely, orientation toward external health locus of control is associated with greater likelihood to delay seeking medical attention (O'Carroll, Smith, Grubb, Fox, & Masterton, 2001). In hindsight, "sudden" cardiac death is often not as sudden or unpredictable as doctors and family members might wish. Many people have symptoms of heart disease but fail to recognize them as such. With a half million people in the United States alone dying of sudden cardiac death annually, there is a need to prospectively investigate the variables that are associated with medical help-seeking and examine whether these factors are implicated in greater likelihood of fatality. Because it is only possible to investigate cardiac denial in people who have survived the event, these types of studies are more difficult to design; however, understanding how people interpret symptoms is important for the prevention of sudden cardiac death.

ASSESSMENT OF ANXIETY

Selection of an anxiety measure depends very much on the type of anxiety that is of interest. In this chapter, measures are selected to assess anxiety conceptualized as a personality trait (trait anxiety) or as a result of external conditions (state anxiety), a symptom, or a disease-specific measure for ICD recipients.

State–Trait Anxiety Inventory

The trait form of the State–Trait Anxiety Inventory (STAI; Spielberger, Gorsuch, & Lushene, 1968) consists of 20 statements assessing how the respondent generally feels (e.g., "I worry too much over something that doesn't really matter"). Each statement is rated on a 4-point scale. Given that cardiac patients often demonstrate a number of somatic symptoms that can be mistaken for anxiety (i.e., respiratory changes, tachycardia), the trait form of the STAI is particularly useful with this population, because it is less sensitive to fluctuations in mood and immediate physical experiences. More specifically, trait anxiety refers to a relatively stable personality construct, whereas state anxiety measures an individual's emotional status at a given moment and is subject to fluctuations and variations in intensity. Whereas the state form of the STAI has been shown to be sensitive to external stressors and transitory emotional states, trait anxiety scores are shown to remain essentially unchanged in response to external events. In addition, the trait form of the STAI assesses cognitive symptoms of anxiety (e.g., worry, feeling overwhelmed, and presence of disturbing thoughts) as opposed to physical symptoms, which can be mistaken for anxiety among cardiac patients. The STAI is widely used and has shown good psychometric properties. Furthermore, the STAI has been used in previous research with cardiac populations (Frasure-Smith, Lesperance, & Talajic, 1995a; Keren, Aarons, & Veltri, 1991; Wilk & Turkoski, 2001). Clinicians might use the trait form of the STAI when they are interested in trying to understand whether the patient has a longstanding tendency toward anxiety and do not want the assessment to be muddied with somatic symptoms of anxiety.

Hospital Anxiety and Depression Scale

The Hospital Anxiety and Depression Scale (HADS) is a 14-item self-report measure (7 of the items assess anxiety) that takes less than 10 minutes to complete (Zigmond & Snaith, 1983). As the name suggests, this measure was developed for use with hospitalized medical patients. Its strengths include ease of use, especially for clinicians working in an inpatient setting. There is evidence that the HADS is sensitive to change over time on both the depression and anxiety subscales in a cardiac population (Johnston,

Foulkes, Johnston, Pollard, & Gudmundsdottir, 1999). The HADS has also been used as a psychological screener for cardiac rehabilitation patients (Harrison, 2005). There is some evidence in a medical population that the anxiety subscale of the HADS does not discriminate well; that is, it is highly correlated with the depression subscale (Golden, Conroy, & O'Dwyer, 2006). Thus, although the HADS has been used for both research and clinical purposes, clinicians are cautioned that this measure can be helpful as a brief screener but that definitive diagnosis cannot be made without a clinical interview.

Florida Shock Anxiety Scale

People with ICD may have specific fears and worries associated with the implantation of the device. Disease-specific measures can be helpful in clinical practice because such tools can pinpoint the patient's concerns and guide the clinical intervention. The Florida Shock Anxiety Scale (FSAS; Kuhl, Dixit, Walker, Conti, & Sears, 2006) is a brief 10-item measure with items that include the following: "I do not get angry or upset because it may cause the ICD to fire," "I worry about the ICD not firing sometimes when it should," "I have unwanted thoughts of my ICD firing," and "I do not engage in sexual activity because it will cause my ICD to fire." Responses are scored using a 5-point Likert scale from 1 (*not at all*) to 5 (*all the time*). This measure comprises two factors: the consequences associated with being shocked and the presumed triggers of shock. Because the FSAS was only recently published, its psychometric properties have not yet been extensively studied, although the internal validity of the measure is good with Cronbach's alpha of .91, and it correlates well with a measure designed to assess fear of death. The tool has considerable face validity and can serve as an easy screening tool for behavioral cardiology clinicians. The developers of the FSAS suggest that a high score on the test might indicate the benefit of developing a "shock plan" to help patients increase their confidence and belief in their ability to cope with and react to the firing of the ICD.

PSYCHOTHERAPEUTIC TECHNIQUES FOR LOWERING ANXIETY

Psychotherapy with anxious cardiac patients might combine psychoeducation, relaxation techniques, biofeedback, and psychotherapy. Basic psychoeducational counseling techniques can lower anxiety in both cardiac patients and their partners (Johnston et al., 1999).

In a study of inpatient and extended cardiac counseling for anxiety with 100 male cardiac patients and their spouses, Johnston et al. (1999) randomized participants to receive either cardiac counseling in the hospital or extended counseling (which added on additional sessions for up to 6 weeks after discharge from hospital or normal cardiac care). Anxiety levels were found to be very high among spouses, particularly while the patient was still in the hospital. The study found that cardiac counseling from the nurse counselor lowered anxiety in both patients and their partners and prevented an increase in anxiety after discharge. The benefit of cardiac counseling on anxiety levels endured for 1 year. Both patients and their spouses responded well to this intervention, which was designed to decrease distress and improve quality of life.

Central to treating anxiety in cardiac patients is the appropriate assessment of symptoms. Cardiac patients may have a full-blown presentation of any anxiety disorder or enough symptoms that they might be called subclinical manifestations. Regardless of the presentation, the therapist's goal is generally to help the patient reduce symptoms of anxiety, develop a greater sense of internal control, and cope adaptively with fears. Because many cardiac patients are novice therapy seekers, a therapist's relational stance that is warm, engaged, and attuned goes a long way toward calming the anxious cardiac patient.

Cognitive Techniques to Reduce Symptoms of Anxiety

The mind runs amok when anxiety mounts. There is seemingly no end to the distorted thoughts and skewed cognitions stimulated by fear. Cognitive therapy is based on a theoretical model that hypothesizes that by changing beliefs and thoughts, people will shift perspective and become less anxious. In particular, therapists hone in on understanding a patient's automatic thoughts or instant judgments that occur in response to an event or situation. In addition, cognitive therapy also focuses on identifying core beliefs or ingrained, rigid, overgeneralized conceptions about the self or other people.

Clinical Example

Linda was a 54-year old White female executive who had recently undergone open heart valve replacement surgery and then sought out psychotherapy for stress management. In the first session, Linda's speech was pressured as she described her insomnia, difficulty concentrating, fear of speaking in public, and inability to stop thinking about work. Often she would wake in the middle of the night and check her e-mail for the next day or be unable to tear herself away from the office at the end of the day. A review of her life history confirmed that she met criteria for generalized anxiety disorder and had probably had it for more than 2 decades with predictable exacerbations during stressful times. Her heart surgery convinced her that she was no longer able to effectively manage her stress, but she found it very difficult to stop ruminating about her symptoms. Not surprisingly, the more she thought about her insomnia, concentration problems, worries about public speaking, and work, the worse her anxiety became. The cycle was difficult to break. Linda laughed at the idea of trying meditation or diaphragmatic breathing. She liked to exercise but often found herself too tired and overworked to get to the gym. Therapy with a cognitive focus was an excellent starting point for her because it built on one of her strengths—the ability to think logically about a problem to solve it. A focus on Linda's cognitions revealed the following thought process: "Since being out of work from the heart surgery, I have so many things on my plate. I can't possibly get to them all. I have to make a presentation and I'm not prepared. If I screw it up, I will look foolish in front of other senior officers at the meeting. I don't know if I can keep going like this. I have so much going for me but I can't enjoy it. I'm worried about losing it all."

Linda was high functioning and did not avoid anxiety-provoking experiences such as public speaking, but her inner world was unusually chaotic and negative. Verbalizing her thoughts helped her to gain some perspective. She grasped how her judgments ratcheted up her anxiety until a cascade of negative thoughts flooded her. Linda's automatic thoughts seemed to spring from a core belief that if she did not strive for perfection, she would surely overlook something crucial and suffer a humiliating failure. Looking back, as long as she could remember, she had felt inordinate pressure and fear of failure. Her father had declared bankruptcy during her adolescence, and she noted that since that time, she had always had a deep fear of being fired and a general sense of pressure.

Initially, Linda was able to verbalize more adaptive thoughts only in therapy sessions, such as the following: "There will always be more things to do than I can possibly get to. I have been very successful in my career. Even if I miss something important, I'll have to forgive myself and move on. I'm fortunate to have the support of my family and my health." Over time, Linda's perception of herself became more realistic, and she showed more resilience in her ability to deal with adversity. As she practiced replacing automatic thoughts with more compassionate and rational cognitions, she grew in confidence and self-esteem. Behavior change soon followed. She spent more time on self-care and made getting to the gym a priority. She was able to limit her time at work, yet reported feeling more productive at the office.

Linda was treated with about 30 sessions of therapy over 18 months. During the early phase of therapy, she experienced a significant reduction in anxiety symptoms. By the end of therapy, she appeared to experience a deeper, more profound, long-lasting relief from the feeling of pressure and worry that had plagued her since adolescence. The early focus on cognitive behavioral strategies was very useful, and she often returned to these techniques when she became overwhelmed with stress.

When cognitions follow a logical process, specific relaxation techniques can be extremely useful. The next section examines various techniques for relaxation.

Relaxation Techniques

Relaxation therapies include breathing techniques, meditation, mindfulness, visualization, and progressive muscle relaxation. Some psychotherapists are comfortable with teaching relaxation techniques whereas others are not. Many practitioners and laypersons in the community excel at relaxation techniques. In addition, there is a wide proliferation of books, DVDs, and audiotapes on this topic. It is important that therapists understand what relaxation therapies are and how they can be helpful to the patient, even if the therapist is not proficient in using the technique. The relaxation response is hypothesized to be the physiological polar opposite of the stress response. Whereas the sympathetic nervous system increases the stress response, the parasympathetic nervous system relaxes the muscles and slows heart rate, stress hormone production, and respiration. Virtually all relaxation techniques are built on a foundation of proper breathing.

Breathing

Diaphragmatic breathing refers to deeper breathing and is the foundation of most relaxation techniques. This type of breathing is evident when the abdomen rises and falls in response to each breath. By contrast, more shallow breathing is called *chest breathing*. A focus on the breathing pattern is usually the starting point in eliciting feelings of relaxation. A simple example of diaphragmatic breathing is as follows:

- Place a hand over the belly button;
- Relax the stomach muscles;
- Inhale a slow, deep breath through the nose, causing the abdomen to rise;
- Exhale through the mouth, noticing that the abdomen falls; and
- Continue this for as long as desired or until feeling more relaxed.

Meditation

Meditation refers to focusing the mind on an activity, such as the breathing technique just described, such that the person becomes more inwardly focused. Of course, everyone meditates naturally at times. The regular practice of intentional meditation is an effective and widely used method of inducing feelings of relaxation.

The following is a meditation technique. Find a comfortable place to sit. Begin by using the breathing technique described earlier. Use a focus word or phrase to accompany the breathing. For example, most people have seen examples of meditation on TV or in the movies using the classic mantra *Om* as the focus. However, any word or phrase can be used to focus breathing. When thoughts or images come to mind, the person is reminded to focus on the word or phrase and his or her breathing and simply let that thought go. Meditation is usually recommended for at least 20 minutes to achieve relaxation, but any amount of meditation can be beneficial and calming.

Mindfulness

Mindfulness refers to the practice of staying in the moment with thoughts, feelings, and senses (Kabat-Zinn, 1991; Kabat-Zinn et al., 1992). Mindfulness can be practiced through meditation that is directed at keeping the senses focused only on the present. Mindfulness can also be demonstrated with patients by asking them to eat a raisin (or other food), and eating it with full awareness of each nuance of the sensations of sight, sound, touch, smell, and sight. Mindfulness is as much a philosophy as it is a relaxation technique, with the overall goal of helping people to achieve a better ability to stay in the present.

Visualization

Visualization, also called guided imagery, is the process of imagining things that elicit a feeling of relaxation. Usually, as with all relaxation techniques, a focus first on breathing may be helpful, followed by the visualization technique:

- Imagine that you are in a place that makes you feel very relaxed;
- Focus on the sights in this place to see the details;
- Notice the smells of your place and how they make you feel;
- Focus on the sounds that you hear, such as the wind or water; and
- Notice the sensations of your body, such as the grass under your feet.

Visualization is progressive, and so the patient usually feels more deeply engaged as the exercise moves along. At the end of a visualization exercise (as is true in all relaxation exercises), the patient is slowly and gradually brought back into greater awareness of their current surroundings.

Progressive Muscle Relaxation

People with tense, tight muscles can find much relief through practicing progressive muscle relaxation. The process, as it suggests, consists of contracting and then relaxing all the muscles from the top to the bottom of the body. The process begins with the basic breathing technique and awareness of any areas of tension in the body.

- First, focusing on the muscles in the forehead, tighten for a few seconds, then release the muscles;
- Moving down to the eyes, tighten and release those muscles;
- Tighten, then release, the muscles of the jaw;
- Tighten, then release, the muscles of the neck;
- Tighten, then release, the muscles in the spine;
- Tighten one shoulder, then relax those muscles; and

- Moving down from that shoulder, tighten, then relax, the muscles of the upper arm.

This process is repeated for the entire body, moving from one region to another in a progressive fashion (i.e., first the left shoulder and arm, then the right).

Techniques that focus on regular, slow breathing and muscle relaxation generally are the foundation of all relaxation methods. A great deal of evidence from the cardiac rehabilitation literature supports the integration of these types of techniques into the treatment of anxious cardiac patients. Many cardiac patients who have high anxiety levels come to therapy complaining of muscle tension, headaches, back pain, sleeplessness, and high blood pressure. Therapists who are comfortable with relaxation techniques can incorporate any one of a number of strategies to help patients to learn diaphragmatic breathing, visualization, or progressive muscle relaxation. However, these strategies are also widely available to the lay public through yoga, meditation, and self-help tapes and books. It may not be the best use of therapy time to focus on relaxation strategies because such techniques can be taught by other qualified people. However, there are certainly occasions when patients might benefit from a demonstration, if the therapist is comfortable with this. In contrast, demonstrating techniques in cardiac rehabilitation groups is a useful way to segue into a discussion of mind–body connection. Relaxation methods work. Patients often find it truly helpful to spend time outside of therapy trying out different techniques and learning what helps their body to become calm.

It is extremely difficult for people to practice relaxation techniques when they are acutely anxious. Thus, the most important aspect of relaxation is to practice under nonstressful conditions. Lamaze classes are taught during pregnancy and well before delivery, so that during childbirth the laboring mother and her partner can remember how to control breathing and calm anxiety. Similarly, people with high anxiety levels may not get much out of trying to learn to meditate or breathe slowly when they are acutely anxious. Instead, the techniques must be learned and practiced regularly to have a substantive effect. Alice Domar of Harvard Medical School advocates using mini relaxation exercises or brief, 10-minute relaxation exercises throughout the day to practice (Domar & Dreher, 1996).

Biofeedback

Biofeedback refers to the process of providing patients with information on their own physiological parameters (e.g., heart rate, skin temperature, muscle tension, sweat response) by attaching sensors to measure these involuntary responses. The personal computer has brought biofeedback to home users who can see their physiological signals on a laptop computer or a stand-alone biofeedback device. For example, through use of a finger pulse sensor and software, information on heart rate variability can be transmitted to a computer. The software itself can be used as a relaxation tool rather than simply relying on audiotape, videotape, or DVD. Therapists can use biofeedback to demonstrate to patients that positive emotions and relaxation techniques are readily evident in their effect on their heart. Patients can purchase or borrow the equipment to practice between sessions. Biofeedback can be practiced in sessions as short as 20 minutes or as long as 1 hour and can be used to lower anxiety by providing direct feedback on physiological signs of stress. Heart rate variability biofeedback software is becoming more popular in behavioral cardiology practice and has great potential as a tool to increase the personal relevance of techniques to increase relaxation and positive emotion (McCraty & Tomasino, 2006).

Exercise

People who do not want to try relaxation techniques to lower anxiety may find that exercise provides tremendous stress relief. Aerobic exercise that increases heart rate has been shown to decrease anxiety and depression. Aerobic exercise increases endorphin levels, which improves mood and provides a different method to relax tight muscles. Aerobic exercise is effective in treating diabetes and high blood pressure, which generally improves physical health and metabolism and thus might indirectly reduce physiological symptoms of anxiety. The type of exercise provided in a 12-week cardiac rehabilitation (brisk walking on a treadmill) has also been shown to have beneficial effects in terms of relieving stress, depression, and anxiety as well as improving physical well-being (Lane, Carroll, & Lip, 1999; Roviaro, Holmes, & Holmsten, 1984). When patients remain distressed despite valiant attempts on the part of the clinician, it may be time to consider whether to shift focus to underlying feelings, as described next.

Affect-Focused Therapy

Anxiety itself is a symptom, not necessarily a pure emotion such as fear. Affect-focused therapy techniques are aimed at identifying conflicted emotions. Some theorists have analogized that anxiety is to underlying emotion as smoke is to fire (Magnavita, 1997). That is, the anxiety is merely the sign of an underlying emotional conflict. To eliminate the smoke (anxiety), the source must be identified and expressed adaptively.

Affect-focused techniques can be extremely helpful for anxiety-ridden cardiac patients because therapy techniques that incorporate emotion may have a greater chance to penetrate the anxiety. Emotion is stimulated in a different part of the brain (the amygdala) than is cognition. Every therapist has had an instance when an anxiety-ridden patient could not respond to efforts to shift into more rational thinking. In such cases, greater emphasis on identifying emotions that are inhibited by the anxiety may yield more benefit.

Clinical Example

Joan was a 54-year-old paralegal with a recent heart attack. She identified work-related stress as her primary problem. She lived alone, and her
fellow employees were "like family," although on further examination it
sounded remarkably similar to the dysfunctional family of her youth. She
described how she would lie awake at night worrying about the next
day's projects. At work, she would sometimes become panic stricken and
leave work for the day after her anxiety mounted to an unbearable level.
Joan's boss was about a decade older than her, and they had worked together for more than 15 years. She described him as exacting, hot tem-
pered, and liable to scapegoat her when he was down. At the same time,
she recognized that he also had the capacity to be kind and he valued her
over the other staff. Joan had no difficulty recognizing that she was angry
with her boss. However, she never expressed anger directly toward him
but instead described her "stress, worry, and migraines" to any willing
listener, intimating that her boss was the cause of her heart attack. He
ignored her complaints, and she became increasingly resentful over time.

Joan's anxiety dissipated when she was able to identify her anger in
the moment and express it adaptively with her boss. On one occasion, he
blamed her because he missed a court hearing and called to castigate her
over the phone. In the therapy session the day before, Joan had described
similar behavior, and the therapist and Joan had role-played some ways
that she might handle it. When her boss arrived at work with the benefit
of an hour to cool down, Joan was able to appropriately express her anger
that she was being unfairly blamed. She was surprised that her boss was
able to take responsibility and apologize for his bad behavior. Over time,
their relationship shifted in tone toward a more positive, healthy partnership. Joan's anxiety dissipated, and she was far better able to assert
herself appropriately with authority figures.

Affect-focused techniques are aimed at identifying underlying emotions
and helping the person learn to express feelings appropriately (McCullough
et al., 2003). McCullough et al. wrote a treatment manual that uses the cognitive behavioral language of systematic desensitization or exposure and response prevention as a primary method in working with affect. Systematic
desensitization is a behavioral technique used in the successful treatment of
phobias. In this model, the goal of therapy is to expose the patient to the
feared affect, to discourage the maladaptive avoidant response (response prevention), and to decrease anxiety in both the exposure and response prevention (anxiety regulation). The premise of the manual is that people learn to
develop inhibition or avoidance of emotion. McCullough explained,

> We are all born with all the emotional capacities we need in life. But we
> lose those natural spontaneous capacities. Babies wail when they are
> hungry, tired, or wet, but later learn to inhibit crying. Toddlers vigor-
> ously stomp their feet and say no, but learn through punishment to in-

hibit their defiance. Young children run with open arms to their parents to seek nurturance but later to inhibit those loving feelings. (L. McCullough, personal communication, February 23, 2007)

The therapist's task is to expose the patient to the feared affect gradually, until the inhibitory response is eliminated and the patient is desensitized to the feeling and can express it appropriately. McCullough, as well as most good therapists, aims to regulate the level of anxiety so that it is neither so high that the person is immobilized nor so low that the patient has no motivation to change.

There are a multitude of methods that therapists might use to decrease anxiety about expressing feeling and increase adaptive expression of affect; thus, the following list is not comprehensive.

- Use of fantasy or role play. Example: Overcoming patients' avoidance of affect by asking them to imagine in detail what would happen if they were to confront a feared situation.
- Recognition of disconnection between verbal and nonverbal expression of emotion. Example: "You are laughing as you describe what it was like when you were held helpless on the intensive care unit, but it doesn't sound like you are amused at all. What are you feeling as you recall that time?"
- Reinforcement of appropriate expression of emotion within the therapeutic relationship in an effort to help the patient tolerate intense affects. Example: "You have had some difficulty letting yourself get close to people, so I'm really touched that you are giving me this holiday gift. You must have a lot of positive feeling toward me."

Perhaps the most difficult aspect of focusing on emotion is to know whether the emotion that is being expressed is adaptive. McCullough described the differentiation between adaptive emotions (emotions to increase) and inhibitory emotions such as shame or guilt (emotions that therapists do not want to increase). For example, when grief is expressed, it is cathartic and patients feel relief. However, McCullough warned against encouraging the expression of defensive, inhibitory feelings. Affect-focused techniques have not received as much attention in the research literature as cognitive and behavioral strategies. The goal of focusing on affect is not to flood the patient with more emotion than he or she can handle but to gradually expose the patient to increasing doses of the feared affect, thus diminishing anxiety. An emphasis on affect would be contraindicated when a patient has a score on the *Diagnostic and Statistical Manual of Mental Disorders, Fourth Edition, Text Revision* (American Psychiatric Association, 2000) global assessment of functioning score of less than or equal to 50 (McCullough et al., 2003). Patients who are not functioning well "would not have the strength to guide and direct affects in an adaptive way. They need building of defenses, coping ability, support, and strengthening of human connection first," noted McCullough (personal communication, February 23, 2007). From McCullough's perspective, signals of improved functioning include when avoided feelings are more easily expressed, previously conflicted relationships are closer and more gratifying, and one feels more compassionate about the self.

SUMMARY

Anxiety is the most prevalent form of psychological distress in all populations, including cardiac patients. There is much to be learned about the effect of anxiety on cardiovascular prognosis. Some people with heart problems adjust more poorly to cardiac events because of an underlying predisposition to anxiety, and others develop anxiety as a reaction to a clear precipitant, such as the firing of an ICD. It is clear that treating anxiety improves quality of life, and most of the therapeutic strategies outlined in this chapter can be used to reduce symptoms of anxiety.

6

ANGER AND HOSTILITY

One of the basic human emotions, anger is universally experienced across cultures. Anger has been described as a negative, activating feeling that generates high levels of sympathetic arousal, occurs relatively frequently, lasts longer than other affective states, is more likely to lead to verbal expression with more effect on tone and volume than other emotions, and is more likely to negatively effect other interpersonal relationships compared with other affective states (DiGiuseppe & Tafrate, 2007). Anger can serve as an adaptive response to assert one's needs or to stop an undesired action (McCullough et al., 2003), but it may also have health consequences. Anger becomes a problem when it cannot be expressed adaptively. Maladaptive expression of anger falls into one of two categories: disinhibition (temper tantrums, rages) or overinhibition (silent seething or resentment). By contrast, hostility has been viewed as a personality trait in that it incorporates cognitions, behaviors, and emotions into a habitual pattern of relating to others with mistrust, pessimism, contempt, antagonism, and a propensity to react to frustrating situations with resentment or irritation (Barefoot, 1992). Aggression refers to both verbal and physical behaviors with the intent to hurt or injure another person (Smith, Glazer, Ruiz, & Gallo, 2004).

HISTORICAL RESEARCH ON ANGER

From the time that Hippocrates first described the four humors, it has been recognized that there is a link between anger and bodily response. According to Hippocrates, the choleric person was thought to have an excess of yellow bile and to be easily angered. Psychoanalyst Franz Alexander was one of the first contemporary psychiatrists to suggest a link between heart disease and hostility (French, 1964). Alexander was known as the "father of psychosomatic medicine" for his recognition that emotions were linked to physical illness. Nearly 70 years ago, in the first issue of the first volume of the journal *Psychosomatic Medicine*, Alexander (1939) suggested that repressed anger was responsible for elevations in blood pressure. Alexander observed that, of course, not all people with high blood pressure are hostile and theorized that essential hypertension could develop when other neurotic symptoms that serve to drain off pent-up hostile impulses are absent.

Twenty years later, Rosenman and Friedman launched scientific investigations into the relationship between anger and heart disease in a research endeavor called the Western Collaborative Group Study. This epidemiological study of more than 3,000 men in California began in 1960 and followed them over 8½ years. The Western Collaborative Group Study showed that Type A behavior pattern (TABP)—a clustering of behaviors including a competitive, goal-driven approach to daily activities, aggressive behaviors, hyperarousal of emotional and physical alertness, and hostile affect—doubled the risk of developing coronary heart disease (CHD), even after controlling for cardiac risk factors, in a sample of healthy men ages 39 to 59 (Rosenman et al., 1975). Findings of an association between TABP and CHD in an initially healthy population also supported these findings (Jenkins, Rosenman, & Zyzanski, 1974), as did the longitudinal evidence from the Framingham Heart Study (Haynes, Feinleib, & Kannel, 1980). The Framingham Heart Study is a federally funded longitudinal study that began in 1948 and recruited more than 5,000 men and women from Framingham, Massachusetts, with follow-up assessments every 2 years. The Framingham Heart Study is ongoing with more than 5,000 participants in the second generation (children of the original cohort and their spouses) as well as more than 4,000 enrolled from the third generation.

What became puzzling about the Type A research is that studies of people with established risk factors for CHD did not show a relationship between TABP and heart disease. People who were already at risk for heart disease by virtue of the fact that they had one or more risk factors and also had TABP were no more likely to have a subsequent heart attack compared with those who did not. Multiple large, randomized clinical trials failed to show a relationship between TABP and first major coronary events (Cohen & Reed, 1985; Shekelle et al., 1985). These puzzling results led to many post hoc analyses of the original studies that measured TABP (Matthews, Glass,

Rosenman, & Bortner, 1977). Only hostility was confirmed as being predictive of increased risk of death in healthy subjects (Hecker, Chesney, Black, & Frautschi, 1988) and increased risk of recurring heart disease in people with CHD (Goodman, Quigley, Moran, Meilman, & Sherman, 1996; Koskenvuo et al., 1988).

RECURRENT CORONARY PREVENTION PROJECT

The Recurrent Coronary Prevention Project (RCPP) was a trial of counseling designed to alter Type A behavior (Friedman et al., 1986). The RCPP study was completed in the mid-1980s and included 862 post–myocardial infarction (MI) patients who were randomized, between 1978 and 1979, using a ratio of two to one into the control condition (cardiac counseling; n = 270) or the experimental condition (cardiac counseling plus Type A counseling; n = 592). A third comparison group was a convenience sample of 151 men who declined random assignment but agreed to be followed in the research study. Study participants were predominantly male (92%) and averaged 53 years of age. All counseling was provided in a group format. Cardiac counseling was provided by cardiologists who met with patients twice a month for 3 months, then monthly for 3 months, then once every 2 months for the entirety of the study. Type A counseling was provided by a psychiatrist or psychologist, and participants in the experimental group met weekly for the first 2 months, twice a week for the next 2 months, and monthly for the remainder of the study. Type A counseling was designed to promote relaxation and reduce time urgency, competitiveness, and hostility. TABP was assessed using videotaped clinical interviews as well as using self-report ratings, spouse-completed ratings, and ratings completed by a work colleague. TABP significantly declined in the group treated with Type A counseling, and this change was maintained at 4.5-year follow-up. More than one third (35%) of the intervention group had a reduction in Type A behavior equal to one standard deviation, compared with less than 1 out of 10 participants (9.8%) in the cardiac counseling group. The cumulative 4.5 cardiac recurrence rate was 12.9% in the experimental group, significantly less than the 21.2% in the control group or the 28.2% of the group that was followed without treatment. Although the difference between groups was noteworthy, other behavioral cardiology researchers did not enthusiastically embrace the findings. The findings were published at a time when a number of negative studies were published that failed to confirm a relationship between Type A and risk of recurrent heart disease in patients with established cardiac disease (Shekelle et al., 1985), and the methodology was criticized for the subjectivity inherent in rating videotape of TABP (the dependent variable). Consequently, this type of treatment was never widely adopted in the clinical community. Dreher (2001) pointed out that the RCPP is a "sleeper" study because the scientific community has largely overlooked the results. The sample of 863 in the RCPP study is 10 times larger than that of Spiegel's widely known study (Spiegel, Bloom, Kraemer, & Gottheil, 1989) that tested the value of psychosocial intervention for women with metastatic breast cancer. Indeed, it is an irony that the field of oncology has translated a far smaller base of psychosocial research into widely adopted clinical practice at a far more rapid pace than behavioral cardiology. Most hospital oncology programs offer a multitude of support groups for cancer patients, but few cardiology programs offer treatment services similar to the model provided by Friedman et al. (1986).

The use of a large-scale clinical trial to alter a personality trait is a unique characteristic of the RCPP trial, and the magnitude of difference between the treated and untreated groups was equal to one standard deviation. By comparison, the Canadian Cardiac Randomized Evaluation of Antidepressant and Psychotherapy Efficacy trial, designed to test interpersonal therapy for depression in cardiac patients, showed no difference between the psychosocial treatment and control conditions, and the Enhancing Recovery in Coronary Heart Disease trial, designed to test cognitive behavioral therapy for depression in cardiac patients, produced a difference of about 10 percentage points that disappeared in the long-term follow-up (Berkman et al., 2003; Lesperance et al., 2007). A return to the focus on altering personality traits might prove fruitful in behavioral cardiology. A personality theorist, Jeffrey Magnavita, stated,

> If we conceptualize personality as a more fluid concept, then we can postulate that everyone's personality can, under stress, enter into a state of dysfunctioning. Some individuals experience this as a chronic state while others may episodically experience symptom outbreaks. The reluctance to initiate more psychotherapy treatment trials designed to alter personality may arise from the ill-conceived notion that personality characteristics are immutable. (personal communication, March 7, 2007)

Although the "Type A" description still resonates with many people, propelling them to seek treatment for stress management, no large-scale clinical trials have since tested psychological treatments for hostility in the last 2 decades.

Clinical Example

> The cardiac rehabilitation staff referred Clarisse, a French Canadian woman in her early 60s. She had increasing bouts of angina 5 months ago and was treated with a four-way coronary artery bypass graft operation (CABG). During this same time period, Clarisse was worried about her daughter, Monique, who had small children of her own and was going through a divorce. Clarisse provided child care three times a week for her grandchildren, but her relationship with her daughter was stormy.

They had frequent control battles over how the children were dressed or disciplined. Clarisse did not discuss her cardiac problems with her children, declaring that she did not want to worry them. Her daughter brought her to medical appointments, but Clarisse refused to share details of her prognosis, leaving Monique to wonder whether her mother might die imminently. Clarisse martyred herself, pushing well beyond her physical limits to care for her grandchildren and feeling resentful that her daughter seemed to fail to appreciate the sacrifice.

Clarisse's therapy consisted of about 60 sessions and lasted more than 3 years. She dropped out once for several months, but she soon returned and recounted a number of blunders by the therapist that had led to her departure. Clarisse initially presented her primary stressors in terms of her worry about her daughter, her inability to care for her grandchildren, and her worry that she might die too young. Her relevant family of origin data included the loss of her own mother, who was in her early 50s when she died of sudden cardiac death. At that time, Clarisse's children were very young, and she buried her grief to continue to function as a stay-at-home mother. Clarisse recognized that she was angry with her children and considered her feelings justified.

In the first session, Clarisse went on at length, ignoring the therapist's efforts to try to gently end the session to meet with another waiting patient. She rose from her chair on her own timetable (about 10 minutes after the session should have ended). In the following session, she shifted course and left 15 minutes early before the session was over. She waggled her fingers at the therapist dismissively, saying she would see the therapist next week.

Clarisse's therapy was long term by current standards. She was easily hurt, and it took more than a year before she could freely admit that the therapist had inadvertently angered her at times. It was another year before she could empathize with her daughter's perspective. To her credit, she remained an attentive and loving grandmother even when she felt injured by her daughter. Her turning point came after she dropped out of therapy for several months but returned with an improved ability to verbalize her intense feelings. After testing out her ability to express anger constructively, the quality of her communication with her children began to improve. Clarisse focused on her open heart surgery at the beginning and end of therapy. Toward the beginning, she felt very hurt that her children were not as attentive following her surgery as she would have preferred. At the end of therapy, she freely admitted that the surgery had left her feeling terrified of depending on others. She struggled with difficulty trusting that her children and, to a lesser extent, her doctors, would take care of her in a time of need. Clarisse's therapy focused on changing longstanding predisposition toward hostility by addressing her fears of dependency, her need to exert control over others, and her inability to express anger adaptively with her loved ones.

Dreher (2004) suggested that effective psychotherapy treatment for a cardiac patient needs to address not only psychological reactions to the cardiac event but also the patient's characteristic coping style and the origins of the symptoms. The tendency to ruminate angrily, after a provocation, is an example of a characteristic coping style that is ripe for the development of psychological intervention.

ANGRY RUMINATION

Rumination is a trait that refers to the tendency to focus on negative interpretations or aspects of one's self. Angry rumination (Gerin, Davidson, Christenfeld, Goyal, & Schwartz, 2006) refers to the tendency to think obsessively about a situation after anger provocation, similar to Clarisse's case discussed earlier. Angry rumination might explain one pathway connecting depression to cardiovascular disease. Multiple laboratory studies have demonstrated that people with a tendency toward angry rumination tend to have a prolonged cardiovascular reaction following anger provocation. Gerin and colleagues conducted a laboratory study with 60 men and women, measuring their tendency toward trait rumination and asking them to remember situations from the past year that were upsetting and still upset them to think about, a task that is associated with elevations in blood pressure (see Figure 6.1). Participants were then divided into a distraction condition, in which magazines, puzzles, or small toys were available that could provide distraction, or a no-distraction condition, with nothing else to focus on.

As hypothesized, people scoring high on trait rumination who had no distraction had the poorest blood pressure recovery. Theoretically, it is not cardiovascular reactivity itself but the inability to take the body off of its state of "red alert" that is detrimental to the heart. People with an angry ruminative coping style may become afraid of getting angry after a cardiovascular event for fear that anger will trigger a heart attack, and the suppressed anger might lead to other psychological sequelae, such as depression (Dreher, 2004).

CONTEMPORARY PERSPECTIVES ON HOSTILITY AS A PREDICTOR OF CARDIAC MORBIDITY AND MORTALITY

The field of research on hostility as a predictor of cardiovascular morbidity has a rich and often confusing history. A review by Smith et al. (2004) on this topic noted six, large-scale prospective studies published between 1996 and 2002 that have shown that trait anger and hostility predict cardiac morbidity in initially healthy people. One study, the Atherosclerosis Risk in Communities Study, enrolled more than 13,000 Black and White men and women and found that trait anger predicted increased risk of CHD over a follow-up period of 4.5 years (Williams, 2000). However, at least two large-

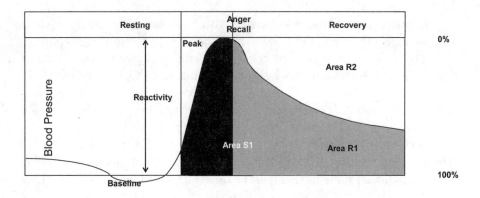

Figure 6.1. Blood pressure recovery from angry rumination. The method for analyzing blood pressure recovery was previously described in "Psychological and Physical Stress-Induced Cardiovascular Reactivity and Diurnal Blood Pressure Variation in Women With Different Work Shifts," by K. Kario, J. E. Schwartz, W. Gerin, N. Robayo, E. Maceo, and T. G. Pickering, 2002, *Hypertension Research, 25,* 543–551. From "The Role of Angry Rumination and Distraction in Blood Pressure Recovery From Emotional Arousal," by W. Gerin, K. W. Davidson, N. J. Christenfeld, T. Goyal, and J. E. Schwartz, 2006, *Psychosomatic Medicine, 68,* p. 67. Copyright 2006 by Lippincott Williams & Wilkins. Reprinted with permission.

scale studies have reported null findings (Eng, Fitzmaurice, Kubzansky, Rimm, & Kawachi, 2003; Sykes et al., 2002). It seems likely that hostility and anger may increase risk for cardiovascular events in people with an underlying vulnerability. For example, anger provocation can trigger MI in vulnerable people (Mittleman et al., 1995), and researchers can induce myocardial ischemia in people with CHD in lab experiments simply by asking them to recall a previous anger-provoking incident (Boltwood, Taylor, Burke, Grogin, & Giacomini, 1993; Ironson et al., 1992). Anger can also trigger arrhythmia in people predisposed to heart rhythm problems. Rachel Lambert, an electrophysiologist at Yale University, conducted a study with 42 patients who have implantable cardioverter defibrillators (ICDs). The study participants were given diaries to record their mood and physical activity during time periods that preceded spontaneous ICD shocks as well as control periods 1 week later. Feelings of anger were more likely to precede shock than the control periods. Feelings of anxiety, worry, sadness, or happiness were not predictive of shock (Lampert et al., 2002).

HOW DO ANGER AND HOSTILITY AFFECT THE HEART?

There are a number of intriguing somatic consequences to anger provocation that, in turn, are linked to CHD (Compare, Manzoni, & Molinari,

2006). Anger provocation is associated with increased sympathetic arousal. That is, anger can trigger increases in heart rate, blood pressure, epinephrine, and cortisol levels as well as increase levels of C-reactive protein and the expression of proinflammatory cytokines (Sinha, Lovallo, & Parsons, 1992; Suarez, 2004; Suarez, Lewis, & Kuhn, 2002). People with a greater tendency toward trait anger may have neurological differences from those who do not score highly on this measure, as evidenced by the fact that trait anger is associated with greater left frontal cortical activity (Harmon-Jones, 2007). Anger arousal has been shown to precede heart rate variability in people who have arrhythmia problems (Lampert et al., 2002). In addition, people with a greater tendency toward angry and hostile affect are more likely to be socially isolated or have unsatisfying interpersonal relationships and more likely to engage in health risk behaviors such as smoking (Brummett et al., 1998, 2002, 2005), which in turn have a negative impact on health. Although there is much to be learned about the pathophysiological mechanisms connecting anger and hostility to CHD, it is clear that the human body tends to react strongly to the inability to express anger in a healthy way.

ASSESSMENT OF ANGER AND HOSTILITY

Many measurement tools assess anger and hostility, but only four measures are presented here. These are chosen because they are easy to administer and can be incorporated into clinical practice. Although there are several interview rating methods to assess hostility, these require extensive training and have been validated primarily in studies with White, higher socioeconomic status males. Self-report measures of anger and hostility do have the disadvantage of being influenced by social desirability (Harris, 1997) and so must be interpreted in the context of other relevant information obtained in the clinical setting.

Aggression Questionnaire

The Aggression Questionnaire (AQ) was developed by Buss and Perry (1992) and is a 29-item self-report measure that taps four domains: physical aggression (e.g., "I have threatened people I know"), verbal aggression (e.g., "I often find myself disagreeing with people"), anger (e.g., "I sometimes feel like a powder keg ready to explode"), and hostility (e.g., "I wonder why sometimes I feel so bitter about things"). The psychometric properties of the AQ are well established, and people who score high on this measure also have been shown to have higher levels of risk with respect to a number of markers of cardiovascular disease (Bernstein & Gesn, 1997; Diamond & Magaletta, 2006; Gallo & Smith, 1998; Harmon-Jones, 2007; Harris, 1997; Hillbrand et al., 2005). The AQ is relatively easy for clinicians to administer and provides specific examples of behaviors and attitudes that can be addressed therapeutically. When cardiac patients present for treatment asking for help with anger management, this questionnaire can provide an excellent starting point that can guide the treatment goals.

Anger Rumination Scale

The Anger Rumination Scale (ARS) is a 19-item self-report questionnaire that measures the tendency to ruminate or brood about anger episodes (Sukhodolsky, Golub, & Cromwell, 2001). One mechanism by which rumination appears to exert its effects on the heart is by maintaining blood pressure elevations well beyond the precipitating event (Gerin et al., 2006). The ARS measures the tendency to engage in unintentional reoccurring thoughts about anger episodes. The scale consists of four factors: angry afterthoughts, thoughts of revenge, angry memories, and understanding of causes. The ARS has adequate internal consistency (α = .93) and test–retest reliability (r = .77) and has shown good convergent validity with other measures of anger and negative affectivity (Sukhodolsky et al., 2001). The ARS can be particularly helpful to guide interventions designed to alter the cognitive patterns that are associated with angry rumination.

Spielberger State–Trait Anger Expression Inventory

The State–Trait Anger Expression Inventory—2 (STAXI–2) is a 57-item self-report questionnaire that takes about 10 minutes to complete and is appropriate for adults and for teens over the age of 16 (Spielberger, 1999; Spielberger, Reheiser, & Sydeman, 1995). The questionnaire measures the intensity of anger as an emotional state (state anger) and the tendency to experience angry feelings as a personality trait (trait anger). The instrument consists of six scales measuring the intensity of anger and the disposition to experience angry feelings. The scale also measures (a) *anger expression–out*, the expression of anger toward other persons or objects; (b) *anger expression–in*, holding back or suppressing angry feelings; (c) *anger control–out*, controlling angry emotions by restraining the expression of anger; and (d) *anger control–in*, controlling suppressed anger by cooling off or calming down. Although the STAXI has been primarily a research tool, it can be used as a clinical measure for those patients who seek help with adaptive expression of anger (M. Burns, Bird, Leach, & Higgins, 2003). For example, patients who have difficulty finding adaptive mechanisms for expressing their anger may find it helpful to pinpoint more specifically which dimensions of anger are most problematic, as measured by the subscales. DiGiuseppe and Tafrate (2007) suggested that therapists can incorporate standardized measures of anger therapeutically by offering to provide nonjudgmental feedback about the individual's score relative to norms in the population. This approach is an adaptation of the motivational interviewing methods that W. R. Miller and Rollnick (2002) have used to address problem drinking.

Cook–Medley Hostility Scale

The Cook–Medley Hostility scale is a 50-item self-report scale from the Minnesota Multiphasic Personality Inventory (MMPI), which uses true–false questions (Cook & Medley, 1954). There is a 27-item abbreviated version (Barefoot, Dodge, Peterson, Dahlstrom, & Williams, 1989) that has been more closely linked with CHD compared with the 50-item version. The Cook–Medley Hostility scale has been shown to predict acute MI (Barefoot, Larsen, von der Lieth, & Schroll, 1995) as well as survival in cardiac patients (Barefoot et al., 1989). In particular, the subscales of cynicism, hostile affect, and aggressive responding have been shown to be better predictors than the full scale (Barefoot et al., 1989). An ancillary study from the Heart and Estrogen/Progestin Replacement Study trial has also provided evidence that the Cook–Medley Hostility scale predicts recurrent coronary events in postmenopausal women (Chaput et al., 2002). This measure has been used primarily for research purposes. To the extent that a clinician is already competent and familiar with administering and interpreting the MMPI, this scale could be used in clinical practice.

Summary of Assessment Measures for Anger and Hostility

Each measure described is useful in certain circumstances and can inform clinical practice. The AQ, ARS, and STAXI–2 are somewhat easier to interpret and sensitive enough to intervention that a psychotherapist could use them to examine change over time. These measures are also commonly used in research studies. However, because it is not socially desirable to endorse angry feelings, thoughts, or behaviors, there are some drawbacks to using self-report measures of anger and hostility. In clinical practice, paper-and-pencil measures need to be combined with a thorough clinical interview to uncover the array of personality traits, behaviors, attitudes, beliefs, cognitions, and emotional states associated with anger and hostility. Paper-and-pencil measures can help a psychotherapist to have good operational definitions of the patient's anger problem, so that it can be easily explained and become a point of therapeutic focus.

PSYCHOTHERAPEUTIC TECHNIQUES FOR ADAPTIVE EXPRESSION OF ANGER

Working effectively with anger is a challenge for most therapists. Because there is widespread awareness among the lay public about TABP, it is not uncommon that cardiac patients will present for therapy treatment with the belief that anger (a.k.a. stress or irritability) plays an etiological role in their heart disease. More often than not, patients will present with the hope that some type of stress management or relaxation therapy will rid them of their pent-up anger. Sometimes traditional relaxation therapies such as those discussed in chapter 5 of this volume can be beneficial for such patients. Some of the leaders in behavioral cardiology have even targeted the lay public directly with self-help strategies. Redford Williams, author of the book *Anger Kills* (Williams & Williams, 1993), has written prolifically on the toxic effect that anger and hostility have on the heart. Williams, along with his wife, Virginia, have developed a videotape educational module and a workshop series titled "Williams LifeSkills" aimed at teaching techniques and coping strategies to improve quality of life. The challenge for mental health professionals who practice behavioral cardiology is to offer something to patients beyond what they can find in the self-help section of the bookstore or the many how-to articles on psychological health in most women's magazines (e.g., how to stop controlling others, how to avoid getting angry).

Accurate Identification and Differentiation of Anger

The ability to identify anger is a necessary first step for patients. Overt displays of aggressiveness or tantrums are not difficult to recognize as maladaptive expressions of anger. However, patients and therapists can find it difficult to recognize and identify the emotion behind the many more subtle covert expressions of anger or hostile traits. Hostility is a complex construct that has cognitive, behavioral, and affective dimensions. The cognitive aspects of hostility include pessimistic attitudes, cynicism, and the tendency to mistrust others. Behavioral expressions of anger are threatening gestures or actions (e.g., punching walls) or silent withdrawal and isolation. Affective experience of anger is often reported as an intense, visceral feeling (e.g., "I feel like there is a volcano about to explode inside").

Some cardiac patients have difficulty recognizing and expressing anger appropriately, whereas others have trouble controlling anger outbursts. In either case, the goal of treatment focuses on improving ability to adaptively express anger, but the therapeutic approach for the former involves greater elicitation and activation of anger, whereas the approach for the latter includes greater use of methods to refocus, control temper, and defuse negative emotion using strategies such as those described in the "Hook" technique (Powell, 1996), described subsequently. If there were a triaging system for this therapeutic focus, the most important first step would be to help people who are violent or aggressive learn to practice effective methods of impulse control. Cardiac patients who seek counseling or stress management or psychotherapy often present with examples of rage that is deflected, such as pulling a phone out of a wall or cutting off another driver in traffic. These behavioral expressions of anger are ubiquitous and do not necessarily require the focus on impulse control that, for example, a person with a domestic violence history would need. In general, cognitive approaches are good for people who need to learn to dampen and defuse their anger response. Psychodynamic and affect-focused approaches are good for people who have difficulty admitting that they are angry and expressing it constructively. Both techniques are critically important to help patients become more aware of the experience of anger and to learn to control their reaction and express their feelings adaptively.

Cognitive Behavioral Approaches to Treat Maladaptive Anger

In their 1996 book, *Heart and Mind: The Practice of Cardiac Psychology*, Robert Allan and Stephen Scheidt included a chapter by Linda Powell called "The Hook: A Metaphor for Gaining Control of Emotional Reactivity." The metaphor of the hook refers to the tendency to become angry in response to provocation, and this psychoeducational approach focuses on helping people to identify their triggers of anger and to avoid being baited or "hooked." The treatment model was developed through the RCPP and is essentially a cognitive behavioral treatment to avoid reacting with anger to provoking stimuli by changing the perception of the trigger. The hook is a useful technique in that each step is operationally defined. To begin, the clinician asks patients three questions:

- What is behavior modification? Answer: *Keeping control by changing the way you think about others.* The group of patients is introduced to the theory that people influence each other with their actions, and they come to understand that changing the way they respond to a provocation is the essence of behavior modification.
- What is impatience and irritation? Answer: A *quick response to a small and unexpected stressor.* In a group situation, the clinician might at this point demonstrate how people are "hooked" by accusing one or more of the participants of not paying attention. The goal of this step is to point out that the typical thought runs to the injustice of the stressor and that this cognition precedes the emotion of anger.
- What can we (you) do about it? *At this point, the clinician typically draws a picture of a hook, as well as a light bulb.* The correct answer is that people should correctly identify stressors as hooks, and that the labeling process itself will defuse the level of emotional arousal elicited by the stressor. (Powell, 1996, pp. 318–322)

The technique of teaching cardiac patients the Hook to control emotional reactivity is useful, particularly in settings such as cardiac rehabilitation groups. This psychoeducational technique could also be considered in individual therapy to strengthen a client's self-control capacities. However, the Hook technique will not necessarily help people who genuinely do not have a good understanding of the emotion of anger. A discussion of this follows.

Psychodynamic Techniques to Treat Maladaptive Anger

There is a generation of short-term dynamic psychotherapy (STDP) therapists who have made great use of dynamic and gestalt techniques to increase awareness of emotional inner states and increase a client's capacity to tolerate angry feelings (Davanloo, 1978; Magnavita, 1997; McCullough et al., 2003; Sifneos, 1981). Therapists will often "de-repress" feelings by encouraging a patient to recall an anger-provoking incident in detail, with special attention to the bodily experience of the emotion. *Forced fantasy* goes a step further by asking the patient to imagine, "What would have happened if . . ." (e.g., "you really let go and have him have it?" or "you could have said exactly what you wanted to say?"). This type of vivid imagery can help people to recognize the intensity of the angry feeling in a safe environment and become more comfortable with the fact that anger is a normal human emotion. Clinicians who practice STDP tend to make frequent use of interpretation and even interruption of psychological defenses. For example, the therapist might interrupt a patient on a tangent and help the patient examine his or her reaction to being interrupted. STDP therapists may be more likely than therapists in other modalities to interpret nonverbal defenses, such as laughing when describing a situation that would provoke anger or hair twisting when describing rage. This class of defense restructuring techniques has been termed *challenge and pressure* by Davanloo (1980). A benefit of this therapeutic modality is that this type of relatively intensive intervention can penetrate defenses against anger very quickly, thus activating patients sufficiently to see an effect. A downside of this type of technique is that it requires extensive training and has the potential for iatrogenic effects if it is misused and the patient is left feeling emotionally aroused, with no relief from the anger.

Clinicians might consider STDP techniques for people who seem angry but do not recognize it. It is not particularly difficult for therapists to help cardiac patients to stop acting out aggressive behaviors, but it is somewhat more challenging to assist patients to recognize silence, withdrawal, isolation, tone of voice, and facial expression as behavioral communications of anger. Again, the anger itself is not the problem; instead, the mode of communication is ineffective and maladaptive.

Clinical Example

Rona, a hardworking mother of four who had recently undergone valve replacement, described her exasperation with her adolescent son. "I work

50 to 60 hours a week and he cannot even pick up his clothes off the floor." Her eyes narrowed, her voice became even softer, but her rage was evident and barely restrained. "My parents beat us and I swore I would not beat my kids, but I want to knock this kid into the next room." Although Rona easily recognized her anger, she felt impotent to do anything constructive with it. She spent some effort in therapy determining what she wanted to communicate (i.e., the consequences of failure to live under house rules) and how she wanted to communicate it (i.e., with a firm and authoritative but not hostile manner).

Effective communication of anger requires more emotional maturity than most of us, including therapists, have, and thus there is almost always room for improvement in this area. Effort expended tends to correlate well with improved relationships with others.

Affect-Focused Approaches to Treat Maladaptive Anger

Underlying attitudes of mistrust, pessimism, or cynicism take time to untangle in therapy. One such therapeutic approach that focuses primarily on emotion and has direct relevance to the treatment of anger is affect-focused therapy. As mentioned in chapter 5 of this volume, affect-focused therapy conceptualizes problems with feelings as "affect phobias" (McCullough et al., 2003) and is based on the theory that conflict about feeling (affect phobia) is a key etiological contributor to major depression that occurs in cardiac patients. By helping patients to experience conflicted feelings and desensitize them, they are better able to respond adaptively, that is, are less anxious or ashamed about the emotions that drive depressive symptoms.

Therapeutic gains from an affect-focused therapy may last longer because emotion-laden interaction is more memorable and easily retrievable in times of need (Dornelas & Magnavita, 2001). Emotional information is better remembered than neutral information, probably because the information is encoded using the amygdalar–hippocampal network, whereas neutral information is encoded using the prefrontal cortex–hippocampal network (Dolcos, LaBar, & Cabeza, 2004). Laboratory studies support this hypothesis. For example, in a study conducted by Dolcos, LaBar, and Cabeza (2005), participants were showed 180 pictures that were equally divided into pleasant, neutral, and unpleasant images while they were undergoing functional magnetic resonance imaging (fMRI). One year later, the participants were rescanned with fMRI and viewed the old images plus 90 new images again. Participants remembered emotional pictures more easily than neutral ones. Thus, it is not a huge leap to speculate that therapies that address angry emotion directly, rather than merely attempting to alter the angry thoughts and behaviors, might be more effective and memorable. Interventions that incorporate a direct focus on emotion may also engage patients more quickly because affect is a primary motivator of behavior (Tomkins, 1984).

McCullough et al. (2003) hypothesized that if affect is a primary motivator of behavior, then it should be more explicitly integrated into psychotherapy treatments.

Therapists sometimes worry that anger expression might be dangerous for cardiac patients (e.g., will cause the person to have a heart attack). This fear seems groundless, because the goal in therapy is not to provoke the patient into becoming angry in an uncontrolled manner but to allow the person to express an avoided emotion in a healthy way. Most therapists who specifically focus on affect recognize the need for patients to have both cognitive understanding and emotional experience.

A Word About Countertransference

Countertransference, or the therapist's experience of feelings toward a patient, is almost inevitable when the patient is hostile, controlling, or has difficulty expressing anger. Even as the therapist guides the patient toward mastering feelings of anger, it can be difficult to find something constructive to do with the therapist's own irritation toward the patient. Therapists who are themselves prone to trait anger or are highly controlling might feel particularly challenged. Discussion of cases with peers, clinical supervision, self-reflection, or personal therapy can all be useful ways to use the countertransferential feeling as an opportunity for emotional maturation.

SUMMARY

Helping people to become less hostile and better able to express their anger adaptively can involve any of the techniques described in this chapter. At the minimum, it is essential, but not always easy, to help patients to recognize their own anger. Cognitive behavioral and psychoeducational techniques, such as that demonstrated by the Hook, can be an important aspect of gaining control over cardiovascular reactivity. Because there is a social desirability to not express anger, it is important to recognize and address the defenses that patients have against anger. Finally, work on anger cannot be done in an abstract, intellectualized manner. An effective way to learn to cope with angry feelings is to experience such feelings in the therapy session without negative consequences. Visceral experience is more easily remembered and translated into behavior change in the patient's own outside relationships.

Cardiac patients often have some knowledge about anger and heart health and are very often motivated to change, even if they may refer to "stress" rather than to anger or hostility. Cardiac patients do not have the luxury of waiting until the research community has published more clinical trials to evaluate the benefit of differing therapeutic strategies for treatment of anger or hostility. When patients present for treatment, it is wise to assess and consider whether there is any room for improvement in the adaptive expressive of anger and the extent to which hostility (mistrustful attitudes, cynical beliefs, aggressive behaviors, or bodily experience of anger) is a problem for the patient. If so, anger may be worthy of therapeutic focus in the treatment.

7

INTERPERSONAL RELATIONSHIPS
AND SOCIAL SUPPORT

Social support, similar to the constructs of depression, anxiety, and anger discussed in previous chapters, is a large umbrella term with a variety of different meanings. Multiple studies of cardiac patients have demonstrated that lack of social support, whether evidenced by the number of social ties or the quality of the relationships, is related to depression, anxiety, and poor cardiac prognosis. Low levels of social support predict initial coronary heart disease (CHD) incidence and subsequent mortality. High levels of social support buffer the effects of the cardiac event. Social isolation and lack of emotional support predict death after heart attack (Barefoot et al., 2003; Frasure-Smith & Lesperance, 2000).

HOW DO INTERPERSONAL RELATIONSHIPS
AFFECT THE HEART?

Why is it that people with no emotional support are more likely to develop heart disease and to die after a heart attack? Social isolation is a strong predictor of cardiac mortality. A study by Brummett et al. (2001) of

103

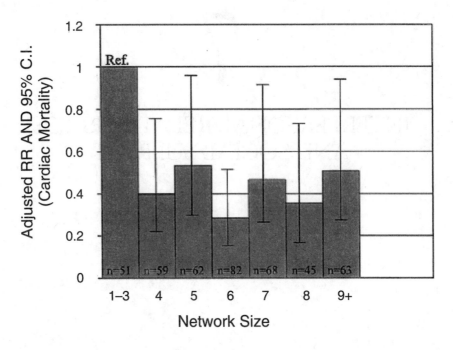

Figure 7.1. Adjusted risk of cardiac death associated with network size ($N = 430$, number of events = 120). Analyses were adjusted for number of diseased vessels, left ventricular ejection fraction, presence or absence of congestive heart failure, age, and comorbidity. RR = relative risk; C.I. = confidence interval. From "Characteristics of Socially Isolated Patients With Coronary Artery Disease Who Are at Elevated Risk for Mortality," by B. H. Brummett et al., 2001, *Psychosomatic Medicine, 63,* p. 269. Copyright 2001 by Lippincott Williams & Wilkins. Reprinted with permission.

430 patients with significant coronary artery disease showed that cardiac patients with few or no supports are at elevated risk for recurrent events and death (see Figure 7.1).

Figure 7.1 demonstrates that the risk of mortality for people who have the fewest social ties was significantly higher, even when age and disease severity were controlled in the statistical analysis. Brummett et al. (2001) found that the most socially isolated cardiac patients scored higher on a hostility measure, had lower incomes, and were more likely to be cigarette smokers, compared with those with more social ties. However, when these variables were adjusted for in the analysis, social isolation remained a robust predictor of mortality. Berkman (1995) reviewed the social support literature and noted that lack of support is linked to suppressed immune function; this conclusion is supported by research on bereaved spouses and caregivers of chronically ill spouses. In addition, Berkman also underscored that primate studies are consistent in their findings that isolation and lack of affiliation in groups are linked with impaired neuroendocrine function. Overall, the distress associated with loneliness and relational problems has been proposed to affect the heart through the three primary physiological pathways described in chapter 3 (this volume): general sympathetic arousal, autonomic balance as reflected in heart rate variability, and inflammation. Of course, social relationships may also affect cardiovascular health as a result of nonadherence. People who have no support, perceive that they have no support, or have poor relational quality may also find it very difficult to comply with health care provider instructions. Socially isolated people may face a variety of barriers, from the obvious (e.g., getting a ride to a cardiologist appointment) to the less straightforward (e.g., feeling motivated to stick to a diet without any supportive help from family or friends).

The hormonal response to positive relationships has been less studied but may represent another physiological pathway by which interpersonal relationships affect heart health. Human beings are inherently social creatures, driven to attach and connect with others. The effects of positive, secure relationships seems likely to have a beneficial effect on the heart. Increases in positive affiliative behaviors are associated with reductions in sympathetic activity and increases in oxytocin levels. Oxytocin is the neuropeptide associated with maternal behavior and attachment bonding (Insel, Gingrich, & Young, 2001). It is plausible that cardiovascular risk could actually be improved through the presence of positive interactions rather than simply the absence of hostile, negative interactions. Although this supposition is speculative, it is based on several strong lines of research on affiliation in both primates and humans. Increases in affiliative behavior have been shown to be associated with improvements in physiological parameters. For example, Light, Grewen, and Amico (2005) demonstrated that women who were hugged by their partner more often showed lower basal blood pressure and higher oxytocin levels. Other research from this group has provided support that relational quality, partner support, and warmth of the contact are associated with lower cardiovascular reactivity in both men and women, Caucasians and African Americans (Grewen, Anderson, Girdler, & Light, 2003; Grewen, Girdler, Amico, & Light, 2005; Grewen, Girdler, & Light, 2005). Oxytocin has been called one of the "antistress" hormones because it reduces blood pressure and cortisol levels and promotes feelings of trust, which dampen pain and fear reactions (Light, Grewen, Amico, Brownley, et al., 2005).

Perhaps the most compelling animal studies on the effects of affiliation and contact comfort are those that came from Henry Harlow's primate laboratory at the University of Wisconsin more than a half a century ago (Blum, 2002). In a series of experiments, Harlow showed that infant monkeys consistently seek out soothing through physical contact with soft, cloth surrogate mothers rather than wire surrogate mothers outfitted with the necessary nutrition supplied by bottles of milk. Harlow's research was consistent with observations, particularly by leading psychiatrist René Spitz, that human infants raised in foundling orphanages with adequate nutrition but inadequate holding, soothing, and affection were more likely to become sick and even die compared with infants raised in more nurturing environments. Late in his career, Harlow built what he termed a *pit of despair*, a vertical chamber designed such that the monkey would be able to struggle up the sides with great difficulty to peer out but would quickly grow exhausted and, within several days, would listlessly crouch, unmoving, at the bottom of the device. The stress caused by several days of isolation in the pit catapulted the monkeys into what the researchers interpreted as deep despair and left them socially isolated when returned to their peers, without the ability to engage in normal behavior. As Blum (2002) pointed out, this model for inducing depression was shockingly effective. Later experiments designed to reverse the effects of the isolation demonstrated that the contact comfort from non-threatening, baby monkeys who cuddled and clung to the isolated outcasts gradually healed the traumatized monkeys such that they were able to engage their peers and were no longer showing signs of depression (Blum, 2002; Harlow & Suomi, 1974).

In summary, satisfying, connected interpersonal relationships are shown to have a robust relationship with heart health and longevity. Proposed pathways linking relationships to cardiovascular response have included the increased sympathetic arousal, heart rate variability, and inflammatory responses that accompany distress incurred as a result of poor or nonexistent social relationships as well as the negative effects that lack of support can have on compliance with treatment. However, research on the hormonal tie between affiliative behavior and heart health, although still nascent, perhaps has the most important implications for psychotherapists who use the human connection as their primary therapeutic tool.

GENDER DIFFERENCES WITH RESPECT TO SOCIAL SUPPORT

Social support and companionship are important for both men and women, but there are important differences in the health-related significance of living alone and marital quality for women compared with men. In general, women suffer more than men, in terms of their health outcomes, when they are in bad marriages (Kiecolt-Glaser & Newton, 2001). Poor marital quality has been shown to predict mortality in both men and women with congestive heart disease, but the effect was shown to be strongest in women, meaning that women in distressed marriages had the worst cardiac prognosis (Coyne et al., 2001). Similarly, Orth-Gomer et al. (2000) showed that marital stress in women ages 30 to 65 with CHD who were married or living with a partner predicted recurrent cardiac events among subjects enrolled in the Stockholm Female Coronary Risk Study. A subsequent report from the same cohort indicated that marital stress in female cardiac patients was more likely in women who felt a lower sense of belonging and less tangible support (Blom, Janszky, Balog, Orth-Gomer, & Wamala, 2003).

The Pittsburgh Healthy Heart Project (Janicki, Kamarck, Shiffman, Sutton-Tyrrell, & Gwaltney, 2005) evaluated 250 healthy, older adults to examine the effect of marital quality and amount of interaction on intima–media thickening (IMT), a measure of subclinical atherosclerosis and an important risk factor for CHD. Overall, both men and women in good marriages had better cardiovascular risk profiles as assessed by IMT, but the results were qualified for women. Women in good marriages who had the highest rates of interaction with their spouses also had the greatest IMT progression. Janicki et al. suggested that women in good marriages might be more likely to become overinvolved in caretaking, such that they do not take care of their own health and thus increase their risk for heart disease.

Shelley Taylor described a theoretical model connecting stress with caretaking. The *tend-and-befriend model* (S. E. Taylor et al., 2000) hypothesizes that from an evolutionary perspective, women are biologically hardwired to protect their young when faced with life-threatening danger. The pregnant prehistoric woman would have greater ability to propagate the species by protecting the young and unborn rather than fighting the attacker or fleeing to save herself. Taylor argued that, under stress, men's cardiovascular reaction might be best characterized by the fight-or-flight response, whereas women may be more likely to seek interpersonal connections or engage in caretaking behaviors.

Other evidence suggesting that women's cardiovascular response to the dynamics of social support may be different from men's came from the Montreal Heart Attack Readjustment Trial (M-HART; Frasure-Smith et al., 1997). Participants in the M-HART were 1,376 cardiac patients (903 men, 473 women) who were randomized to either usual care or a psychosocial nursing intervention, which included monitoring over the telephone and supportive in-home visits by nurses for patients who were distressed. The results indicated that this type of intervention did not substantively improve depression or anxiety; moreover, there was a nonsignificant trend showing that women randomized to the intervention arm had higher cardiac and all-cause mortality. That is, women who were more distressed and received the intervention were also most likely to die from any cause during the study. Although the results should not be overinterpreted, these findings underscore the likelihood that support in important relationships affects the health of women differently from men (Frasure-Smith et al., 1997). The finding also underscores the need to investigate whether the outcomes of psychological interventions vary when delivered by providers from different disciplines (e.g., nurses vs. mental health clinicians).

DO PERSONALITY FACTORS AFFECT RELATIONSHIPS AND CARDIOVASCULAR FUNCTIONING?

There are an infinite number of permutations in relational structure and quality. Some cardiac patients have a rich history of social support that has faded with age, such as a widow who has children who live far away. Others have an enviable network of friends and relatives but lack some aspects of functional support, such as rides to physician visits or enough money to pay for prescriptions. Sometimes, people have a support network available but seem not to derive benefit from these interpersonal relationships. A 2005 review in *Psychosomatic Medicine* differentiated between structural support (the quantity and type of social ties) and functional support (roles that serve functions such as financial, emotional or task-oriented; Lett et al., 2005). As Lett and colleagues noted, some theorists have questioned whether personality factors play a role in influencing perceptions of social support. Overall, the review by Lett and colleagues concluded, the empirical evidence has shown that personality measures do correlate with perceptions of support and do not correlate with measures of functional support, thus providing some evidence that personality factors are related to perceptions of support. Social dominance and social inhibition are examples of personality factors related to heart health.

Social Dominance

People who tend to be more dominant may have more intense cardiovascular responses when they become stressed. Some of this research has come from the original studies of Type A behavior pattern. The Western Collaborative Group Study (Rosenman et al., 1976) data analysis continued several decades after the study completion, and scientists were able to investigate the Type A construct further. They showed that male subjects who score high on dominance, that is, those who interrupted the interviewer, gave quick verbal responses, or attempted to control the interview, had higher risk for death from any cause over the next 22 years compared with men who were not dominant (Houston, Chesney, Black, Cates, & Hecker, 1992). Dominance was an independent predictor of all-cause mortality in this sample, even after baseline measurements of hostility, blood pressure, cholesterol, and cigarette smoking were included as covariates (controlled for) in the analysis. A growing number of studies have shown that dominance is an independent risk factor for CHD (Siegman, Kubzansky, et al., 2000; Siegman, Townsend, Civelek, & Blumenthal, 2000).

Dominance has also been studied in animal models, particularly with primates. Such research has consistently demonstrated that when highly dominant male primates are subjected to the stress of repeated social reorganizations, they develop more atherosclerosis compared with nondominant primates (J. R. Kaplan & Manuck, 1999). However, there is a sex difference with respect to social dominance. Subordinate female monkeys subjected to the stress of social reorganization produce less estrogen and develop more atherosclerosis than do dominant females (J. R. Kaplan & Manuck, 2004). Siegman, Townsend, et al. (2000) suggested that dominance is a manifestation of aggressiveness that is differentiated from anger-driven aggression because it lacks the intent to hurt others. The primate model suggests that dominance might have been adaptive from an evolutionary perspective. However, when people high in dominance suffer stressors (e.g., job loss, forced subordinate status), they may be more prone to a cascade of stress hormone responses that lead to atherogenesis.

Social Inhibition

Social inhibition might be the direct antithesis of dominance (subordination) and may be related to heart health. Social inhibition (manifested by difficulty making conversations, talking to strangers, feeling comfortable in social interactions, or getting close to other people) and negative affect (manifested by often feeling down, irritable, gloomy, anxious, or worried) are characteristics that have been shown to cluster together and have been termed Type D personality (Denollet, Pedersen, Ong, et al., 2006). The theory of Type D personality posits that some people are characterized by a tendency to experience negative emotions more often and to inhibit the affect while avoiding social interaction with others (Denollet, 2005). Type D predicts long-term cardiac events in patients with CHD, independent of concurrent stress levels (Denollet, Pedersen, Vrints, & Conraads, 2006), is associated with poorer health in patients with heart failure (Schiffer et al., 2005), and predicts mortality in cardiac populations (Pedersen & Denollet, 2003).

An interesting aspect of behavioral cardiology research is that, similar to any other field, dominant views and strongly held beliefs influence the translation of research into clinical practice. The Type D construct is conspicuous by its absence in most of the publications of the North American behavioral cardiology researchers. Most of the research on Type D published thus far has come from Denollet and his colleagues. Leaders of major clinical trials in behavioral cardiology in the United States have continued to conceptualize depression and social support as two independent and separate constructs that predict CHD and have not conceptualized social inhibition as a personality trait that mediates heart disease. However, outside of the field of behavioral cardiology, a wealth of research has previously demonstrated a strong link between rejection sensitivity and depression and has shown that people with avoidant tendencies score lower on perceptions of social support (Berry & Pennebaker, 1993; Downey, Freitas, Michaelis, & Khouri, 1998; Eng, Heimberg, Hart, Schneier, & Liebowitz, 2001). Thus, it is plausible that a characterological predisposition toward social inhibition, avoidance, and rejection sensitivity might incur greater risk for lifetime depression, which in turn is linked to greater lifetime risk for heart disease.

Is the Type D construct "old wine in new bottles," as critics have claimed, or has Denollet helped the behavioral field to inch forward in its level of sophistication by integrating parallel lines of research to derive a more nuanced understanding of the propensity for development of depression among cardiac patients? Pedersen and Denollet (2003) argued that Type D is emphatically *not* old wine in new bottles but instead is a valid construct derived from both personality theory and empirical evidence. Clinicians have reason to be enthused regardless of whether they are swayed by one camp or another. To the extent that personality traits are amenable to psychological intervention, there is potential for psychotherapeutic intervention to improve these domains.

Clinical Example

Bob was referred for therapy by his wife. He was an accountant in his late 40s with a lifelong history of irritable, depressed mood. He had no history of heart disease but did have noteworthy cardiovascular risk factors, including high cholesterol and blood pressure, as well as general dissatisfaction in his relationships at work and home and a sedentary lifestyle. He sought therapy to reduce the amount of stress he felt at home and work. Bob described himself as extremely ill at ease in social situations. Although he was accomplished in his job, he dreaded any situation that would cause him the potential for interpersonal conflict. He would endure bad food at a restaurant or damaged merchandise from a retailer rather than assert himself with another person. Whether he was at the holiday Christmas party or an event at his children's school, social occasions caused him stomach-churning distress. In contrast to other patients who are shy but engaging when approached one to one, Bob came across as hard to warm up to, and he typically had a negative, irritable demeanor. He took an antidepressant but had a relatively dim view of the mental health field as a result of his own longstanding problems.

The therapist's formulation of Bob's presenting problem was that he was at the core fundamentally insecure, with an avoidant style of attachment and a high-strung temperament. Even as a child he had been avoidant in peer relationships and easily embarrassed. As an adult, he was self-defeating. In therapy, he often asked the therapist to help convince him that people could change, when he was certain that he could not.

This would not be a true or realistic book if every clinical example tied up neatly and rapidly into a positive ending. In Bob's case, he was helped by 9 months of individual therapy, and he did develop a good alliance with the therapist. The therapist worked with him on overcoming his beliefs that other people were judging him socially, greater assertiveness when he was being mistreated, and improved ability to recognize and communicate his anger adaptively at home with his family. His wife also pursued her own individual therapy, and their communication improved. Despite this, the therapist had hoped that Bob would make an even more substantive change, such that he would present his best side socially and have the sense of belonging and security that he had always craved. The therapist wished that Bob's chronic dysthymia would remit to a greater degree. Although this did not happen under the therapist's care, it was a pleasure when Bob stopped by the therapist's office in the hospital, 5 years after his treatment had ended. He reported that he and his wife had seen a wonderfully astute couples therapist for about 2 years. He felt a greater sense of secure attachment to his wife, as well as more confidence in most social situations. Bob looked a decade younger and reported that he took far more pleasure in life and was happier at that stage than at any other point in the past.

Bob exemplifies many aspects of Denollet's Type D personality. It is likely that Bob's prior mental health treatments, combined with greater emotional maturity, support from his wife, and a clinically savvy couples therapist, all contributed to moving him along the path to personality shift. Bob's story illustrates that the characteristics associated with Type D personality are not terribly difficult to recognize but can be complex and challenging to treat.

IMPLICATIONS OF AFFILIATION RESEARCH FOR THERAPIST STANCE

The complex interplay in relational dynamics and the resultant effects on heart health is the subject of a chapter by Ruiz, Hamann, Coyne, and Compare (2006) titled "Interpersonal Risk and Resilience in Cardiovascular Disease." Ruiz et al. cited Timothy Leary's (1957) interpersonal circle (later renamed a circumplex), which posits that social behaviors vary along the dimensions of *affiliation* (ranging on a continuum from warmth and friendliness to coldness and hostility) and *control* (ranging from dominance to submissiveness).

The schema of the interpersonal circumplex is guided by two important principles about how people relate to each other, according to Ruiz et al. (2006). The first is the notion that relationships between people are guided by the principle of *reciprocal determinism*, meaning that people influence each other with their interactions. The second is the principle of *complementarity*, meaning that there are predictable responses to social interaction such that affiliative interactions elicit similar behaviors and controlling behaviors "pull" for reciprocal responses. In therapist parlance, dominance pulls for submissiveness, warmth is met with greater engagement, and coldness is responded to with distancing.

Clinical Example

A male patient described his mother as a dominating and relatively cold woman who frequently made him feel humiliated as a child. After a heart attack, he was paired with a female psychologist still in training who was competent but relatively neutral in her demeanor. The patient perceived her to be cold, aloof, and uncaring. The therapist correctly interpreted this as a projection, but the interpretation only made the patient combative. In supervision, she noted that her therapeutic stance had worked very well in her previous setting as a trainee in an inpatient psychiatric service. As she watched herself on videotape, she noted that her impassive demeanor precipitated control battles, argumentativeness, and agitation from the patient. In subsequent sessions, a warmer, friendlier stance from the therapist was (not surprisingly!) met with a considerably better response from the patient. Hence, the cold and dominating mother begat the patient's expectation that attachment figures in dominant positions would be hostile. The mismatched therapeutic stance elicited controlling behavior on the part of the patient. In turn, the patient's expectation that his therapist would perceive him to be a difficult patient was self-fulfilling.

Ruiz et al. (2006) presented a convincing argument that personality factors interact with interpersonal dynamics to influence how people perceive and relate to each other. The relevance for heart disease, in the example described earlier, is that the stress of a mismatched stance with the patient's personality characteristics, prior history, and expectations would be associated with increases in cardiovascular reactivity.

It follows then that clinician stance can improve or worsen a patient's sense of isolation. Theorists at the Stone Center in Wellesley College, Massachusetts, have advanced a relational model of psychotherapy. The Stone Center principles dovetail with the research cited earlier. One of the center's founding members, Judith Jordan (1997), has suggested that a traditional, nonexpressive, neutral, uninvolved, analytic stance is iatrogenic when it causes the patient to feel isolated and disconnected from the therapist. The following are some of the ideas proposed by the Stone Center:

- People grow through and toward relationships throughout the life span.
- Movement toward mutuality rather than movement toward separation characterizes mature functioning.
- Relational differentiation and elaboration characterize growth.
- Therapy relationships are characterized by a special kind of mutuality.
- Mutual empathy is a vehicle for change in therapy.
- Real engagement and therapeutic authenticity are necessary for the development of mutual empathy. (Jordan, 2000, p. 1007)

The Stone Center model posits that mutual empathy is a curative change agent in psychotherapy. Jordan (2000) described this model of relational therapy as more about therapist responsiveness and less about technique. This idea is congruent with the principle of reciprocal determinism (i.e., interpersonal interactions are always bidirectional and influence each other) and complementarity (i.e., coldness pulls for distancing and more coldness; friendliness pulls for greater warmth and sense of interpersonal connection).

Virtually all clinicians agree that therapist involvement with the patient is critically important. If psychotherapy for distressed cardiac patients is eventually shown to be beneficial in improving heart health as well as psychological dysfunction, the match between the patient's personality tendencies on dominance and affiliation and the therapist's ability to adjust stance accordingly and to be fully present in the therapy may prove to be an important moderator of cardiovascular outcome.

ASSESSMENT OF SOCIAL SUPPORT AND SOCIAL INHIBITION

The types of measures that are used to assess social support vary widely, and most have been used for research rather than clinical purposes. The three measures selected for this chapter are chosen for their relevance to individual psychotherapy and ability to tie the items to therapy goals. It is expected that many other indices of support network (e.g., living alone, number of friends, marital distress) would be assessed in the context of an initial clinical interview.

Multidimensional Scale of Perceived Social Support

The Multidimensional Scale of Perceived Social Support (MSPSS) is a 12-item scale that measures perceived social support from family, friends, and significant others (Zimet, Powell, Farley, Werkman, & Berkoff, 1990). The MSPSS, which is also sometimes referred to by its original 24-item name (Perceived Social Support Scale), was used with patients with CHD in the Enhancing Recovery in Coronary Heart Disease or ENRICHD study (P. H. Mitchell et al., 2003). MSPSS scores have been shown to buffer the effect of depression on cardiac mortality (Frasure-Smith et al., 2000). This measure has been validated extensively in cardiac populations (Blumenthal et al., 1987). The items are clinically relevant (e.g., "I have a special person who is a real source of comfort to me") and can be used as a guide to developing therapy treatment goals.

Social Inhibition Subscale of the Type D ("Distressed") Personality Scale

The Type D Personality Scale is a 14-item self-report measure that has been studied over a 10-year period (Denollet, 2005). The social inhibition subscale of Type D correlates highly with extraversion ($r = .68$), and the negative affect subscale correlates highly with neuroticism ($r = -.59$). This measure is internally consistent with Cronbach's alpha score of .89 and multiple validity studies (Denollet, 1998; Pedersen & Denollet, 2004). This questionnaire uses a 5-point Likert scale ranging from *false, less false, neutral, less true*, or *true* on items such as "I make contact easily when I meet people" to "I am often down in the dumps." A review on this topic suggested that Type D might represent either temperament factors or habitual behaviors that are associated with poor health, including predisposition to cardiac events, higher cortisol levels, and impairments in hypothalamic-pituitary-adrenal axis function (Sher, 2005). The Type D Personality Scale is the type of questionnaire that includes items that, in therapy, could be viable goals for change (e.g., "I would rather keep people at a distance"). For this reason, it is worth considering for use by behavioral cardiologists who provide direct service. The items of the social inhibition subscale of Type D are similar to those that define avoidant personality disorder measured by the *Diagnostic and Statistical Manual of Mental Disorders, Fourth Edition, Text Revision* (American Psychiatric Association, 2000) and also have some overlap with Spielberger's Trait Anxiety Scale.

Inventory of Interpersonal Problems–32

The Inventory of Interpersonal Problems–32 (IIP-32; Barkham, Hardy, & Startup, 1994, 1996) is a 32-item self-report measure that is admittedly not a social support measure; however, it is included in this section because it focuses on interpersonal domains. The IIP includes eight scales: (a) *hard to be assertive*, (b) *hard to be sociable*, (c) *hard to be supportive*, (d) *hard to be involved*, (e) *too caring*, (f) *too dependent*, (g) *too aggressive*, and (h) *too open*. The scale structure of the IIP-32 was well replicated in a confirmatory factor analysis. Furthermore, the IIP-32 has good internal consistency (α = .86) when administered to clients presenting for individual psychotherapy, with alpha coefficients for the eight scales ranging from .71 to .89. The measure also demonstrates good sensitivity to change from pre- to posttreatment (Barkham et al., 1996). There are multiple versions of the IIP, and at least two versions have been used in research studies involving medical populations (Lackner & Gurtman, 2005; Monsen & Havik, 2001). In these studies, medical patients were shown to have interpersonal styles characterized by nonassertiveness and social inhibition when compared with healthy reference samples. So although the IIP has not been commonly used in behavioral cardiology research, it is included because it is often used by clinicians and converges well with common goals for psychotherapy.

PSYCHOTHERAPY TO IMPROVE INTERPERSONAL FUNCTIONING

At the most basic level, efforts to intervene in social support systems can help by remediating social deficits through the intervention itself (e.g., meeting other people in a support group), by helping people to improve their ability to reach out and communicate productively with others already in their social network, or by assisting a person to disengage from a relationship that is particularly destructive. This section focuses on therapeutic approaches for cardiac patients that (a) provide support through self-help modalities, (b) improve functioning in a dyadic relationship, (c) restructure family dynamics, (d) help to process feelings about the loss of an important other person, and (e) provide general principles for deciding on how to combine or sequence therapy modalities.

The psychotherapy models referenced in earlier chapters (cognitive behavioral, interpersonal, and affect-focused) are also appropriate for individual therapy with people who are socially inhibited or isolated. However, the National Institute of Mental Health Depression Collaborative Research Program cautions that people whose therapy focuses on interpersonal deficits are less responsive to interpersonal therapy (IPT) than those whose therapy focuses on one of the other typical IPT foci (role transitions, interpersonal role conflicts, or grief; Elkin et al., 1989). The therapeutic techniques in the following sections are appropriate for cardiac patients with social support concerns but, as in all other chapters in this book, could also be appropriate for other presenting problems such as depression, anxiety, or inability to adaptively express anger.

Support and Self-Help Group Therapy

Patients who feel isolated in their experience with heart disease or generally are lonely can be greatly helped by the clinician who assists them to expand their social network. There are often a plethora of resources available to meet other people with heart disease through a cardiac rehabilitation program, by joining public health advocacy groups such as the American Heart Association, or attending support groups such as Mended Hearts (http://www.mendedhearts.org). Mended Hearts may offer the widest network of self-help support groups for cardiac patients in the United States, with partnerships with more than 400 hospitals. Mended Hearts volunteers make hospital visits to cardiac inpatients and outpatient visits to family members and caregivers. The chapters of Mended Hearts typically offer monthly support and education groups. Members can receive a quarterly newsletter. Similarly, local chapters of support groups are often available for people with pacemakers and implantable cardioverter defibrillators (ICDs). Paradoxically, some of the people who feel most isolated because they have less common conditions (e.g., young adults, people with congenital heart problems) typically cannot find peers with similar conditions in cardiac rehabilitation or support groups, and thus they can sometimes feel even more isolated.

People with rare conditions who use the Internet may find greater availability of support and education groups through the online community. For example, the Sudden Arrhythmia Death Syndromes Foundation (http://www.sads.org) is dedicated to the education and support of patients, families, and professionals about the risk for sudden cardiac death in young adults and children. The National Coalition for Women With Heart Disease (http://www.womenheart.org/) was founded by three women in their 40s who had a heart attack and were interviewed about their experience. Although these women lived in different states, they stayed in touch and eventually formed a powerful and highly respected patient advocacy organization. One of the more poignant testimonials on the Web site is from a woman who had a heart attack at a young age and stated that she wished she were an alcoholic, simply because then she might have someone else to talk with about her problems. The quality of self-help support groups and online education/support groups varies widely. Therapists should check out online sites before recommending them to patients. The provision of support and education is important, but support groups typically fall into the "self-help" category of therapeutic techniques. Berkman (1995) suggested that therapies that focus on restructuring naturally occurring interpersonal networks may have greater efficacy than self-help groups. However, clinicians who want to start a support group for cardiac patients can benefit from some of the simple planning tips in the next section.

Though starting a support group is not difficult, it can be surprisingly time-consuming. Before undertaking such an endeavor, clinicians should research the need, purpose, and focus of the group. Perhaps one of the more difficult aspects of beginning a support group for cardiac patients is the decision about who to include: Anyone with cardiac disease? Only patients with certain diagnoses, such as ICD recipients, survivors of cardiac arrest, people who have undergone coronary artery bypass graft operations (CABG)? Limitations on age or gender? Only the person with the disease versus caregivers, spouses, or adult children?

Once the target audience is determined, the focus and purpose of the group should be identified. The time frame for meeting (weekly, monthly, or quarterly) should be established. Some clinicians find it helpful to form an organizing committee prior to running a group. A strong support group may take time to become established, and it is important to meet at the same time, in the same location, using an easily identifiable name to establish the group.

Unstructured support groups can quickly lose a sense of focus. Group facilitators need to develop, explain, and enforce group rules regarding confidentiality, respect, and observation of time limits. Identification of one or more volunteers early on in the process can be most helpful, to assist with developing a flyer, identifying a location, recording contact information for group members, and dealing with the large number of questions from prospective members (e.g., providing directions, answering questions, arranging refreshments).

Professional facilitators also need to determine whether the group is provided for a fee and, if so, to determine their state requirements and ethical obligations in terms of medical record keeping or documentation. In short, support groups can be very rewarding but also require a surprising amount of work and dedication.

Couples Therapy

Sometimes spouses fare worse after a hospitalization for heart problems than patients themselves! A study of more than 400 patients hospitalized for heart attack or angioplasty and their spouses showed that the nonpatient spouses had greater anxiety and depression, as well as lower levels of perceived control, compared with patients themselves (Moser & Dracup, 2004). In turn, poor adjustment by a spouse predicts worse prognosis for the patient with the heart condition. Clinicians can help spouses to feel more in control and less distressed by routinely providing information and support. However, because a heart attack may be just one more negative life event in the trajectory of a stressed relationship, it is important to have some history of the quality of the relationship prior to the cardiac event. It is not unusual that patients seek out therapy because they had a heart attack that occurred after their relationship dissolved through separation or divorce. The effect of a near-death experience on an already distressed relationship brings intense emotions to the surface. The therapist who treats a couple will ask about the cardiac event itself and can evaluate the couple's communication style even as they talk about the event. John Gottman, a leader in the field of couples therapy (Gottman & Levenson, 2002; Gottman & Notarius, 2002), has referred to four particularly negative communication patterns that are readily evident in his videotapes of couples: *criticism* (e.g., "It is not surprising that you had a heart attack since all you do is smoke cigarettes"), *defensiveness* (e.g., "I wouldn't smoke so much if you weren't such a nag"), *contempt* (e.g., "You contribute nothing to this family, my mother has been telling me to throw you out for years"), and *stonewalling* (e.g., "This conversation is ended, I have nothing to say to you"). Although all of these communication patterns crop up from time to time in healthy relationships, it is the escalation of these toxic patterns paired with the absence of positive interactions that signals the need for relational intervention. In particular, an increase in contempt typically signals the death knell for a relationship (Gottman & Levenson, 2002). In the terminology of the interpersonal circumplex, contempt conveys coldness as well as dominance, eliciting both submissive and cold behavior from the other spouse.

Clinical Example

Fern and Gerry were both in their late 50s. Gerry had suffered a stroke 3 years ago, followed by a massive heart attack the following year. He had previously been the primary breadwinner as a manager in the insurance industry. He was on medical disability and would not return to work. He ambulated with difficulty, spoke with a slight speech impediment, and had severe vision problems. Fern had previously been a homemaker with a part-time job, but following Gerry's stroke she found full-time employment. Although she enjoyed her job, she felt distressed and resentful at often coming home to find Gerry sleeping on the couch. Fern felt that Gerry was depressed and said that he withdrew into his study and only emerged when she made dinner at night. She felt enraged as the person responsible for earning the income as well as doing virtually all the household chores. Gerry, for his part, was genuinely physically disabled but admitted he felt "lazy" and extremely unmotivated to take up household responsibilities. Without the structure of getting up for work or having anyone at home most of the day, he often resorted to watching TV, sleeping the day away, and spending time on the Internet. Fern complained, "He was never a lazy man. He worked 60–70 hours a week. But now he doesn't want to do anything. I would appreciate just a little help in the house or even a 'thank you' once in a while."

As Fern described it, their marriage of 35 years had been very good, with structured roles of primary breadwinner and stay-at-home mother and part-time worker. Gerry had never been very demonstrative or well able to verbalize his emotions, but he felt that his "actions spoke louder than words" and he was a reliable, kind, loyal husband and father. Fern had yearned for greater affection and more closeness, but overall, she considered that she had been relatively content prior to Gerry's stroke. For the first 6 months following his stroke, both partners described themselves as having been traumatized. Fern had been a devoted caregiver. After Gerry's heart attack 12 months later, they both feared that he had little time left. As more months elapsed, Fern needed to go to work to support the family. Gerry fell into a deep depression but was not particularly psychologically minded and felt that Fern's urges to seek help amounted to telling him that "it is all in my head." Gerry was originally seen for 3 sessions of individual therapy, followed by 20 conjoint sessions with his wife. In couples therapy, the sessions focused on both Fern's resentment that her husband seemed to make no effort to take care of himself, their relationship, or household chores and Gerry's sense that he got no validation for anything he did right and little acknowledgment that he was genuinely physically impaired. In therapy, Fern frequently criticized Gerry, and he usually responded with stonewalling. Treatment primarily focused on strengthening the ability of each partner to empathize with the perspective of the other, encouragement of more supportive and positive communication cycles, and expression of the intense feelings of fear and loss that they both felt as a result of Gerry's deteriorating health. The course of Gerry's illness was marked by progression of disease and increasing hospitalizations. They made contact with the therapist by phone or e-mail from time to time, and after Gerry's death, Fern wrote to express her appreciation and feeling that therapy had helped them both to cope with Gerry's illness.

Emotionally Focused Couples Therapy

Skill development and communication changes are an important focus of couples therapy. A different model for couples therapy is emotionally focused couples therapy (EFT; Greenberg & Johnson, 1988). This format of therapy is time limited (less than 20 sessions) and has been used with both couples and families (Kowal, Johnson, & Lee, 2003; Walker, Manion, Cloutier, & Johnson, 1992). The adaptation of this model for use with cardiac patients was outlined in a chapter titled "Hanging on to a Heartbeat: Emotionally Focused Therapy for Couples Dealing With the Trauma of Coronary Heart Disease" (MacIntosh, Johnson, & Lee, 2006). EFT is distinguished from other therapies by its assumption that faulty attachment patterns cause couple conflict and that affective expression can improve the attachment patterns in the couple. The goals of EFT include creating a more secure attachment between the partners; improving the quality, emotional tone, and frequency of communication; and altering the patterns of emotional communication such that intimacy is increased and satisfaction with the relationship improves. Distressed relationships are those characterized by a poor quality of bond with behaviors such as clinginess or withdrawal.

The EFT model proposes that treatment occurs in three stages: deescalation (e.g., defusing a negatively charged relational pattern), changing (altering the relational patterns), and consolidation and integration (strengthening and reinforcing the new positive communication patterns of the couple). Each phase of this model of therapy comprises multiple stages. *Deescalation* consists of (a) assessing core issues and conflicts using an attachment framework, (b) identifying problem attachment patterns, (c) increasing awareness of underlying or unacknowledged emotions, and (d) reframing the conflict using the language of attachment and affect theory. *Changing* comprises the steps of (a) helping a patient to recognize unacknowledged aspects of the self (e.g., fear of dependency) such that those important parts of the person's development can be brought into the relationship, (b) deepening the experience (e.g., increasing levels of intimacy through empathic acceptance of emotion and improved trust in the relational bond), and (c) facilitation of the ability to adaptively express desires and emotions. The last stage of *consolidation and integration* emphasizes (a) the exploration of new solutions to old relational conflicts and (b) the consolidation of new attachment patterns.

Susan Johnson has been an active proponent of EFT and has published multiple studies showing that it is an effective therapy for distressed couples as well as those dealing with physical illness or a sick child (Johnson & Williams-Keeler, 1998; Kowal et al., 2003; Walker et al., 1992). In the application of EFT to heart disease, the cardiac event, hospitalization, or procedure is conceptualized as a potentially traumatizing event. Couples with less secure attachment styles are thought to be less resilient in the face of the trauma of a cardiac event, leading to loss of affect regulation in one or both partners. A great many people live with less than optimal marriages. The framework for understanding the cardiac event as a trauma may have the side benefit of destigmatizing couples therapy for patients who would otherwise be resistant to seek out treatment.

Sexual Functioning

Sexual functioning is a common concern of cardiac patients that often goes unaddressed by health care professionals. It can be difficult for therapists to determine whether the sexual dysfunction is a result of psychological factors, heart disease, a side effect of medication, or other factors. Among people who were sexually active prior to myocardial infarction, half resume sexual activity within 1 month, but a significant number of patients do not resume activity (H. A. Taylor, 1999). A comprehensive review of this topic for patients is available from Sotile and Cantor-Cooke (2003). Half of people with heart failure experience lower levels of satisfaction with sex after diagnosis (Jaarsma, 2002; Schwarz et al., 2008). Similarly, a substantial number of people who have ICDs report decreases in satisfaction, and it is common to worry that the device will fire during sexual activity. Many patients and their spouses fear dying while having sex. It is reassuring to learn that of the approximately 300,000 sudden cardiac deaths that occur annually in the United States, less than 1% occur during sex (Muller, Mittleman, Maclure, Sherwood, & Tofler, 1996). The elevation in heart rate during sexual intercourse is very similar to heart rate levels during other normal everyday activities such as grocery shopping, leisure walking, or cleaning the house (Jackson et al., 1999). This type of factual information can be helpful to patients. The primary exception is anal sex, which can be dangerous for cardiac patients because it stimulates the vagus nerve, which in turn lowers blood pressure dramatically (Sotile & Cantor-Cooke, 2003). People with uncontrolled hypertension, unstable angina, severe congestive heart failure, very recent (< 2 weeks) myocardial infarction, high-risk arrhythmias, and severe forms of valve disease are those who are considered to be in the high-risk category according to a consensus statement in the *American Journal of Cardiology* (DeBusk et al., 2000), and these patients should consult with their cardiologist about the safety of sexual activity. It is easy to display the American Heart Association's brochure on sexual functioning for cardiac patients among other patient education materials, to normalize the topic and create an environment in which questions are welcome (American Heart Association, 2001).

Strategies for Working With Clients Who Are Very Controlling

There is not enough empirical evidence to translate the literature on dominance into clinical practice, but people who are highly controlling seem to gain some improvement in quality of life and relationships when they relax their controlling ways. Accordingly, addressing this issue can be a fruitful focus of therapy.

Clinical Example

Leon, age 61, was referred by a colleague who is a warm clinician with a track record of referring very difficult-to-treat cases. Leon was severely sick with congestive heart failure, and he was widely regarded as irritating and noncompliant by the medical team. Leon knew no other way to relate to others than by interrupting, controlling, and dominating them. He told the therapist that, in the past, he had greatly enjoyed nearly a year of therapy with a therapist who let him talk, uninterrupted, to his heart's content. He currently lived alone, with few supportive relationships. His primary community of friends was found in his online relationships.

With effort, the therapist drew out a history of a failed marriage, one adult son who was estranged from him, and a once-promising artistic career that stalled in his early 30s and never restarted. Leon himself loved to talk about anything, including art, music, travel, and his medical illness, but he adroitly changed the focus when the therapist made efforts to deepen the process or attempted some affective contact. He controlled the therapy process, and the therapist grew frustrated with the inability to help him and began to wish that Leon would drop out and that his social worker might take over his care. Stubbornly, Leon never missed a session. After 6 months of what felt like unendurable boredom on the therapist's part, Leon made reference to Jacob, his son. As Leon had frequently talked about the many transgressions of his only son, Elliot, the therapist questioned the reference to Jacob and came to learn that more than 35 years ago, Leon also had a son, Jacob, who died in a house fire at only 16 months of age. In his grief, Leon's marriage dissolved, he began to abuse alcohol, and, over time, he became estranged from his other son. In therapy, Leon's need for control was exceedingly effective at blocking him from building any relationship with the therapist as well as keeping his grief contained. The therapist's ability to empathize with Leon returned, and his therapy was productive, although, sadly, he died from his heart failure within the year.

From the perspective of affect-focused therapy, Leigh McCullough (personal communication, February 23, 2007) noted that the therapist might help the controlling patient to build the missing affective capacities:

- A controlling person may be unable to put trust in others or believe that others will help carry the load.
- Control may cover for the inability to ask for help or lean on others, thus leading to excessive caregiving or chronic feelings of self-pity or loneliness.
- Control might cover up patients' lack of self-compassion for their failures or lack of self-confidence or self-worth.

- Control could be a defense against anger at others, trying to force others rather than negotiating what is needed.
- Control could block grief ("If I keep other feelings in line, then I won't cry").
- Control can keep people at a distance, if there is discomfort about closeness.

Some people benefit from identifying how many relationships in their life consist of dominant–subordinate pairings versus true partnerships. For many people, the relationship with the therapist might represent one of the first opportunities to make a decision to engage in a true partnership. When people exhibit controlling behaviors in session, a comment in a direct but friendly, nonaggressive way can be effective. For example, "When you act like that (give example), it seems like you are trying to take control. Do you know what I mean?" It usually takes multiple repeated examples before a person can recognize his or her own efforts to control others, even in a highly structured situation such as therapy. Patients will often attribute this to an innate characteristic of their personality that cannot be changed (e.g., "That is just the way I am"). However, to the extent that the therapist can form a positive partnership with the client, it is possible to observe the degree of malleability of this trait. For example, "You seem to relax in therapy and aren't so controlling. What happens at work that makes you feel like you need to keep such a close eye on the folks you supervise?"

Many cardiac patients readily see their controlling habits and even worry that the constant stress of trying to micromanage their spouse, children, boss, or subordinates is wreaking havoc with their heart health. Some people experience obsessive or perfectionistic tendencies and try to make others conform to their own rigid beliefs about the right way to do something (e.g., clean a house, write a memo). Because control, perfectionism, and obsessiveness are subjective qualities that exist on a continuum, it is difficult to develop hard-and-fast therapeutic strategies. However, if the client perceives control to be a problem or if other important people in the client's lives are recommending that they get help, then there is some room for improvement on how to relate to other people without controlling them.

Attempts to control others are not necessarily linked to anger. The emotions associated with control might be just as likely to have more do with inhibitory affects such as fear or shame (e.g., about perceived judgments of others). Control is often a way to cope with anxiety (e.g., things will fall apart at work or home without extensive efforts to control others).

Sequencing of Therapy Modalities

Patients with relationship problems or support deficits might be treated with any or all of the different therapy modalities described in the preceding pages. If a clinician has decided to recommend more than one therapy modality, the next obvious question is whether therapies should be conducted concomitantly or sequentially. Some therapies such as self-help groups are natural choices to be paired concomitantly with other modalities. However, a decision about the sequencing of most therapies is not so intuitive, and there has been little research available to guide the decision. Cardiac patients with marital conflict may benefit from a sequential approach to therapy, whereby they first increase their ability to adaptively express emotions in individual therapy, then bring in their partner for conjoint sessions or couples counseling. Although not all therapists are comfortable or sufficiently trained to practice each modality, Magnavita (2005) recommended that clinicians should be at least familiar enough that they can make an informed decision about the right modality to use, even if the patient is ultimately referred to another practitioner for treatment.

SUMMARY

This chapter has provided some examples of the many different ways that the construct of social support has been conceptualized in the behavioral cardiology research literature. The unit of measurement varies widely but might include the patient, a significant other, family members, or a wider network of people in the person's environment. Perhaps more than any other aspect of behavioral cardiology research, this field is wide open for the development of new psychotherapy treatment options. In chapter 8, the focus is on living with chronic cardiac disease, a condition that affects both the patient and all who are in the patient's social network.

8

COPING WITH CHRONIC HEART DISEASE

Cardiovascular disease, by definition, is progressive and thus typically follows a chronic course, with effects on both the individual and the caregiver. People who have had heart attacks, complications resulting from cardiac surgery, congenital heart disease, arrhythmia, or any of a variety of other heart-related conditions can manifest with a chronic progressive or refractory disease that is disabling and worsens quality of life. Psychologist Ron Levant, past president of the American Psychological Association, suffered from atrial fibrillation for nearly 2 years. He was treated with medication and ultimately underwent two ablation procedures. He commented,

> I was unhappy with the quality of my life. I took anticoagulants, which made me bleed from mundane tasks, like gardening or shaving. The symptoms of atrial fibrillation, as well as the treatment for it, were very difficult. For example, the arrhythmia was very distracting. I had always been very active but now I could not do things like ride a bike. I had trouble tolerating the medications. Beta-blockers slowed me down and made me dizzy when I stood up. The treatment seemed to be as bad as the symptoms. (personal communication, February 28, 2007)

More than 2 years after treatment, Levant's quality of life had improved immensely. "Now I appreciate my health more than before. I garden all the time. I feel so much more empathy for people suffering from chronic illness after having experienced it" (personal communication, February 28, 2007).

Depending on the severity of the cardiac event and the patient's premorbid physical and psychological functioning, a diagnosis of cardiovascular disease may have substantial impact on day-to-day functioning or, conversely, may seem to have little impact at all. Although some elevation in symptoms of depression and anxiety is normative, most people resume normal functioning within a month or so following an initial diagnosis of heart disease. Many people are retired by the time they have a first diagnosis of heart disease, but a substantial number of people are still working.

GOING BACK TO WORK

The majority (80%) of people who are employed return to their previous jobs after a cardiac event (Bhattacharyya, Perkins-Porras, Whitehead, & Steptoe, 2007). Attitudes and expectations about returning to work play a critical role. Some patients cannot or do not want to go back to work. Factors that medical professionals consider in weighing whether and when to recommend a return to work include the following: the job requirements from both the physical and the mental perspective (e.g., "My boss is very supportive but I have to sit for long periods of time as a truck driver"); the patient's perspective (e.g., "I don't think I can work again, when I think about it I get completely undone"); the workplace environment (e.g., "No one at my job puts in less than 70 hours a week"); age (e.g., "I'm so close to retirement already, what is the point?"); and potential barriers at the workplace (e.g., "The secondhand smoke at work aggravates my asthma, I am coughing all the time").

Therapists can play a critical role in the patient's decision about returning to work. Variables that can be explored include the patient's expectations about the level of disability, attitudes about the job, and the level of support from family, colleagues, supervisor, and physician. In general, a constellation of psychosocial factors (e.g., socioeconomic status, depression) greatly influence the decision on whether to return to work (Cay & Walker, 1988).

People contemplating medical disability often face a difficult choice between improving health versus financial ruin. Most therapists who treat medical patients are often asked to complete disability forms even though the overt reason for disability is a medical problem. The potential untoward consequences of medical disability can be explored as part of the therapy process. These conversations cover issues such as being bored at home, feeling a loss of purpose, reducing social ties, increased dependence on the spouse, or pressures from financial burdens. Clinicians have some ability to provide support, help patients regain a sense of purpose, or help them improve relationships, but unfortunately clinicians cannot protect patients from the financial ramifications of ceasing work.

Clinical Example

Fernando, a 52-year-old Latino blue-collar worker, had two bypass operations. His physician stated unequivocally, "You cannot do this job. You have to find a job that does not require heavy labor or go on disability." He referred himself for therapy after seeing a brochure in his cardiologist's waiting room. Fernando's high school education and 25 years of experience as a laborer did nothing to prepare him for a career change. He was forced at 52 to "retire" on a medical disability that provided him less than one third of his annual income. With two teenage kids and a mortgage, he attempted to make the best of it by increasing his cash flow with small painting and home repair jobs, but over time his financial burden sank him into a deep depression. His wife rose to the occasion, becoming the primary breadwinner and scaling back their already modest lifestyle to live within their means.

Therapy gave Fernando some support and strengthened his coping skills, and he came for 25 sessions over 2 years. Fernando's resilient personality made him better able to deal with his disability than many people. He described himself as the product of two loving parents and, as an immigrant to the United States, he had learned to deal with adversity at a young age. As his ability to provide income to the family decreased, he found contentment in mastering household chores, learning to cook, and spending time with his adolescent children. Although he had only the most rudimentary computer skills, he took a keyboarding class at the local library and became an avid Internet user. Nineteen months after his bypass operation, his oldest child headed off for college with a solid financial aid package, a labor of love created from Fernando's hours of collegiate financial aid Internet research. Fernando's distress was primarily related to his external stressors, and his strong support system and flexibility helped him to cope successfully. He was excited and enthused at the termination of therapy, particularly because he noted that, unlike himself, his children would go to college and would not have to depend on physical labor to earn a living.

Depression among physically disabled cardiac patients is common, perhaps because there are so many obvious situational reasons to be distressed. Yet even so, disabled patients respond well to treatment. Patients similar to Fernando can benefit when the focus of therapy is on adjustment to heart disease. People usually seek therapy because they want to obtain a quality of life that is as good or better than it was before their cardiac event. A diagnosis of congestive heart failure is one of the most common indicators that a cardiac patient is coping with a severe, chronic, progressive illness. Perhaps the most difficult aspect of living with heart failure concerns the inability to predict the future.

COPING WITH PROGNOSTIC UNCERTAINTY FOR HEART FAILURE PATIENTS

Congestive heart failure (described in chap. 1, this volume) refers to a constellation of problems caused by an inability of the heart to pump properly, causing fluid to back up into the lungs and accumulate throughout the body. Heart failure is a complication of other types of heart disease and represents a progression of the disease process. Predicting end of life is an inexact science in all areas of medicine, but especially in cardiology. Although the 5-year mortality rate of 50% is much higher than that for all types of cancer except lung cancer (Agency for Health Care Policy and Research, 1994), the perception of heart failure is generally that of a chronic disease rather than one with high mortality rates. By comparison, the 5-year survival rate of women with breast cancer is 89% and for men with prostate cancer is nearly 100% (American Cancer Society, 2007). Heart failure is predictable in its unpredictability. At least half of the people diagnosed with heart failure simply die suddenly of arrhythmia or an infection. Paradoxically, people with less severe heart failure are at higher risk of sudden cardiac death (Willems, Hak, Visser, & van der Wal, 2004). Patients with heart failure have often already survived serious heart disease, and the course of illness is characterized by periods of relative stability. Perhaps because they cannot easily predict the time course of disease progression for any given individual, it may be understandable that most doctors provide patients with ambiguous information about their prognosis (Lynn, Harrell, Cohn, Wagner, & Connors, 1997). Patients may not have adequate knowledge of their own condition such that they can understand the importance of adherence to the medical regimen. Cardiologists rarely communicate survival rates or prognostic information to patients diagnosed with congestive heart failure (Lynn, Teno, & Harrell, 1995). A qualitative study of 31 people hospitalized with advanced heart failure indicated that patients tend to think about death or end of life only during exacerbations of the disease, such as during hospitalizations (Willems et al., 2004).

Clinical Example

Charlie was a huge teddy bear of a man, imposing in appearance but gentle and well liked in the community. In his 40s, a virus attacked Charlie's heart, putting him in the hospital for nearly 2 months. He recovered with considerable damage to the heart muscle and was diagnosed with heart failure. Charlie entered therapy a few years later, at the request of his cardiologist, to better cope with stress and find more motivation to lose weight. He was more than 100 pounds overweight. He viewed himself as a man who was a survivor. Over the course of a year, Charlie was successful at reducing his stress level at work but had great difficulty in adhering to the diet necessary for people with heart failure. He reasoned that he would eventually be successful in losing weight. At the time, gastric bypass surgery was relatively new and he eagerly attended informational sessions on the procedure, but given the severity of his illness, he was not a candidate for this type of surgery. In therapy, Charlie resonated with the metaphor that, similar to the phoenix, he had successfully risen out of the ashes, multiple times over his life. However, he agreed that he might have used up the number of times he could rise out of the ashes. Despite all that the therapist knew about the capriciousness of heart failure, the therapist was shocked and saddened on learning that Charlie had died from sudden cardiac death early one morning. He left a young family, all of his siblings, his parents, and many friends mourning his loss. In retrospect, the therapist was still left to wonder, was there more that could have been done to help Charlie? He was in an advanced stage of heart failure when he entered therapy and had far less time than either he or the therapist realized. Even if he had acknowledged that he was at very high personal risk for death from heart failure and been successful in making major dietary change, it is impossible to know whether his life would have been prolonged by making behavior change at that point.

It is unlikely that most people with heart failure are completely unaware of their prognosis, because most studies of quality of life show significant psychological distress among this patient population. Cardiologist David Waters had the following to say:

Not recognizing the high mortality rate is often denial, or patients just haven't been told the risk. When heart failure patients truly understand their poor expected survival, they often become depressed or anxious. Beating them over the head with their prognosis is often counterproductive, because they can then feel worse and even give up. On the other hand, some patients with heart failure don't comply with their medications or continue to use the agent that caused their disease, alcohol for example. In those cases it is often very useful to get them to understand how serious their prognosis is. (personal communication, February 1, 2007)

Depression has been the focus of many studies of heart failure patients. Depression is associated with poor prognosis and higher mortality rates for people diagnosed with heart failure (Jiang et al., 2004). Major depression exists in about one out of five people with heart failure and is twice as common among the most severely ill heart failure patients (Freedland et al., 2003). More than one third of people diagnosed with heart failure have increases in anxiety 12 months after diagnosis (Artinian, 2003). Patients with heart failure are at greater risk for impaired cognitive function with deficits in memory and attention, thus producing another factor that might influence how cardiologists impart information about the course of the disease.

A qualitative study of 40 patients with heart failure in Sweden provided important information about knowledge and attitudes of congestive heart disease (Agard, Hermeren, & Herlitz, 2004). The results indicated that patients themselves do not necessarily seek out or want prognostic information about their disease. Some patients feel that it would make them more depressed, lose hope, or feel fatalistic (e.g., "There is nothing I can do, why think about it?"). Other patients prefer to understand the nature of the disease, feeling that they have a right to the knowledge and from a practical perspective want to "put their affairs in order." Because the prevalence of heart failure increases with age, some patients simply see dying as a result of getting older, not necessarily relating that specifically to heart failure. Agard et al. concluded that patients have both "the right to know and the right to choose not to know about their prognosis" (p. 224) and that prognostic uncertainty might actually be a source of hope for some patients.

Male gender and younger age predict better emotional adjustment to heart failure (Evangelista et al., 2002). Poor marital quality predicts mortality among patients with congestive heart disease, especially for women, and even over a period as long as 8 years (Coyne et al., 2001; Rohrbaugh, Shoham, & Coyne, 2006). Women generally report greater disability from heart failure and may derive less benefit from therapeutic treatments. A qualitative study of five women concluded that heart failure affects all aspects of a woman's life and requires a great deal of adjustment in day-to-day functioning (Rhodes & Bowles, 2002).

Families and caregivers tend to suffer when their loved one is diagnosed with congestive heart disease. Caregivers may contend with providing personal care, helping dispense medications, assessing the patient's symptoms, managing household tasks, coping with the financial effects of the disease, providing a liaison to physicians, providing transportation to doctor appointments, and providing emotional support to the patient. The cumulative effects can leave caregivers, and particularly younger caregivers, burned out, with feelings of little control and elevated psychological distress (Dracup et al., 2004; Rankin, 1992).

EFFECTS OF CHRONIC HEART DISEASE ON THE FAMILY

Chronic heart disease can take its toll on both the patient and family members. Heart disease in one family member can greatly elevate anxiety through the family system. There are many circumstances in the lives of cardiac patients in which family therapy might be considered. The following are some examples of patients who might have family members who are particularly affected.

- Cardiac intensive care unit patients: Family members of patients on the intensive care unit have disproportionately high levels of anxiety and depression compared with relatives of people with cardiac surgery. (E. Young et al., 2005)
- Pregnant patients with heart disease: About 1% to 3% of all pregnant women have heart disease. Cardiac illness in pregnancy is so serious that is responsible for 10% to 15% of maternal mortality. (Arafeh & Baird, 2006)
- Patients who have died unexpectedly from cardiac arrest: Among people who die from sudden cardiac death, more than one out of five will have inherited cardiac disease, with important implications for the other family members.

Families have strongly held beliefs and values that influence how a patient might die (Vig, Davenport, & Pearlman, 2002), whether a cardiac patient will enroll in a cardiac rehabilitation program (Jones, Farrell, Jamieson, & Dorsch, 2003), and even whether a patient understands his or her risk for heart disease (Momtahan, Berkman, Sellick, Kearns, & Lauzon, 2004). Family members of cardiac patients are increasingly asked to become trained in cardiac resuscitation, but this request can have profound effects. Long after the clinician has withdrawn from the patient's life, the family will remain a constant (Titone, Cross, Sileo, & Martin, 2004). Therefore, it is important to recognize the circumstances under which family members should be assessed and treated, particularly when the patients themselves are hospitalized or the family adjustment to the event is dysfunctional.

CAREGIVER STRESS

Caregivers are most often family members, and it is a truism that people with chronic heart disease will have increasing need for caregiver support, especially during exacerbations of the disease. Caregivers who are most successful in coping are those who are older, such that age is congruent with a greater expectation of taking care of one's family (van den Heuvel, de Witte, Schure, Sanderman, & Meyboom-de Jong, 2001). Families with strong coping abilities beforehand will deal with caregiver stress better than families with a poor level of functioning. Spouse or partner caregivers typically have different needs from other family caregivers such as children or other relatives. Spouses may also be dealing with their own health problems or may be adversely financially affected by the patient's illness. In contrast, some children, grandchildren, or siblings may not be as accepting of the caretaking role. It may be that the role is not congruent with their stage of life (caregivers in young adulthood or with young children of their own), or they did not have any expectation of taking care of the patient (e.g., the patient is difficult or isolated and no one else will step forward to assume the role). It is not uncommon that a family member will propel the patient to the therapist's office declaring that "we really need some help," only for the therapist to determine that the patient is not appropriate (e.g., too fatigued and sick) to be treated with individual therapy but the caregiver is feeling overwhelmed. When the identified "patient" is really the family unit, the treatment might be best conceptualized as medical family therapy (McDaniel, Hepworth, & Doherty, 1992), discussed in more detail later in this chapter.

Clinical Example

> Linda and Russ attended a cardiac rehabilitation group on stress management and stayed after the session. Linda explained that she was terribly concerned about her husband because his heart condition had worsened a great deal over the previous 6 months. She was still working part time but had recently retired for good, to take care of Russ full time. She was overwhelmed with trying to monitor his fluid intake, cook with a low-salt diet, and motivate him to walk daily, and she was demoralized that they canceled a planned vacation to celebrate their 40th wedding anniversary. She worried about the cost of his prescriptions and whether she would be able to stay in their home if his health care costs escalated. Russ did not want therapy for himself but was fully supportive of Linda's efforts to seek counseling. Through the course of 2 years, Linda came intermittently for therapy sessions. At times, she needed support for the many day-to-day stressors that she dealt with. On occasion, she reviewed her life ruefully and expressed regret that she still felt resentful at Russ for things he had done early in the marriage. Russ's death, 9 months into therapy, was a shock to her, even though she had realized that his prognosis was very poor. She actively grieved and was accepting of support from her children, siblings, and friends. About a year after Russ's death, Linda seemed to have made a good adjustment. She had renewed old friendships, made changes to her house, was traveling more, and reported that she was feeling sad but considerably less stressed as compared with when she had originally sought out therapy. She terminated treatment on a positive note and appeared to have resolved the issues that originally led her to seek therapy.

ASSESSMENT

When working with patients who have chronic heart disease, clinicians should give careful consideration to the purpose of the assessment. Often, patients are referred to a therapist because there is a wish to improve his or her quality of life. Sometimes it is the caregiver, rather than the patient, who is in need of intervention. In this section, only two of many possible assessment measures were selected to give the reader illustrative examples specific to measuring quality of life in heart failure patients and measuring stress in caregivers.

Minnesota Living With Heart Failure Questionnaire

The Minnesota Living With Heart Failure Questionnaire (LHFQ) is a commonly used questionnaire with this patient population (Rector, Kubo, & Cohn, 1993). The questionnaire is a 21-item self-report measure that assesses the impact of heart failure on quality of life on several domains. The questionnaire asks, "Did your heart failure prevent you from living as you wanted this month by . . . ?" There are 21 statements and respondents are asked to score their answers on a Likert scale from 0 (*no impact*) to 5 (*most negative impact on health-related quality of life*). There is substantial evidence for the reliability and validity of this measure (Middel et al., 2001; Rector et al., 1995). The questionnaire has also been translated into Spanish and generates a total score and subscale scores for physical and emotional domains. Cronbach alpha for the total and subscale scores are above .80 and can discriminate between the New York Heart Association functional classification groups (Heo, Moser, Riegel, Hall, & Christman, 2005). The New York Heart Association devised a classification system that is commonly used as a measure of functional status and severity of heart failure (Hurst, Morris, & Alexander, 1999). The classification system ranges from I to IV with Class IV representing those patients with the most severe symptoms and limitations. People with Class I heart failure typically have no physical limitations; those with Class II may feel fatigue, difficulty breathing, or chest pain upon exertion or ordinary physical activity; people with Class III heart failure are usually comfortable at rest but mild activity may bring on fatigue, difficulty breathing, or chest pain; and people with Class IV heart failure often have symptoms of heart failure even at rest and greater severity of symptoms with increased activity. The LHFQ is typically used for clinical purposes in heart failure clinics. There is little information available about how psychotherapists might use this measure, but it may be useful for therapists who are providing interventions specifically directed at improving quality of life in this patient population (Heo, Moser, Lennie, Zambroski, & Chung, 2007).

Caregiver Strain Index

The Caregiver Strain Index (CSI) is a brief screening measure that can be used in the clinical interview to assess the level of caregiver burden (Robinson, 1983). Although there are multiple measures of caregiver burden, most are disease specific and cannot easily be adapted to multiple patient populations. The CSI is a 13-item questionnaire that gives a point for each positive response and asks the respondent to provide an example. The questionnaire uses the stem, "I'm going to read a list of things that other people have found to be difficult. Would you tell me if these apply to you?" Items include the following: "Sleep is disturbed," "It is a financial strain," "Feeling completely overwhelmed," and "There have been emotional adjustments." A score of 7 positive items is indicative of the need for further assessment and consideration of intervention. This measure is helpful because of its simplicity and can be a reminder of the domains that might be potentially screened in caregivers of people with chronic cardiac conditions (M. T. Sullivan, 2002, 2003; Thornton & Travis, 2003).

There are many other potential areas that might be assessed with patients diagnosed with chronic heart disease. The clinician might consider symptom-specific measures that have been covered earlier in this book, such as the Beck Depression Inventory or Brief Symptom Inventory, or assessment of family functioning or couple functioning. However, patients with heart failure and their families will often not have the energy for long questionnaires. Within 8 years of being diagnosed with congestive heart failure, 80% of men and 70% of women under age 65 will die (American Heart Association, 2005). This patient population should not have to go through extensive psychological assessment without good reason. Brief, specific measures that have face validity are more likely to be completed by people who are coping with a serious chronic illness.

PSYCHOTHERAPEUTIC STRATEGIES TO IMPROVE COPING WITH CHRONIC HEART DISEASE

There is a need for research on psychological treatments for people with chronic heart disease. Lane, Chong, and Lip (2005) reviewed psychological interventions for depression in heart failure and were not able to identify any randomized controlled trials. With the population of heart failure patients rapidly growing, clinicians do not have the luxury of waiting until the empirical results are in. All the psychotherapy treatments that have been the focus of previous chapters on depression, anxiety, anger, and social support should be considered for their appropriateness for people with chronic heart disease. Chapter 9 examines the role of the therapist in helping patients to talk about end-of-life issues, and this too might be appropriate for people with chronic heart disease. However, this section focuses primarily on two areas that come up frequently in working with people diagnosed with chronic heart disease: medical family therapy and strategies to decrease nonadherence.

Medical Family Therapy

Susan McDaniel and others have written extensively on working with health care providers, medical patients, and the patients' family members

(McDaniel et al., 1992). Medical family therapy refers to a biopsychosocial approach that integrates family therapy and family medicine in a collaborative approach to treatment of individuals and families who are coping with medical problems. Medical family therapy uses a systems approach to therapy, and thus the medical family therapist might be more likely to use a genogram at the initial consultation, to examine the family's structural configuration and map the mental health and medical history data.

A summary of some common terms used by family therapists may be helpful by noting the work of Murray Bowen (1913–1990), a psychiatrist who developed one of the best known theories about how families function (Bowen, 1978). Bowenian theory views a family as a system of connected and interdependent individuals. From an evolutionary perspective, families that were cooperative and cohesive were more likely to work well together to propagate the species by feeding and sheltering the family. Family interactional patterns occur in predictable ways. Bowen is credited with the development of several principles that underlie family interaction. The concept of *triangles* refers the fact that dyadic relationships tend to be unstable, and adding a third party can diffuse tension and stabilize a shaky dyad. *Differentiation* of self refers to a process by which a person manages individuality and togetherness in relationships such that they are able to assert themselves appropriately yet recognize and accept a healthy dependence on others. The *multigenerational transmission process* refers to the concept that people tend to pick partners who are about at the same level of differentiation as themselves and perpetuate similar relational patterns through each successive generation. In general, Bowen (1966, 1974) provided many examples of how families with highly differentiated members thrive with stability and productivity, whereas poorly differentiated families are turbulent and unhappy. Psychologically healthy families have more emotional resources to cope with chronic heart disease, whereas families that function more poorly have less ability to manage anxiety and deal with the inordinate levels of stress that cardiovascular illness can elicit.

Medical family therapists can help families coping with chronic heart disease to communicate and cope more effectively by processing feelings of loss and providing practical assistance in navigating the medical system. The medical family therapist might help the family identify decisions that need to be made, provide psychoeducation about the disease process, and help caregivers to express negative feelings such as anger, guilt, shame, and loneliness. When no effective treatment is available, caregivers and families may have grief associated with the anticipated loss of the patient. Adult children may have fears or concerns about their own ability to give increasing amounts of care as the disease worsens or can have worries of their own, as they reach an age at which their parent developed the disease. Spouse caregivers can become overwhelmed at living with the uncertainty surrounding progression of the disease. Some techniques that are helpful in treating caregivers are included here.

Practical matters
- Discuss financial or legal matters (e.g., advance directives).
- Provide information and resources about the disease.
- Help families to talk about potentially embarrassing topics (e.g., caring for a parent who has become incontinent).
- Identify resources for support (e.g., groups, respite care, home health aides).

Generally supportive techniques
- Normalize the response of each member.
- Ask the patient to describe helpful versus unhelpful behaviors (e.g., most patients do not like overprotective behavior from family).
- Encourage communication.

Caregiver-focused approaches
- Examine emotions that the caregiver may have difficulty with, such as resentment toward the patient, other family members, or guilt.
- Help the caregiver prioritize self-care activities (e.g., time for self, pleasurable activities, obtaining support).
- Help the caregiver to mourn the loss of the person that the patient once was and anticipate his or her gradual decline or sudden death.

In summary, families have varying responses to coping with heart disease, and medical family therapy can be an extremely helpful treatment modality for both chronic and acute conditions. Even one family consultation can be extremely informative and helpful for the psychotherapist, other members of the treatment team, family members, and the patient. The availability of periodic consultation from a medical family therapist can be comforting to patients as they navigate the path of progressive and chronic heart disease.

Techniques for Addressing Nonadherence to Medical Regimens

The psychotherapy literature traditionally labeled people who did not adhere to treatment as *resistant*, a term that is easy to use but does not necessarily provide a constructive guide to clinical practice. Within the field of behavioral cardiology, many if not most patients with heart disease will be nonadherent to some degree. Even for relatively healthy people, it is very difficult to stick with a heart healthy diet, follow medication schedules, and keep appointments for blood work and medical visits. As people develop more serious and progressive illness, they face a number of psychological and logistical challenges to adherence. A useful article on behavior change for heart failure patients comes from two nurses affiliated with the College of Nursing at the Medical University of South Carolina (Paul & Sneed, 2004). In this article, the authors underscore the importance of tailoring the intervention to stage of change. The following strategies translate well to individual therapy with patients who have any chronic heart problem and are excerpted from the work of Paul and Sneed (2004).[1]

Precontemplation: Strategies aimed at promoting greater awareness.

- Ask the patient to describe the experience of the disease in his or her own words.
- Solicit comparisons of how the person felt emotionally, physically, and socially before the diagnosis of heart disease versus now.
- Elicit thoughts, feelings, and experiences of the family members since diagnosis of heart disease.

Contemplation: Approaches that try to "tip the scale" toward behavior change.

- Role play a scenario in which behavior change would be required (e.g., refusing unhealthy food at a family holiday).
- Fantasize or imagine what their body parts might say if they could talk. In particular, Paul and Sneed (2004) used the example, "What would swollen feet say if they could talk?"
- Visualize what will happen to the body if no lifestyle change is made? Or, alternatively, what will life be like if the patient is successful at making this difficult change?
- Review documents such as quality-of-life questionnaires or dietary records with the patient to better understand his or her perspective.

Preparation: Strategies that help the patient "get ready" to change.

- Write down several thoughts or beliefs about cardiac illness.
- Complete a written contract between the patient and clinician.
- Purchase necessary equipment (e.g., walking shoes, bathroom scale, 1-week pillbox) or complete needed education (label reading).
- Change the environment (e.g., post the medication schedule, develop a shopping list, remove tempting things that might trigger nonadherence, such has potato chips).

---

[1]From "Strategies for Behavior Change in Patients With Heart Failure," by S. Paul and N. V. Sneed, 2004, *American Journal of Critical Care, 13,* pp. 305–313. Copyright 2004 by the American Association of Critical-Care Nurses. Adapted with permission.

Action: Therapeutic approaches that help patients to stick with the change.

- Engage support from others at a cardiac rehabilitation or other support group.
- Identify specific rewards for goals attained.
- Continue educational efforts (e.g., avoidance of restaurants that serve heavily salted and high fat food such as fast-food).

Maintenance: Strategies that reinforce long-term success

- Compare quality-of-life questionnaires or food diaries from beginning of treatment with the present time.
- Encourage patients to join the local heart association chapter or provide a testimonial at a support group to help motivate others.
- Provide specific support for the attainment of goals. Often patients remark that they get a great deal of support in the early stages of behavior change but particularly appreciate it after many months of difficult effort.
- Identify situations in advance that might place the person at risk for "falling off the wagon."
- Continue to remain available as a resource for patients who want to check back in the future if they need additional support.

Clinicians who become proficient at improving patient adherence have no shortage of referrals from cardiologists, nurses, nutritionists, and exercise physiologists. Inevitably, people who are referred for treatment nonadherence are a challenge to treat. If the patients readily adhered to treatment, the other provider would not have referred them in the first place! Guidelines that have proved useful in my efforts with noncompliant patients include the following. Assess and begin to treat psychological distress as the first priority over behavior change. Assess readiness to change the behavior(s) in question, and use an approach that is congruent with the person's stage of change. Do not forget that personality factors may come into play with nonadherent patients. For example, people who are highly dominant may not benefit from an unstructured approach and might like the structure imposed by completing food diaries and questionnaires. Alternatively, the same patient might exert control by refusing to self-monitor behavior. One particularly memorable example from Wayne Sotile's (1996) book is "I didn't use the forms you gave me to keep the food diary. I made up my own form" (p. 122).

The clinician's ability to recognize personality dynamics and adjust response accordingly is typically a key factor to reduce the shame or combative tendencies that can crop up with some noncompliant patients. The following examples are similar to some proposed by Sotile (1996). The therapist might compliment the patient's strengths and appeal to his or her logic, for example, "A person at your level already has a great knowledge about how organizations work; our work together will help to take skills that you already have and apply them to improving your health." A person resistant to behavior change might be asked, "You seem like the kind of person who will really do something once you make up your mind." Over the past decade, I have never met anyone who disagreed with this statement. Or the therapist could say, "So many people depend on you, I think it is wise that you are learning how to focus your energy on the most important issues rather than to react to every single hassle." One intervention that I have found so well phrased that it can only be directly quoted concerns the need to make amends with other important people: "Illness and crisis lead wise people to take a new look at what life is all about. People important to you probably need for you to be strong and wise enough to be the one to start building bridges of connection with them. Now, more than ever, they are afraid and in need of your help in connecting with you" (Sotile, 1996, p. 122).

SUMMARY

Psychoeducation, supportive counseling, and family medical therapy can be effective in helping patients and their caregivers adapt to a diagnosis of chronic heart disease. Clinicians who provide support as well as practical help are often extremely appreciated by patients. Any of the therapeutic approaches that are described in this book can be adapted to work with a geriatric and medically comprised population. As medical technology continues to improve, more patients with chronic heart disease will have devices, medications, and interventions that provide longer survival and better quality of life. However, despite these efforts, many people do not respond or have inadequate response to medical therapy for chronic heart disease. Thus, facing end-of-life issues is an inevitable stage of the progression of chronic heart disease, and this is the focus of chapter 9.

9

EXISTENTIAL ISSUES, HEART TRANSPLANT, AND END-STAGE CARDIAC DISEASE

Virtually all cardiac patients wrestle with existential issues related to their disease. Existential issues are most prominent when patients face end-stage heart disease. This chapter focuses on existential issues and highlights issues related to heart transplant. Although only a very small minority of people will become candidates for heart transplant, it is important to cover this topic in detail for several reasons. Heart transplant candidates provide an excellent illustration of how cardiac patients grapple with existential issues. Furthermore, even though heart transplant candidates constitute just a tiny fraction of the total cardiac population, every psychotherapist who works with cardiac patients is highly likely to encounter multiple pre- or posttransplant patients. Because transplant has such profound psychological impact on the individual, such patients are referred often for counseling and are very receptive to psychological intervention.

HEART TRANSPLANT

The Road Leading Up to Heart Transplant

Some people have a slow progression of heart disease that leads to heart failure, whereas others have an acute, life-threatening injury to the heart that occurs unexpectedly. The typical transplant candidate has severe heart failure with disease that has not responded to other available medical therapies. To be a transplant candidate, the patient usually has a grim prognosis, such that he or she has a low (usually < 25%) likelihood of survival for another year without transplant (Cai & Terasaki, 2004). People who are at very high risk for sudden cardiac death and who have arrhythmias that do not respond to other forms of treatment may be put on a transplant list. Many people are not considered for heart transplant, particularly those with severe pulmonary, liver, or kidney disease; active cancer; systemic infections; pulmonary hypertension; HIV/AIDS; drug, alcohol, or tobacco addiction; peptic ulcer; severe and unmanageable psychiatric disease; or history of noncompliance or inability (e.g., cognitive impairment) to adhere to the posttransplant protocol. Heart transplant candidates are grouped in terms of severity of illness and can spend on average anywhere from 2 to 10 months waiting for a heart transplant. About 800 men, women, and children die every year while waiting (United Network for Organ Sharing, 2007). It has been about 3 decades since the first human heart was transplanted. There are heart transplant recipients who have lived nearly that long, though on average, most transplanted hearts last about a decade. Today, there are medical devices designed to help the failing heart.

Advances in Medical Technology for the Failing Heart

The implantable cardioverter defibrillator (ICD) is the most commonly used device technology to treat end-stage heart disease. Psychologist Sam Sears clarifies, "The fact that there are end-of-life issues is the success story of the ICD. Heart failure was traditionally thought of as the oncology of cardiology" (personal communication, March 2, 2007). Other devices are also used to treat end-stage heart disease, primarily in hospitalized patients.

Mechanical hearts were also originally developed in the 1960s when the first transplants were conducted. However, artificial hearts were not tested in earnest on humans until the 1980s with the advent of the Jarvik artificial heart (Jarvik, 1981). Soon after, a device called the ventricular assist device (VAD) was developed. A VAD is an external pump that helps the left ventricle of the heart to contract. The VAD can be used as a bridge to transplantation. The heart is a muscle, and like any muscle it gets bigger when it gets overworked, leading to an enlarged heart. A VAD helps to rest the left ventricle, which sometimes allows an enlarged heart to return to normal size. There are some people who are placed on a VAD for a temporary length of time and recover much of their heart function. People who are large in size can have an implantable VAD, but those who are smaller can only be helped with an external device. Current efforts are underway to make new, smaller VADs. Although these devices extend life for many people, the mortality rate on the VAD is high, and sometimes there are disagreements over when a VAD should be withdrawn from a patient. Over time, completely artificial hearts may take the place of donor hearts.

Cardiac Transplant Surgery

During transplant surgery, a patient's heart may be left in place to support a donor heart, but usually the heart is removed. Traditionally, donor hearts were removed from the body and packed in ice. Newer technology can allow a heart to keep beating during the transition by using a machine that allows oxygenated blood to flow through it. Surgery usually lasts 4 to 7 hours. The primary risk following transplant surgery is the risk of rejection of the heart. Drug therapies, such as cyclosporine, have substantially reduced that risk. After a successful transplant, most people can resume normal functioning and go back to work 3 to 6 months after transplant.

In the years following transplant, patients are regularly subject to heart biopsy, in which a tube is inserted in the neck or groin and threaded to the heart to extract a heart tissue sample. This procedure is both painful and psychologically difficult. Similar to cancer survivors who must endure the fear that their cancer will return, organ transplant recipients know that eventually their heart function may decline or their other organs, such as their kidneys, may fail because of the effects of immunosuppressive therapy.

Waiting on the Heart Transplant List

Waiting for a transplant is highly stressful for patients as well as caregivers and family members. The waiting period can be a rollercoaster of emotion with hopeful highs and devastating setbacks. The fear of dying while waiting on the transplant list or dying during the surgery itself is common. Transplant candidates often report that they worry as much or more about their family as about themselves.

Clinical Example

Ravi had congenital heart disease that worsened considerably in his late 30s. His father died from a similar condition in his early 40s. By the time he was 42, Ravi had been on a heart transplant list for several months and been on disability for 6 months. As the oldest son, according to traditional Indian culture, his mother lived with him after his father passed away. His wife worked, but her income alone was insufficient to support the couple, their two young children, and his mother. Ravi agonized about the fate of his family should he die while waiting for the heart transplant. He was aware that he looked very ill. Fluid was congested throughout his system, and his face was distorted and puffed up. He made every effort to gather his strength in the presence of his family and rapidly collapsed when the last member walked out the door. It seemed as though he would die before a donor match was made, but in the end, he held on just long enough. Ravi's family provided considerable support during his hospitalization, and he recovered quickly from the surgery. Within several months, he had returned to work, felt very well, and was jubilant about his good fortune. He recalled in hindsight that his greatest fear was that he would leave his family with inadequate means of support and not have the opportunity to see his children grow up. He said, "If I can have 10 good years, I will be so grateful and will use this time to secure their future."

The fears of transplant candidates are not unfounded. Approximately one third of people do die waiting for transplant, and about 10% of transplant recipients die within the first year (Cai & Terasaki, 2004). Family members suffer immensely with the uncertainty of not knowing whether to prepare for death or to hope for a second chance. A study of 41 patients who underwent implantation of a VAD followed by transplantation showed that 23% of the partners but none of the patients themselves met criteria for posttraumatic stress disorder (Bunzel, Laederach-Hofmann, Wieselthaler, Roethy, & Drees, 2005). Generally, patients who have a VAD implanted report comparative improvements in physical and emotional quality of life (K. Miller et al., 2004), and a VAD tends to offer hope to patients when it is viewed as a "bridge to transplantation."

End-stage heart failure patients usually indicate an extreme sense that they have lost control over their life, health, and death (Evangelista, Doering, & Dracup, 2003; Kaba, Thompson, & Burnard, 2000; Kaba, Thompson, Burnard, Edwards, & Theodosopoulou, 2005). Psychotherapy is underused in the care of pre–heart transplant candidates, perhaps because the patients are often so sick that they are not ambulatory. Some patients spend months in the hospital awaiting heart transplant, but in the United States only a minority of clinicians provide psychotherapy in a medical inpatient setting. Those who do provide such services are in high demand. In-hospital medical social workers are often are so stretched that they cannot provide individual therapy. Patients who are waiting for transplant can derive a great deal of benefit from psychotherapy if they are motivated. Often, however, transplant candidates are so medically fragile that it is difficult for them to participate in individual therapy. By contrast, the same patient, after undergoing a successful transplant procedure, can literally look like a different person and may be better able to process his or her feelings in therapy about the transplant, after the fact.

Posttransplant Adjustment

Adaptation and adjustment to heart transplant are understandably more psychologically complex than any other type of cardiac intervention such as open heart surgery, angioplasty, or cardiac ablation. A number of qualitative studies have suggested that heart transplant recipients often feel some guilt regarding the donor's death. A qualitative study found that patients made statements about feeling grateful, while at the same time expressing regret that someone had die so that they would receive a heart (Kaba et al., 2005).

Clinical Example

Patient: I think about the donor every day. He was young and killed in a car crash. It seems so arbitrary, doesn't it? My family thought I would die and I'm alive. His family probably never considered his death, and now they lost their son.

Therapist: I wonder there is some peace in knowing that his death was not in vain?

Patient: Yes, I think so. If it were my son, I would feel glad that a part of him lived on in some way. (Patient starts to cry.) I would feel better that something good came out of a tragic situation. I know I didn't cause his death but . . .

Therapist: But what?

Patient: I guess I'm just feeling so guilty as though it were my fault. But the guilt is no good for me. (Patient laughs a little.) You think I have survivor guilt?

Every patient is different. Some may avoid thinking about their transplant or detach themselves by thinking of the heart as "a pump," similar to replacing an engine part on a car. Others may find themselves inordinately preoccupied with thoughts of the donor.

A topic that is taboo among many behavioral cardiology researchers but of great interest to patients is whether transplant recipients can acquire personality characteristics associated with their donor. Multiple qualitative studies have established that patients can have overt or covert feelings that they might have acquired personality characteristics of the donor. Some patients reported personality change that they attributed to the donor heart (Bunzel, Schmidl-Mohl, Grundbock, & Wollenek, 1992; Kaba et al., 2005; Kuhn, Davis, & Lippmann, 1988). Of course, the notion that a life-threatening event such as heart transplant could change one's personality is not at all unreasonable. However, there are a fair number of reports in the lay media regarding a change undergone by transplant recipients such that their preferences for food, physical activities, choice in music or art, habitual patterns, artistic abilities, and the like are substantively altered following transplant. For example, there is a popular press report of a man with no artistic ability who received the heart of an artist and developed the ability to draw following transplant (New York Organ Donor Network, 2007).

Cellular Memory Hypothesis

The idea that personality traits, abilities, or habits might be passed from donor to recipient is based on the premise that some traits are encoded at the cellular level throughout the body in all organs. The cellular memory hypothesis states, in essence, that all systems of the body (not just the neural and immune systems) have feedback loops that store information (Pearsall, Schwartz, & Russek, 2000). Pearsall and colleagues suggested that some transplant recipients are more sensitive than others to the effects of the transplantation. In other words, some people are more highly attuned or receptive to the cellular memory of their implanted heart. A qualitative study of 10 patients and their donor families found changes following surgery that paralleled with characteristics of the donor (Pearsall et al., 2000). Some transplant recipients even reported physical sensations that seem to parallel experiences of the donor. For example, the authors documented the history of a donor who was killed from a gunshot to the face and the parallel of the transplant recipient who had dreams about hot flashes of light in his face.

Would the cellular memory hypothesis hold true for other transplanted organs such as liver, lung, and kidney? The topic is interesting in that many kidney transplant recipients and some lung transplant recipients also know their living donors, who are often family members. There is far more interest and attention related to the ability of the heart to "remember" than there has been related to the kidney. Perhaps if the cellular memory hypothesis is proven to hold water, the heart will be shown to be qualitatively different from other organs in its ability to encode individual traits. Or perhaps, the heart simply has a rich history throughout the ages and documented in literature and art, such that people readily think of it as being the core of the body's emotional center. Currently, there is limited evidence that supports the cellular memory hypothesis, but the theory is not easily cast aside either. Clinicians would be ill advised to dismiss the beliefs of heart transplant patients who want to talk about their thoughts of whether they have acquired characteristics of the donor and may have even conducted their own research on the topic.

PRESURGICAL PSYCHOLOGICAL ASSESSMENT OF CARDIAC TRANSPLANT CANDIDATES

Sometimes, practitioners of behavioral cardiology are asked to provide a psychological evaluation of a candidate for heart transplant. Multiple protocols have been outlined for this purpose (Norvell, Conti, & Hecker, 1987; Rozensky, Sweet, & Tovian, 1997). As noted earlier in this chapter, contraindications for heart transplant include drug, alcohol, or tobacco addiction; severe and unmanageable psychiatric disease; and history of noncompliance or inability to adhere to the posttransplant protocol. Clinicians need to evaluate the stability of the patient's social support structure, his or her history and current mental health, history and risk for noncompliance, financial resources, and knowledge about the transplant procedure. Medical adherence typically involves the domains of exercise, blood pressure monitoring, medication compliance, following a dietary regimen, attending medical appointments, follow through with blood work, and abstinence from alcohol and tobacco use. The worst prognostic indicators for poor survival of cardiac transplant patients are a history of previous suicide attempts, poor adherence to medical regimens, history of drug or alcohol rehabilitation, and history of depression (Owen, Bonds, & Wellisch, 2006).

The necessary first step in conducting a presurgical psychological assessment is to determine the reason for the referral by talking to the referring clinician. The patient's cardiologist is usually the referring clinician and is the clinician who has a long-term relationship with the patient. By contrast, the cardiothoracic surgeon will have a time-limited relationship with the patient. Sometimes, a transplant coordinator, who is often a nurse, might make the referral for psychological assessment. The logistics of assessment can be complicated if the patient is too sick to have the stamina for a long interview or to complete paper-and-pencil testing questionnaires. Sources of data usually include the clinical interview, behavioral observation, medical chart review, standardized questionnaires, and information obtained from family members and members of the treatment team.

Both informal verbal feedback and a formal written report are given to the treatment team after a psychological assessment. The treatment team is typically looking for concise feedback on psychological or behavioral contraindications to surgery and concrete therapeutic recommendations with respect to psychological and behavioral issues. Effective reports are those that draw conclusions based only on the evidence cited in the report, use terminology correctly, integrate the findings into a cohesive summary, and consider the treatment implications of the report (Rozensky et al., 1997). After the assessment, the results also need to be communicated to the patient, often by the cardiologist, who may want the examiner to be present, or by the examiner, who may want the cardiologist to be present. Who will communicate the results to the patient should be clarified beforehand, so that he or she understands who will provide feedback and in what time frame. If surgery is deemed inappropriate for a patient on the basis of psychological issues, the examiner who performs the assessment has the responsibility to make therapeutic recommendations to the treatment team on how to best manage these issues and to identify treatment resources for the patient.

Only a small number of heart transplants are done in any one center, and formal psychological assessment is not routinely done on all candidates. Therefore, there are few people who work in psychological testing who have done a high volume of assessments of cardiac transplant candidates. However, psychological assessments of cardiac transplant candidates have life-altering consequences for the patient and should not be undertaken lightly or by a practitioner who has experience with cardiac patients but little training in psychological assessment. Most clinicians who practice behavioral cardiology are probably more likely to be called into service to provide psychotherapy for the patient or his family than to conduct a great many psychological assessments of potential heart transplant candidates. However, clinicians who are asked to provide assessment can be extremely helpful to the treatment team but should carefully consider the parameters and limits of their own expertise before undertaking the task.

EXISTENTIAL ISSUES AND END-STAGE HEART DISEASE

Any cardiac patient who is contemplating his or her own mortality might bring up existential issues in psychotherapy. Existential issues concern the questions that humans have struggled with through the ages:

- Why do I exist?
- What happens after death?
- Am I truly alone?
- What is the meaning of my life?

Facing one's own mortality can be distressing but also can be a uniquely gratifying journey. The conceptual material presented in this section is relevant for people awaiting transplant but can also be generalized to all the other patient populations (e.g., post–myocardial infarction [MI] or coronary artery bypass graft operations) that are the focus of this book. Heart disease raises the very real possibility that one's life span will be shortened. Some people search for greater meaning in the face of death. However, the ability to seek transcendence assumes that the dying person is feeling physically well enough to talk, think, or respond to the therapist. In fact, many people are usually too sick at the end of their life to contemplate existential matters. However, most cardiac patients become acutely aware of their own mortality after a cardiac event, and thus there is opportunity for existentially focused therapy in work with most patients.

Wrestling with the major existential questions of life often, but not always, has a spiritual dimension. Spirituality has been studied in many other medical populations, especially people with cancer. Among a subset of depressed cardiac patients enrolled in the Enhancing Recovery in Coronary Heart Disease (ENRICHD) trial, no relationship was found between spirituality as measured by a spirituality questionnaire, attendance at worship services, and frequency of prayer or meditation and health outcomes, namely, death or nonfatal MI (Blumenthal et al., 2007). There is limited literature addressing the role that spirituality may play in helping cardiac patients explore the meaning of their lives. Spirituality is broader than religion in that it does not necessarily require a belief in a deity. Some studies show that an increased sense of spirituality is associated with better coping practices, healthy behaviors, and more optimistic, hopeful beliefs. Some therapeutic modalities, such as Alcoholics Anonymous, are based on a strong spiritual faith.

Many, but not all, people express their spirituality through the practice of religion. Religion is narrower in scope than spirituality in that religious practice involves a community of people with similar beliefs and practices. However, spirituality as a quest for transcendent meaning might take place through religious practice or through myriad other means (e.g., art, music, or philosophical values). Research on how life-threatening experiences such as cardiac events can trigger "stress-related growth" or the maturation through a stressful, traumatic, or difficult experience has been the focus for psychologist Crystal Park, who commented, "Searching for and finding meaning refers to the piecing together of one's worldviews and one's understanding of a particular occurrence, such as a health crisis. Often searching for meaning leads to the identification of areas of growth" (personal communication, February 26, 2007). Her research seems to be supported by the studies of posttransplant recipients, who report that they tried to stay optimistic, maintain some sense of spiritual faith, and come to acceptance of their situation. Following transplant, some people reported that their values had changed, such that they became more altruistic or had changed their life goals in some way as to reflect a greater sense of personal meaning (Kaba & Shanley, 1997).

Aspects of spirituality that arise in facing death include the belief in life after death, the role of forgiveness in the face of death, finding meaning in one's life, and making peace with loved ones or God. Sometimes, deeply religious people are surprised to find that they are afraid of death, despite a belief in an afterlife. Some people experience terrible distress in contemplating death, particularly if they are conflicted about their relationship with God or have fear that they will suffer punishment after dying or will await a punitive judgment (Koenig, 2002; Larson, Larson, & Koenig, 2002).

PSYCHOTHERAPEUTIC APPROACHES TO HELP PATIENTS WITH END-STAGE DISEASE

Any of the psychotherapeutic approaches discussed earlier in this book may also be appropriate for patients facing end-of-life issues. Cardiac patients who come to psychotherapy inevitably touch on their efforts to make meaning out of their life.

Humanistic–Existential Therapy

Existential therapy helps people in their search to understand the major questions of existence. Irving Yalom (1980) organized existential therapy according to the themes of death, freedom, isolation, and meaninglessness. Perhaps the most relevant themes for cardiac patients are those of meaninglessness and death. An ongoing debate among existentialists lies in whether people create meaning or seek meaning, or whether people are driven to do both.

Clinical Example

Patient: I'm 74 now, and I built a wonderful business. I raised a nice family and tried to live a good life. I'm glad, but not sure what those things mean. Every day right now is a gift.

Therapist: Not sure what those things mean?

Patient: Yes, the purpose of it all. I'm not really sure. Sometimes I think about this a lot. After my wife died, I realized that the love you have for a person continues in a lot of ways. I feel very good about my relationship with my kids. I feel sometimes like my role in creating those bonds . . . that was my purpose. My kids picked great spouses and they are fantastic parents to their own children. So, I feel like that my love for my kids made the world a little better.

This type of dialogue as well as the sense of peace that can come from the feeling of having transcended the microscopic level of one's own life is often a critical aspect of facing end of life. Yet at the same time, it is only possible to provide general principles and clinical examples of how a clinician might rely on a humanistic–existential perspective in helping patients grapple with existential themes. Death is perhaps the most challenging of all themes that arise in working with cardiac patients. Rollo May (1983), James Bugental (Bugental & Sterling, 1995), and Irving Yalom (1980) are some of the major figures in the field of existential and humanistic–existential psychotherapy who have written extensively on this topic.

In practical terms, the primary task with patients who are grappling with issues related to their own mortality is to come to some balance, which allows greater appreciation and awareness of death without being paralyzed or terrorized by it. A central theme that life is finite usually is at the forefront of work with critically ill medical patients, so in this respect, the practice of behavioral cardiology fits in well with an existential perspective. Experiencing the emotional, bittersweet poignancy of the reality of death can at the same time bring a more profound appreciation of life. People facing death have strong emotions, but there is not really any psychotherapy manual for how to help another human being wrestle with issues of mortality. In his book *Psychotherapy Isn't What You Think*, Bugental (1999) emphasized the need for psychotherapists to help their clients become more aware of their own mortality so as to live a more satisfying life.

Expressive Writing

James Pennebaker has done considerable research that documents the value of expressive writing as a therapeutic strategy. Expressive writing can be used in cardiac rehabilitation groups or in individual therapy. Expressive writing has been associated with improvements in physical and mental health across multiple populations, ages, and cultures. The assumption is that the construction of a story about a highly painful life event helps people to understand and organize their experience. The technique is relatively simple and is easily adapted for cardiac patients as follows:

> Write about your deepest thoughts and feelings about the most traumatic or worst part of having heart disease. Let go and really explore your deepest thoughts and feelings. Write for 15 minutes without stopping. Do not fix spelling, grammar, or sentence structure.

This technique must be used judiciously because people generally feel worse immediately after writing. Patients who are amenable to writing should be warned that the research shows they might feel immediately worse but that most people feel happier within weeks compared with people who act as control subjects in writing experiments (Pennebaker & Seagal, 1999).

Expressive writing can be used as a therapeutic strategy that is confidential in that the contents of the writing are not shared with another person. However, sometimes sharing the experience of cardiac illness through writing can be therapeutic, as Ron Levant can attest. Levant shared his postings about his "medical odyssey" with atrial fibrillation over 2 years with the members of the American Psychological Association (APA) through listserv postings. He noted, "it was really very therapeutic to get so much support from the members of APA. Often after a posting, I would get fifty to a hundred supportive responses" (personal communication, February 28, 2007).

Writing is also relevant to heart transplant patients, because in the United States, anonymous letters can be sent through a heart transplant coordinator. Expressive writing about the patient's deepest thoughts and feelings associated with the transplant can be a prelude to the formulation of a letter that could be sent to the donor's family. In general, expressive writing can be a useful therapeutic tool for cardiac patients who seek a way to organize their thoughts and feelings about having heart disease. This approach is most appropriate for people who seek a way to make sense out of their experience or come to terms with basic existential issues. It would not typically be appropriate for people who are at the end stage of the dying trajectory. Patients who are dying imminently are often faced with more practical issues, as discussed in the following section.

The Good Death

People who are truly nearing the end of their life within months or weeks usually have no energy or interest in focusing on the purpose of their life. The dying are usually too sick to contemplate such abstract issues. Instead, most people wish for themselves and their family what is usually referred to as a "good death" (Kayser-Jones, 2002). A good death usually involves the hope that

- there is no pain or discomfort;
- what control is possible is retained;
- loved ones are nearby;
- financial affairs and last wishes have been communicated;
- if forgiveness is important, it has been given; and
- inappropriate prolongation of dying is avoided.

Dying is frightening. It is unknown. People avoid the dying. At end of life, the primary purpose of the therapist is not to abandon or avoid the patient and not to let the patient face death alone.

Clinical Example

Shawna was a young woman who had been in individual therapy for 2 years beginning in her early 20s. She had congenital birth defects that affected multiple organ systems, including her heart. Her prognosis was confusing, and she seemed to have been ill all of her life. Toward the end of her life, Shawna had multiple, repeated hospitalizations, and at her request, her therapist frequently saw her at her bedside.

Shawna was developmentally young for a woman of her age, and catastrophic illness caused her to regress further. Early in her treatment, she had talked with the therapist abstractly about the fact that she believed she would die prematurely, but neither could have predicted that her death would be neither easy nor quick. She suffered a great deal in dying, particularly from having a feeding tube and having her lung secretions suctioned out. She did not want these invasive treatments but at the same time was terrified of death. Her parents hoped that she might rally, as she had many times before in her young life. She wanted the therapist to visit her, but she clung to the therapist and became distraught when the therapist had to leave. Not all therapists are in the position to provide therapy to dying medical patients, but those who are face the dilemma of how to act in the patient's best interests. There isn't really any possible training other than experience for how to be helpful to a patient in such situations. In the end, the therapist decided that if her presence was soothing to Shawna and was wanted by Shawna's parents, she would give Shawna the time that she had available. She gave Shawna a transitional object from the office that Shawna had wanted and explained that although she could not be physically with Shawna all the time, she thought of her often. In general, the therapist tried to help Shawna to hold on to a soothing representation of her. After Shawna's death, her mother said that this had been helpful to her.

Medical technology offers life-prolonging potential that can sometimes have untoward consequences, such as the suffering endured by the patient discussed earlier. In an examination of 100 families of ICD patients, researchers found that 27 patients were shocked by their ICD in the month before they died, and one third of those patients were shocked in the last minute of their life (Goldstein, Lampert, Bradley, Lynn, & Krumholz, 2004). This topic received some national attention with a *Washington Post* article titled "Shocks to a Dying Heart" (Stein, 2006). The article highlighted the emotional toll on family members who experience a device firing while the patient is dying and compared it with the ethical dilemma of whether deactivating the device is tantamount to enacting a patient's right to die. An article on quality of death in ICD patients by Sears et al. (2006) provided guidelines for recognizing end of life in this population and considerations about deactivating an ICD. Sam Sears had this to say on the topic:

> The challenge for cardiologists is to decide when the burden of the shock outweighs the potential benefit. It is very hard for cardiologists to give up. The prevailing culture of cardiac care is to "find it and fix it." Cardiologists are the cowboys of medicine who wrestle and fix problems, they never want to give up. (personal communication, March 2, 2007)

Decisions about the use of technology to prolong life and withdrawal of medical care that will hasten death are agonizing for patients, family members, and medical practitioners alike. The optimal solution, to the extent that a solution can be found, is the discussion of such issues and documentation of advance directives well before end of life.

Grief Therapy

When a person dies from heart disease, family members may present for psychotherapy with bereavement issues. Variables that affect response to grief include the cause of death, length of time to prepare (sudden death vs. extended illness), reason for death, availability of a support system to mourn, and the degree to which the death is acknowledged in the patient's social network (Romanoff & Terenzio, 1998). Clinicians have distinguished between various presentations of grief (Schum, Lyness, & King, 2005). Traumatic grief refers to those cases in which the patient has a distressing preoccupation with the deceased and shows signs of trauma, including numbness, sense of meaninglessness, or avoidance of reminders of the deceased for at least 2 months after the death. Complicated grief has been recognized as bereavement that persists longer than 6 months and includes symptoms such as intrusive thoughts, yearning for or searching for the deceased, as well as purposelessness, detachment, numbness, or difficulty acknowledging the death. Within a month after bereavement, 40% of people meet criteria for major depression, and 15% of bereaved individuals are depressed at 1 year (Hensley, 2006).

The goals of therapy that focus on bereavement are to help the patient to remember the deceased, to adjust to life without that person, and to express the grief related to the loss. Grief work follows its own timetable. Patients who report that they have returned to their former level of functioning, are able to talk about the deceased without becoming overwrought, and have remittance in depressive symptoms are considered improved from grief therapy. However, from an attachment perspective, people who have suffered traumatic losses may not easily form an alliance with a therapist. In the wake of a traumatic loss, adults with a history of previous traumatic losses may need more dedicated efforts to form a bond with the therapist.

SUMMARY

Volumes have been written about facing the end of life, but many people facing end-stage heart disease can benefit from the ability to talk with another person about their thoughts and feelings. These are issues that confront all people. As will everyone else, therapists will die (from heart disease or some other cause). By allowing ourselves to think about and experience the emotions associated with facing mortality, therapists provide our patients with an opportunity to live life more fully.

III

SPECIAL TOPICS IN BEHAVIORAL CARDIOLOGY CARE

10

ADDICTIONS TO COCAINE, ALCOHOL, OR CIGARETTES

Addictions and dependence problems stymie psychotherapists and cardiologists alike. Despite the obvious incentives after a health scare such as a heart attack, patients cannot easily change addictive behaviors. In this chapter, alcohol, cocaine, and cigarette smoking are discussed because these are the most commonly encountered substance abuse problems in the cardiac population. Among people who are hospitalized with myocardial infarction (MI), approximately 1% use cocaine (Mittleman et al., 1999) and 33% smoke cigarettes (Attebring et al., 2004), and among people who are admitted to the hospital for any medical reason, 20% to 30% have alcohol problems (Spies et al., 2001). People who drink heavily, cannot stop smoking, or have cocaine dependence are also more likely to have concomitant psychiatric distress, particularly depression and anxiety (Sherbourne, Hays, Wells, Rogers, & Burnam, 1993). Such distress can be both a cause and a result of the problem behavior itself and makes the individual less likely to succeed in treatment programs.

After a cardiac event, relapse to alcohol, smoking, or cocaine can be deadly and will cancel out any benefit of standard secondary prevention measures such a daily aspirin. For example, resuming smoking after a heart attack eliminates most of the benefit of standard cardiac treatments, such as statin medications (Dornelas & Thompson, 2007). Patients with these problems and who have heart disease are truly "walking time bombs" in the sense that their health is very fragile. With patients who cannot stop abusing alcohol, cocaine, or tobacco, their addiction or dependence is the most important risk factor to treat. It is clear that patients who use cocaine or abuse alcohol are also at greater risk for abuse of prescription medications. This chapter does not focus specifically on abuse of prescription stimulants, sedatives, and narcotics in the cardiac population because there has been limited research that is specific to people with heart disease. However, there are excellent articles that provide guidelines on assessing and treating prescription drug abuse in the primary care setting (Finch, 1993), and chapter 12 (this volume) also provides an overview of the use of psychotropic medications in cardiac populations.

ALCOHOL

Excessive alcohol consumption is not uncommon among people with heart disease. About 20% to 30% of people admitted to hospitals are alcohol abusers (Spies et al., 2001); in the general population, alcohol dependence is one of the most common *Diagnostic and Statistical Manual of Mental Disorders* psychiatric diagnoses (Kessler et al., 1994). There are few studies on this topic in cardiac patients, but one has shown that 19% of outpatients with coronary heart disease (CHD) meet criteria for alcohol abuse (Bankier, Januzzi, & Littman, 2004).

Alcohol abuse refers to a pattern of drinking occurring within a 12-month period and characterized by impairment or distress with one or more of the following problems: failure to perform obligations at work, home, or school; use of alcohol in dangerous situations (e.g., driving); legal problems related to alcohol use (e.g., arrests); or continued drinking even when there are severe relationship problems related to alcohol use (e.g., verbal or even physical fights about or related to drinking). Alcohol abuse incurs risk for cardiomyopathy, hypertension, coronary artery disease, arrhythmia, sudden cardiac death, and stroke. Although men drink more alcohol, women are more sensitive to its effects. In general terms, a 12-ounce beer, a 4-ounce glass of wine, and a 1½-ounce shot of 80-proof spirits contain the same amount of alcohol (½ ounce). Three or more drinks a day is associated with poorer prognosis, although some of that risk may be because heavy drinkers are also likely to smoke cigarettes (Spies et al., 2001). In clinical practice, however, assessment of alcohol abuse typically does not focus on the amount of alcohol consumed so much as the effects of drinking. For example, questions from the Michigan Alcohol Screening Test (Hays & Revetto, 1992) include the following:

- Does your wife (husband, parent) ever worry or complain about your drinking?
- Have you gotten into fights when drinking?
- Have you ever gotten into trouble at work because of drinking?
- Have you ever been arrested for drunk driving?
- Have you gone to anyone for help about your drinking?

Patients who are severely addicted to alcohol and then are hospitalized for heart disease may have delirium tremens, characterized by withdrawal symptoms such as shaking, sweating, or auditory or visual hallucinations. This experience makes the cardiac event even more traumatic, and there is only a small window of opportunity to intervene effectively while patients are still hospitalized. Patients with this level of dependence are at the highest level for risk of relapse immediately following discharge and should be discharged to an alcohol treatment program if possible.

Clinical Example

Dan had been married for more than 25 years and, along with his wife, raised two boys to adulthood. He drank beer every night. According to his wife, he went through a minimum of 2½ cases (36 cans of beer) a week. Dan never thought of himself as an alcoholic. He went to work every day, never had a hangover, and had only twice been arrested for driving under the influence. He enjoyed drinking with his friends at the local bar and, moreover, smoked a pack of cigarettes a day. Dan suffered an MI at the age of 52. In the hospital, he became agitated, highly anxious, and unable to sleep. He began to sweat profusely and had auditory hallucinations. Despite all this, he was highly resistant to hearing that he was suffering from alcohol withdrawal. He clamored for benzodiazepines or any medication to "take the edge off" his symptoms. His wife was very distressed and asked for assistance to treat him for his alcohol addiction.

Hospitalization provided the only window of opportunity to present to Dan that he would soon die if he did not change his ways. He saw that the heart attack had finally given him an opportunity to take time off from work and seek treatment for his alcohol use privately, so that no one but his wife would know. He agreed to simultaneously enter a substance day treatment program, a cardiac rehabilitation program, and individual therapy. He was able, over the course of 4 months, to abstain completely from both alcohol and cigarettes. He went back to work 4 months after his heart attack but attended nonsmoking Alcoholics Anonymous (AA) groups three times a week and stayed in therapy for about 2 years. Dan's case is unusual in that most patients do not agree to treatment, but his case does demonstrate that sometimes a heart attack can present an opportunity to change.

Often patients with alcohol problems will challenge practitioners with questions such as, "Red wine is good for your heart, weren't you aware of that?" Indeed, most of the research on alcohol and heart disease has focused on the protective effects of moderate alcohol consumption, not the comorbidity of alcohol abuse with cardiac disease. This line of research on the protective effects of alcohol has shown that alcohol in moderation raises high density lipoprotein, or HDL, cholesterol, makes platelets less sticky, and increases tissue plasminogen activator, a chemical that dissolves blood clots. Red wine, in particular, has flavonoids, antioxidants that also have benefit for the heart. The difficulty with this line of research is that the epidemiologic evidence has only shown that some level of alcohol consumption is associated with protection against CHD, but there is as yet no clarity about what level of consumption, for which people, and what degree of protection is conferred (Wannamethee & Shaper, 1998). Whatever benefit alcohol may provide, such benefit pertains to those cardiac patients who use alcohol responsibly and not the minority who have alcohol abuse or dependence and who are the focus of this chapter.

COCAINE

The prevalence of cocaine use among people with heart disease is unknown. A large study showed that approximately 1% of 3,946 patients with acute MI reported that they had used cocaine before the onset of symptoms (Mittleman et al., 1999). Cardiac patients who use cocaine are likely to be young (mean age of 33 years), male (92%), and cigarette smokers (Amin et al., 1991). Cocaine use can result in coronary vasospasm (i.e., a sudden constriction of the coronary arteries, thus reducing blood flow), heart failure, cardiogenic shock, MI, cardiac arrest, and potentially fatal arrhythmias.

Clinical Example

Wayne, a 31-year-old man who looked like he would fit in on any college campus, was hospitalized only recently. Nothing in his chart indicated a history of drug use. The therapist was called to see him because he was a cigarette smoker. When questioned about his understanding of why he was in the hospital, Wayne disclosed that he had been using drugs for more than a decade, had snorted cocaine the night before, and attributed his heart attack to cocaine, although he had denied drug use when previously questioned by other medical practitioners. During the interview, Wayne said that the heart attack was a "real wake-up call" and that he would like to enter a treatment program. He was seen by the hospital's substance abuse counselor, and a treatment plan was put in place before he was discharged. Four weeks later, when the therapist called to follow up about Wayne's cigarette smoking, he admitted that he had relapsed "in a big way" about a week following discharge and was smoking cigarettes, using cocaine, and drinking alcohol once again. He rationalized that he had "a pretty minor heart attack" and, at 31, wasn't likely to die from cardiac disease anytime soon. Wayne's case is all too common. These are the types of patients who are badly in need of a clinician who can treat multiple and complex addictions.

Cocaine use is usually considered as a cause in a heart attack that occurs in an otherwise healthy young person. Obviously, the major difference between cocaine abuse compared with heavy drinking is that there is no safe or moderate amount of consumption. In contrast to cigarette smoking, cocaine is illegal, and thus there is a considerable element of stigma associated with cocaine that is dissimilar to the abuse of alcohol or cigarettes.

CIGARETTE SMOKING AND OTHER TOBACCO USE

About one out of three cardiac patients in the United States is a cigarette smoker (Attebring et al., 2004; Dornelas, Sampson, Gray, Waters, & Thompson, 2000). By comparison, in the general population about one out of five Americans smokes cigarettes. It may be hard for clinicians who are unfamiliar with smoking cessation to appreciate how deadly and common this habit is among cardiac patients. In fact, one out of three cardiac deaths are caused by smoking (CDC, 2002); 50% of cardiac patients relapse to smoking within 1 year after hospitalization (Dornelas et al., 2000); and middle-aged men and women who smoke a pack a day or more lose 10 or more years of life on average (Sigfússon, Sigurdsson, Aspelund, & Gudnason, 2006). Compared with patients hospitalized for other reasons, people with acute MI have the highest motivation to stop smoking, and one third to one half quit or reduce their smoking habit after hospital discharge (Ockene et al., 1992). Unfortunately, relapse rates are high, and within 1 year of heart attack, the majority of people have resumed smoking again (Rigotti, McKool, & Shiffman, 1994). Continued smoking greatly increases risk of cardiac mortality following MI, whereas cessation can diminish risk by as much as half (Critchley & Capewell, 2003).

IS IT REALLY ADDICTION?

Many people who could change behaviors such as smoking in response to public education campaigns have done so. Among cardiac patients is a subgroup of people who are unable to change behavior, even though the behavior places them at the very highest level of risk for cardiac mortality.

It is necessary to first define some terms to answer the question, "Is it really addiction?" *Tolerance* refers to a decrease in effect, such that increasing doses are needed to produce the effect. *Dependence* refers to the development of withdrawal symptoms when the substance (alcohol, cigarettes, or cocaine) is discontinued. *Addiction* is generally thought of as a loss of control over the drug use and continued use, despite negative consequences. Whether *dependence* or *addiction* is the correct terminology, there is no question that many people are unable to stop using drugs, smoking cigarettes, or drinking alcohol despite life-threatening consequences. People who are hardest to treat (sometimes called hard-core addicts) are those who have made no recent attempt to change or quit, whose substance abuse began at a young age, and who have few supports (Emery, Gilpin, Ake, Farkas, & Pierce, 2000). Addictions rarely occur alone, and the combination of cocaine and alcohol or alcohol and cigarettes together is far more toxic than either substance alone. The majority (7 out of 10) of alcoholics also smoke cigarettes (Batel, Pessione, Maitre, & Rueff, 1995). Patients often present with other types of substance abuse, including abuse of amphetamines, designer drugs, anabolic steroids, and caffeine. However, these cases are not as common as the presentation of abuse of alcohol, cocaine, or tobacco. One of the common denominators for the hard-core addict is the vulnerability to negative affect, thus this topic is covered next.

THE RELATIONSHIP BETWEEN NEGATIVE AFFECT AND ADDICTIVE BEHAVIORS

People with addiction are more likely to have comorbid depression, anxiety, and other psychological difficulties compared with people without addictions. The reverse is also true in that people with mood disorders are also more likely to abuse substances and smoke cigarettes. There is a complex interaction between addictive disorders and mental disorders. Depression is an independent predictor of relapse to smoking for cardiac patients (Brummett et al., 2002). The co-occurrence of smoking and depression is also high in cardiac patients. Prevalence of lifetime depression among people with cardiac disease is 20% to 30% (Carney et al., 1987), but prevalence of lifetime depression among smokers is 46% to 61% (Hall, Munoz, Reus, & Sees, 1993). Similarly, the rates of depression are disproportionately high among alcoholics and cocaine users.

Clinical Example

Roy was 45 when he was hospitalized for a second heart attack. In his younger years, he had abused drugs. Although he stopped using drugs and hard alcohol, he considered beer to be benign and drank six beers a night and about a case on the weekend. He smoked one pack of cigarettes a day. After his first heart attack, Roy's physician impressed on him that his heavy drinking and smoking would kill him. Roy gave every indication that he would not abstain from alcohol and pressed his cardiologist to give him some minimum amount of beer he could drink. He negotiated with his cardiologist that he would limit himself to no more than two beers a day. The day after the Superbowl, Roy was airlifted to the hospital with a third massive MI. He had consumed a case of beer over the course of weekend. He justified this with the following preposterous rationalization: "You told me I could drink 2 beers. So I saved them up. I didn't drink anything these past few weeks so I could party a little over the weekend."

The personality factors involved in Roy's behaviors made him particularly challenging to treat. He was defiant, rebellious, and disinclined to listen to the pleas of his spouse, parents, children, or doctors. In therapy, it did not seem that Roy verbalized a death wish, although his behavior certainly seemed to indicate a disregard for his own life. His treatment consisted of about 16 months of weekly therapy sessions, tapering to twice monthly for the last 5 months of treatment. Roy revealed that he started smoking cigarettes when he was 10 in an attempt to emulate his older brother and cultivate a more sophisticated persona. As a result of an undiagnosed learning disability, he was a poor student, and his parents often berated him for his "laziness." He began drinking beer when he was 12, primarily to impress his peers, and dropped out of high school when he was 17, following a period of intense conflict with his parents. Despite this rough early start, Roy was a successful entrepreneur who built a thriving business and married in his 20s. Unfortunately, he simultaneously developed a cocaine addiction, and by the time he was 30, he had divorced, declared bankruptcy, and entered a treatment program.

By his late 30s, Roy had been abstinent from street drugs and hard alcohol for many years, rebuilt another successful business, and married again, to a woman he described as "the love of my life." Together, they had two children, and by all accounts, his life was very successful at the time he had the heart attack. Roy eventually came to see himself as a man who had many strengths, but he was extremely vulnerable to feeling intense shame at any indication that he was not "measuring up" or failing in some way. He reflexively reached for a beer and cigarettes when he felt ashamed. In social gatherings, he felt extremely self-conscious, humiliated, and anxious when he was not drinking or smoking. Roy responded well to a great deal of positive reinforcement of his many good attributes and gentle challenging of his self-defeating behaviors. He was a devoted father, a hardworking businessman, and a loving husband. He came to view himself as "a man who can do anything once I put my mind to it" and recognized the need that his children had for him to do everything in his power to improve his health. He suffered several setbacks in the first 4 months of treatment, but after that point was able to stop smoking and drinking for good. He stopped drinking before joining AA but found the support helpful. Roy was quite the raconteur and thrived in AA, and he received much support and praise for his abstinence.

ASSESSMENT

There are many tools that can be used for the formal assessment of people who drink too much, use drugs, or smoke cigarettes. However, if the purpose of the assessment is to establish the degree to which the person exhibits characteristics of dependence, a clinical interview with carefully worded questions is also important. Cardiac patients know they are not supposed to use drugs, drink heavily, or smoke cigarettes. The pull to deny or minimize the problem for social desirability is so overwhelming that it is difficult for clinicians to get an accurate sense of the patient's addiction without a clinical interview. The CAGE Questionnaire and the Alcohol, Smoking, and Substance Involvement Screening Test (ASSIST) are both methods of clinical interviewing to assess addictive behaviors. The Fagerstrom Nicotine Tolerance Test can either be used as a paper-and-pencil test or be embedded into a clinical interview.

CAGE Questionnaire

One of the easiest ways to screen for alcoholic dependence is through using the CAGE Questionnaire in a clinical setting, embedded as part of the general health screening (Ewing, 1998; Watson et al., 1995). The acronym CAGE refers to the key words for questions about the use of alcohol: **cut down, annoyed, guilt, eye** opener. These questions are as follows:

- Have you ever felt you should cut down on your drinking?
- Have people annoyed you by criticizing your drinking?
- Have you ever felt bad or guilty about your drinking?
- Have you ever had a drink first thing in the morning to steady your nerves or get rid of a hangover? (eye opener)

A *yes* response is scored 1, and a *no* response is scored zero. A patient with a score of 2 or more is considered to have clinically significant drinking, but this cut point may result in low sensitivities for medical patients and women (Bradley, Boyd-Wickizer, Powell, & Burman, 1998; Watson et al., 1995).

Alcohol Substance Involvement Screening Test

One of the more promising methods of assessment of addiction for cardiac patients lies in the Alcohol Substance Involvement Screening Test (ASSIST) developed by the World Health Organization. This measure is administered through a clinical interview in a primary care setting and has questions on cannabis, cocaine, amphetamines, inhalants, sedatives or sleeping pills, hallucinogens, opiates, and other drugs, as well as questions on alcohol and tobacco. Similar to the CAGE Questionnaire, this screening tool conducts an assessment in the context of general health and lifestyle questions. The concurrent, construct, discriminative, and predictive validity of the ASSIST have been established (Newcombe, Humeniuk, & Ali, 2005). This interview asks about lifetime use and the frequency of any recent use. Similar to the CAGE Questionnaire, the ASSIST also provides an assessment of the degree to which substance use has created health, social, legal, or financial problems; prior history of treatment; and whether friends or relatives have expressed concern. One advantage of this measure is that it provides a single set of questions that simultaneously addresses nicotine, tobacco, and alcohol abuse.

Fagerstrom Nicotine Tolerance Test

The Fagerstrom Nicotine Tolerance Test is a self-administered questionnaire that provides an index of nicotine addiction. In seven out of eight reports examining the relationship between cotinine (a metabolite of nicotine that is excreted in blood, urine, and saliva) and Fagerstrom scores, significant correlations ranging between .33 and .70 were found, providing evidence that this is a valid measure of nicotine dependence (Fagerstrom & Schneider, 1989). This eight-item brief questionnaire is easy to use and score with items such as, "How soon after you wake up do you smoke your first cigarette?" Answers are "Within 30 minutes" or "After 30 minutes." Clinicians who work with cigarette smokers can use this tool in clinical practice for an easy way to determine level of nicotine dependence.

Assessing people with addictive behaviors is difficult. People with addictions are usually guarded in the clinical interview. Nonetheless, these methods of assessment have been shown to be effective approaches that have been tested extensively with medical patients. The multifactorial nature of addiction makes it unlikely that any one approach to assessment will consistently provide all of the necessary information to make an informed treatment decision. Recommendations for treatment usually consider modalities that can address as many of the factors responsible for the development and maintenance of the addiction as possible. Consideration of multiple forms of treatments that vary in intensity and address both the physical and psychological concomitants of addiction is useful.

PSYCHOTHERAPEUTIC APPROACHES FOR TREATING CARDIAC PATIENTS WITH ADDICTIONS

Any of the therapeutic modalities discussed in previous chapters might be appropriate for a patient with one or more addictions. The transtheoretical model of behavior change applies to many types of behavior change and provides a framework for making a decision about what type of intervention to select. In addition, motivational interviewing, supportive 12-step groups, Internet Web sites that provide education and support, and telephone hotlines might be considered when treating this challenging patient population and are described in the sections that follow.

The transtheoretical model (Prochaska, DiClemente, & Norcross, 1992) posits that behavior change is a nonlinear progression through five stages of change. This model was introduced in chapter 2 of this volume. Here, a brief review of the stages of change is provided as a background to a more in-depth discussion of motivational interviewing.

1. *Precontemplation*: General goal is to raise awareness of the problem behavior.
2. *Contemplation*: Approaches to resolve ambivalence about change are used.
3. *Preparation*: Reflective listening to support the patient's confidence in his or her ability to change is useful.
4. *Action*: Solution-oriented strategies are elicited from the patient to increase likelihood of behavior change.
5. *Maintenance*: Relapse prevention strategies help the patient to anticipate high-risk situations.

The therapist's assessment of the stage of change is crucial for developing an effective intervention. An individual in the earlier stages of change needs more motivation and exploration of the factors sustaining the addiction, whereas an individual in the maintenance stage needs to focus on methods to cope with situations or triggers that might make him or her vulnerable to relapse.

Motivational Interviewing

Motivational interviewing is a collaborative approach to psychotherapy developed by W. R. Miller and Rollnick (1991) and originally developed for problem drinkers. Motivational interviewing involves a collaboration or partnership between the therapist and the patient and has been successfully used to negotiate behavior change and alter addictive behaviors in medical patients. Motivation refers to the belief that change is worthwhile (Rollnick, Butler, & Stott, 1997). An assumption of this approach is that virtually all people, at some level, have some degree of wish to alter the behavior in question as well as some reasons that they cannot do so. The assumption underlying this approach to therapy is that the responsibility and capability for change lie entirely within the patient. The therapist's job is to elicit the patient's own intrinsic motivation to change. The following are five principles used in such an approach.

1. *Express empathy:* The patient is viewed with respect, and the primary tool used by the therapist is reflective listening.
2. *Deploy discrepancy:* The therapist makes a consistent effort to highlight the difference between where the patient is now and where the patient says he or she wants to be.
3. *Avoid arguing:* The therapist does not seek to force the patient to accept a diagnostic label. It is the patient rather than the therapist who makes the argument for change.
4. *Roll with resistance:* The therapist does not meet resistance head-on and treats ambivalence as normal and as a topic for exploration.
5. *Support self-efficacy:* The therapist's role is to reinforce a patient's belief and confidence that he or she can change the behavior in question.

Essentially, the goal of motivational interviewing is to resolve ambivalence, which involves eliciting the patient's own reasons for concern about the problem behavior and arguments for change. These are called motivational self-statements. Steven Rollnick and colleagues have described motivational techniques as the exact opposite of advice-giving. For example, commonly a patient will respond to advice to change from the clinician with stubbornness or defiance. This pattern has been described as the *confrontation-denial trap* (W. R. Miller & Rollnick, 1991). As Rollnick, Heather, and Bell (1992) explained, "What appears to be a fairly convincing line of reasoning to the practitioner often seems to fall on deaf ears; patients seem reluctant to launch into behavior change and might even counter the practitioner's logic with arguments of their own" (p. 25). For example, in the case of Roy, a typical exchange with his cardiologist would be as follows.

Clinical Example

Cardiologist: You are lucky you survived after drinking so much, especially because you haven't stopped smoking either. Did you contact the smoking cessation program yet?

Roy: I'll bet you never smoked a day in your life. It isn't that easy, you know.

Instead of this type of nonproductive dialogue with the patient, Rollnick et al. promote use of open-ended questions such as, "How motivated, from 1 to 10 (with 10 being the highest) are you to stop smoking (cocaine/drinking)?" Replies are tailored to the patient's response, for example, "Why a 5 and not a 1? What makes you as motivated as you are?" or "How can I help you move from a 5 to a 10?" Other techniques designed to increase motivation include the following:

- Tell me about a typical day for you. Where does the cocaine fit in?
- What are the good parts about drinking? What are the not-so-good parts?
- Would it be helpful for you if I gave you more information about the health risks associated with smoking?
- What have other people told you about your drinking?
- I assume from the fact that you are here that you are concerned about your smoking. Tell me about that.
- Why do you think you might need to make a change?

It is important to spend time probing for an exhaustive response to each question rather than simply accepting a superficial response at face value. For example, when the therapist asks what a patient likes about smoking, if only a brief response is accepted and the patient is later found to have multiple other reasons to enjoy smoking, it can undermine motivational efforts. Motivational interviewing is appropriate for many patients encountered in primary care settings in that the approach does not require that the patient be motivated to change. Natural problem-solving strategies are elicited from the patient rather than taught by the therapist, and the approach is good for patients who resist highly structured therapies. Lest it be confused with Rogerian approaches to therapy, motivational interviewing is directive and does incorporate the therapist's own feedback when appropriate.

Paradoxical approaches can be used in motivational interviewing (W. R. Miller & Rollnick, 1991). The therapist could say, for example, "Our program requires a high level of motivation that I'm not sure you have. Do you think you are ready for this?" Reflective listening requires a high degree of attunement to the verbal and nonverbal responses of the patient. Videotape recording of therapy sessions makes it easy for therapists to review their ability for empathic listening. For example, when a patient says, "My husband judges me for smoking," a reflective response may be, "I see tears welling up; that must make you very sad." Or if a patient says, "I do drink more beer than my wife thinks I should, but I don't see myself as an alcoholic," a reflective response may be, "So you see some reasons for concern and at the same time you don't want to be labeled as an alcoholic."

Resistance from cardiac patients with addictions seems to be the norm, not the exception. Examples of behaviors indicative of resistance include (a) talking over the therapist, (b) changing the topic or evading discussion of it, (c) challenging or putting down the therapist or the setting or showing open hostility, (d) minimizing the problem or blaming someone else, and (e) refusing to participate in the session or not responding. Reflective strategies can work well to defuse resistance:

Patient: I know I'm not a cocaine addict, but my wife has gotten this idea that I am.

> *Therapist:* So you don't want to get labeled as an "addict."

Shifting focus can also be extremely productive with highly resistant patients:

> *Patient:* You seem really young, probably younger than my daughter. I'm not sure you could help me with my problem.

> *Therapist:* Well, let's not get stuck on that right now, I just want to make sure we make good use of this session so I can really understand your perspective. At the end, you can decide how to proceed and I'll support you. I just want you to get the result that you are looking for.

Rolling with resistance is infinitely less stressful on the therapist than confronting it head-on!

> *Patient:* I have had nothing but bad experiences at this hospital. Coming today was probably a bad idea.

> *Therapist:* Well, it might be at the end that you decide this isn't the right place for you to get treated. That will be up to you, but I want to make sure you get your money's worth today, so let's talk a little more about why you came.

A general goal of motivational interviewing is to elicit motivational self-statements from the patient rather than to give advice on how to change behavior. The outcome data for motivational interviewing show that this approach is effective in a wide variety of patient populations, including cocaine users, cigarette smokers, heavy drinkers, and medical patients encountered in a primary care setting (Carroll et al., 2006; Martino, Carroll, Nich, & Rounsaville, 2006; Rollnick et al., 1992, 1997). Motivational interviewing can be used in conjunction with or as a prelude to virtually any form of psychotherapy. One commonly used and accessible form of treatment for alcohol and drug dependence is 12-step groups available in the community.

Supportive 12-Step Groups

There are support group treatments in most communities for alcohol, cocaine, and, less commonly, cigarette smoking. Groups offer the advantage of social support, structure, and a specific focus on abstinence. Groups are generally effective and increase the odds of success. One of the most commonly available modalities is the 12-step programs offered by local chapters of Alcoholics Anonymous, Nicotine Anonymous, and Narcotics Anonymous. These organizations all have their own Web sites; all offer groups in person, and some also offer groups over the telephone or online. The 12 steps for Alcoholics Anonymous are based on the following general principles (Ferri, Amato, & Davoli, 2006):

1. *Powerlessness:* Admitting powerlessness over the addiction.
2. *Hope:* Believing in a power greater than the self.
3. *Faith:* Deciding to turn will and life over to God (or a higher power).
4. *Moral Inventory:* Making a moral inventory of the self.
5. *Honest sharing:* Admitting to the higher power and others the exact nature of wrongs.
6. *Willingness:* Letting God remove the defects of character.
7. *Humility:* Humbly asking God to remove shortcomings.
8. *Social Housecleaning:* Making a list of people harmed.
9. *Amends:* Making direct amends to such people, except when to do so will injure them or others.
10. *Continuous inventory:* Continuing to take personal inventory and, when wrong, to admit it promptly.
11. *Conscious contact:* Seeking through prayer and meditation to improve conscious contact with God (as God is understood to each person).
12. *Carrying the message:* Having had a spiritual awakening as the result of these steps, the message is carried to others and the principles are practiced in all affairs.

Bill Wilson and Bob Smith established Alcoholics Anonymous in 1935. Wilson originally wrote the 12 steps, and many other programs have adapted the original 12 steps to help people to overcome addictions. The empirical literature has shown that AA is about as effective as other types of treatment for alcohol dependence (Ferri et al., 2006). In general, positive aspects of 12-step programs include the opportunities to have a sponsor, give back to the community, and for daily contact and long-term aftercare follow-up. People who attend 12-step groups more often are those with severe addiction, a history of treatment, and more arrests (B. S. Brown, O'Grady, Farrell, Flechner, & Nurco, 2001). Sometimes clinicians worry that people who are not Christian or are agnostic or atheistic will not be appropriate for 12-step programs, but research shows that this concern may be overstated and less religious patients are just as likely to attend and be helped by such programs (Winzelberg & Humphreys, 1999).

On the surface, motivational interviewing may seem to be the direct antithesis of a 12-step program, in that the former promotes the belief that the responsibility and capability for change rest entirely with the patient, whereas the latter gives up on self-reliance to promote reliance on a higher power. In practice, 12-step programs are often used in conjunction with a wide variety of alcohol and drug programs and as an aftercare resource. Frequent (weekly or more) participation in 12-step programs is associated with abstinence from both alcohol and illicit drug use (Fiorentine, 1999). Patients with a history of addiction often comment on the value of self-help groups in that they offer a wide network of support, a lifelong availability for treatment, and a strong structure, particularly at times when the patient's life can seem chaotic and without structure. In 1995, *Consumer Reports* published the most extensive survey ever on the effectiveness of psychotherapy and mental health treatment ("Mental Health: Does Therapy Help?" 1995; Seligman, 1995). More than 7,000 readers of *Consumer Reports* responded to the survey. Readers who went to AA overwhelmingly endorsed that approach. Although 12-step groups obviously are not suitable for everyone, community groups are widely accessible and often free, and the majority of the *Consumer Reports* respondents who used that modality attested to the fact that they were helped by this approach.

Internet Education and Support

Similarly, the Internet is widely accessible to people with home computers, and there are many Web sites devoted to the treatment of addictions. Research on Web-based treatment programs is limited, but there is no question that these sites offer the advantages of print materials that can be downloaded, links to other Web sites, instant messaging, peer support, and treatment plans that can be individually tailored.

Web sites can provide an online community of support. Internet support and education can be helpful for patients who like using the computer but may be homebound or lack access to treatment resources. The research on effectiveness of Internet-delivered interventions is scarce, and this type of research is difficult to conduct. Research on Internet-based smoking cessation shows that smokers tend to want withdrawal information and individually tailored information rather than expert or peer support (Cobb & Graham, 2006). There is a demand for Internet-based treatment programs, but few Web sites for substance abuse problems actually provide services (Copeland & Martin, 2004; Toll et al., 2003). Internet-based programs tend to appeal to younger people (Cobb, Graham, Bock, Papandonatos, & Abrams, 2005) and would not be appropriate for cardiac patients who are older, who are unfamiliar with using the Internet, or who do not have a home computer (Steinmark, Dornelas, & Fischer, 2006). The following are some useful Internet links:

- http://www.smokefree.gov: information and links for smoking cessation from the National Cancer Institute.
- http://www.na.org or http://www.ca.org: information and links for the national organization for Narcotics Anonymous or Cocaine Anonymous.
- http://www.aa.org: information and links for the national organization for Alcoholics Anonymous.

Web sites can help therapists to provide patients with printed information and can always be considered as a possibility to augment traditional psychotherapy treatment.

Telephone Quitlines and Hotlines

Telephone hotlines are widely accessible and very effective (Lichtenstein, Glasgow, Lando, Ossip-Klein, & Boles, 1996), particularly among smokers who are motivated to quit. For the treatment of alcohol and cocaine use, telephone hotlines usually provide referrals for treatment or as a method of relapse prevention. Smokers have much wider access to treatment through the telephone. The toll-free number 1-800-784-8669 is a single access point for the National Network of Tobacco Cessation Quitlines (National Cancer Institute, 2007). Callers are automatically routed to a state-run quitline, if one exists in their area. If there is no state-run quitline, callers are routed to the National Cancer Institute quitline.

For drug or alcohol abuse, the Girls and Boys Town (http://www.girlsandboystown.org) national hotline offers counseling 24 hours a day, 7 days a week at 1-800-448-3000. Clinicians are often unfamiliar with how to refer clients to telephone hotlines. However, it is worthwhile to know about this valuable resource because it can provide counseling in multiple languages, referrals to local cessation programs, and mailed print materials.

SUMMARY

Cardiac patients with a history of heart attack, arrhythmia, or congestive heart disease are already at heightened risk for death or additional disability. When cardiac disease is coupled with alcoholism, drug abuse, or smoking—or, worse yet, a combination of those risk factors, along with depression—patients can indeed be considered to be walking time bombs. Defusing the time bomb is a laborious process that involves building a collaborative partnership with the patient; increasing motivation; tailoring the approach to the person's readiness to change; assessing comorbid psychological problems, particularly depression; and marshalling access to as many resources to support abstinence (support groups, Web site, peer support) as possible. Most people attempt to alter the problem behavior many times before they are able to change for good. Although many therapists try to avoid treating patients with addictions, it is important to treat this subgroup of cardiac patients because their problems account for a disproportionate amount of medical expenditures and unfathomable diminution of quality of life.

11

MORBID OBESITY

Morbid obesity refers to the most extreme form of obesity, and the most serious cardiac problems result from morbid obesity rather than less clinically severe conditions such as overweight or moderate obesity (Sturm, 2007). The prevalence of morbid obesity is increasing at a much faster rate among adults in the United States than is the prevalence of moderate obesity (Sturm, 2007). Between 1988 and 1994, 2.9% of American adults were morbidly obese, but that rate jumped to 4.9% when measured again between 1999 and 2002 (Hedley et al., 2004). Most morbidly obese cardiac patients who seek psychotherapy (or are referred) have problems (e.g., depression) that may or may not be related to being overweight or physically disabled.

Obesity is measured in terms of body mass index (BMI), which refers to weight in kilograms, divided by height in meters, squared (kg/m^2). Overweight is defined as a BMI = 25 kg/m^2, a category that 65% of Americans fell into in 2002. Obesity is defined as BMI = 30 kg/m^2, and 30% of Americans met this criterion in 2002 (Hedley et al., 2004). Extreme or morbid obesity used to be defined as more than 100 pounds (45.3 kilograms) over ideal body weight but is now defined as a BMI of = 40 kg/m^2.

Obesity is associated with many health risks, including cardiovascular disease, diabetes, hypertension, high cholesterol, reflux disease, sleep disorders, degenerative arthritis, stress incontinence, and liver, renal, and gall bladder disease. Obesity is life threatening. On average, a 40-year-old woman who is morbidly obese lives about 7 years less as a result of the complications caused by excess weight (Peeters et al., 2003). Obesity dramatically increases risk for metabolic syndrome, the clustering of cardiac risk factors that includes high triglycerides, low high-density lipoprotein (HDL) cholesterol, high blood pressure, high fasting glucose, and abdominal obesity. Some ethnic minority groups, such as African American and Mexican American women, are at higher risk for obesity and heart disease (American Heart Association, 2005).

PSYCHOLOGICAL DISTRESS IN MORBIDLY OBESE CARDIAC PATIENTS

People who are morbidly obese are often judged by others to be less attractive, less intelligent, and less disciplined than people who conform more closely to the societal ideal of slenderness (Hebl & Mannix, 2003). Social discrimination and mistreatment on the job are often experienced by people who are very heavy (Carr & Friedman, 2005), so it is not surprising that many people who are morbidly obese report low self-esteem and poor body image. Some cardiac patients who are morbidly obese meet criteria for binge-eating disorder or have characteristics that fit the description of a condition called night-eating syndrome. These topics are discussed next.

Binge-Eating Disorder

Binge-eating disorder refers to a disorder in which a person has two or more binge-eating episodes a week for at least 4 months (Latzer & Tzchisinki, 2003). People who compulsively overeat, tend to eat alone, and eat very quickly may meet criteria for binge-eating disorder. People with binge-eating disorder eat whether they are hungry or full and usually feel ashamed, disgusted, or guilty about their eating (Cargill, Clark, Pera, Niaura, & Abrams, 1999; Jambekar, Masheb, & Grilo, 2003). Cardiac patients who have binge-eating disorder do not purge their food as bulimics do, and this disorder occurs as frequently in men as it does in women (Striegel-Moore & Franko, 2003). Often, this may be overlooked in a cardiac population.

Night-Eating Disorder

A related but different constellation of behaviors, night-eating syndrome is not in the *Diagnostic and Statistical Manual of Mental Disorders, Fourth Edition, Text Revision* (*DSM–IV*; American Psychiatric Association, 2000) primarily because the field has not yet reached consensus on how to define the disorder (Striegel-Moore et al., 2006). Night-eating syndrome was first described more than 50 years ago and has been defined as a circadian delay in food intake, such that more than 25% of daily calories are consumed after the evening meal (e.g., waking up at night to eat) three or more times a week (Stunkard, Allison, & O'Reardon, 2005; Stunkard, Grace, & Wolff, 1955). People with night-eating syndrome favor high-fat and carbohydrate-rich foods (Birketvedt et al., 1999). Many people who are treated by a behavioral cardiology clinician may fit this profile.

WEIGHT LOSS SURGERY

The evolution of surgical intervention for morbid obesity, combined with an increase in prevalence rates, has created new interest in bariatric surgery among patients with heart disease. People with a BMI of $= 40$ kg/m^2 or a BMI > 35 kg/m^2 and the presence of high-risk comorbid medical conditions such as cardiovascular risk factors are eligible candidates for weight loss surgery. Between 1998 and 2004, the number of weight loss surgeries in the United States increased ninefold, to 121,055 surgeries in 2004 (Zhao & Encinosa, 2007). More than one out of four patients who seek bariatric surgery meet criteria for at least one Axis I psychiatric disorder (Rosik, 2005). Accordingly, out of necessity, practitioners in the field of behavioral cardiology typically develop expertise in treating psychological problems of cardiac patients who seek bariatric surgery.

Weight loss or bariatric surgeries are either restrictive (limiting amount of food that can be consumed) or malabsorptive (bypassing parts of the small intestine to prevent nutrient absorption). In the United States, the most commonly used operations are the Roux-en-Y gastric bypass surgery (combination of restrictive and malabsorptive) and adjustable gastric banding surgery (restrictive) to treat morbid obesity (Buchwald et al., 2004). The Roux-en-Y procedure creates a very small stomach pouch and bypasses a portion of the intestine to prevent absorption of calories. Weight loss after the Roux gastric bypass is usually more than 100 pounds (45.3 kg) or about 65% to 70% of excess body weight. Weight loss usually begins immediately following surgery and levels off between 12 and 18 months postsurgery. A less invasive form of bariatric surgery is gastric banding, or the technique of using a band, with an attached inflatable balloon, to encircle the stomach. Inflation of the balloon tightens the band, producing a smaller stomach that holds less food. Gastric banding is a reversible procedure and can be performed laparoscopically. Weight loss after gastric banding is about 50% of excess body weight by 2 years, but in contrast to gastric bypass, weight loss can continue to progress over time. Mortality rates for the 30-day period following surgery were 0.5% for gastric bypass and 0.1% for gastric banding according to a review and meta-analysis of bariatric surgery outcomes (Buchwald et al., 2004).

PSYCHIATRIC DISTRESS IN WEIGHT LOSS
SURGERY CANDIDATES

Many of the studies about psychiatric problems in people who are morbidly obese have been conducted with bariatric surgery candidates and thus are not representative of all people who are extremely overweight. Weight loss surgical candidates are predominantly women; although White men are as likely to be morbidly obese as White women, they are underrepresented in those seeking weight loss interventions. One cohort study of 288 bariatric surgery candidates from a single surgical practice used the Structured Clinical Interview for *DSM–IV* to assess psychiatric distress. The sample was predominantly female (83%) and White (88%), with a mean age of 46 years and mean BMI of 52. In this sample, 24% of weight loss surgical candidates met criteria for a current anxiety disorder, 16% met criteria for a current mood disorder, 16% met criteria for binge-eating disorder, and 38% had at least one Axis I psychiatric disorder. Although one third of the sample had a lifetime history of a substance abuse disorder (primarily alcohol abuse or dependence), less than 2% had a current substance abuse disorder (Kalarchian et al., 2007). It was noteworthy that about one fourth of the sample had diagnosable anxiety at the time of presurgical evaluation, and 37.5% of the sample met criteria for lifetime history of any anxiety disorder. In particular, this group of surgical candidates was most likely to have a history of panic disorder (19%), posttraumatic stress disorder (12%), social phobia (9%), and specific phobia (8%). If Kalarchian et al.'s sample is representative of most weight loss surgery patients, the findings suggest that mental health professionals need to be particularly attentive to the prevalence of anxiety during the presurgical period. Ironically, high rates of depression are associated with greater weight loss following surgery (Averbukh et al., 2003).

Disordered eating among weight loss surgery candidates is not uncommon. More than one fourth of people who are candidates for weight loss surgery report that they binge eat (Lang, Hauser, Schlumpf, Klaghofer, & Buddeberg, 2000), and about 2% to 9% of candidates for weight loss surgery meet criteria for night-eating syndrome, depending on what criteria are used to define this condition (Allison et al., 2006). A study of 552 bariatric surgical candidates who were morbidly obese (mean BMI = 52) revealed five underlying factors associated with morbid obesity: (a) eating in response to negative affect, (b) eating in response to positive affect and social cues, (c) general overeating and impaired appetite regulation, (d) overeating at early meals, and (e) snacking. Each factor, except for eating in response to positive affect, was associated with depressive symptoms (Fabricatore et al., 2006).

It is somewhat difficult to get a true handle on the prevalence of psychiatric distress, even among the well-studied population of people who seek out bariatric surgery, because surgical candidates have considerable motivation to minimize psychiatric distress and eating disorders if they suspect this may rule them out for having the procedure. So the prevalence rates cited may be underestimates, even for the patient population that seeks weight loss surgery. However, it is encouraging that weight loss surgery does seem to be associated with improvements in psychological well-being: Of those who seek weight loss surgery, more than 7 out of 10 people report that they do not feel attractive (Camps, Zervos, Goode, & Rosemurgy, 1996), but following surgery, most people report substantially improved body image (Neven et al., 2002). More research is needed to evaluate the prevalence of psychiatric distress in other morbidly obese patient populations that have not been studied (e.g., men, ethnic minorities, uninsured people, and younger adults).

ROLE OF THE MENTAL HEALTH CLINICIAN

The mental health practitioner has a complex role to play in helping the morbidly obese cardiac patient, with some elements that are distinctive to clinicians with psychotherapeutic expertise and others that are not. Other members of the team of medical professionals treating an obese patient may include a nutritionist, an exercise physiologist or personal trainer, a nurse or case coordinator, and a physician (e.g., cardiologist, internist, and, for patients seeking weight loss surgery, a bariatric surgeon). The mental health professional who has expertise in behavior change may be directly involved in using cognitive behaviorally oriented techniques to effect weight loss, but this can overlap with what a nutritional counselor may do. Mental health clinicians who focus only on psychological factors have a role that is distinct from other members of the health care team. Psychotherapists have the requisite training to help overweight patients explore how their weight has affected their relationships, job, and overall quality of life. The mental health professional has the capacity to work both directly with the patient and as a consultant to the health care team. Other members of the health care team may need consultation from the mental health clinician regarding characteristics such as motivation and ability to alter dietary intake or exercise patterns, level of psychiatric symptomatology, alcohol consumption, and illicit or prescription drug abuse.

Clinical Example

June was a 50-year-old White woman with a BMI of 48 who was referred from the bariatric surgery program. She was treated by her cardiologist for high cholesterol and hypertension. In addition to obesity she had two other significant cardiac risk factors: adult onset diabetes and depression. Secondary to obesity, she had sleep apnea and urinary stress incontinence. Women like June are at very high risk to experience a cardiac event at a young age. Between 2000 and 2002, cardiac mortality increased by 1.5% for women 35 to 54 years of age, a trend that researchers attribute to the increase in the prevalence of obesity and diabetes (Ford &

Capewell, 2007). In contrast to the steady decline in coronary heart disease mortality since 1980, women in this age cohort age are the only group in the United States whose cardiac mortality has increased.

June understood that she already had multiple major risk factors for heart disease and sought gastric banding surgery. She saw a nutritionist for dietary counseling who referred her to a therapist to treat her depression. The nutritionist helped June evaluate her eating patterns, identify healthier food choices, and review food diaries during their once-weekly meetings. Concurrently, the therapist treated June with seven presurgical sessions and 28 postsurgical sessions. During the presurgical period, the therapy focused on June's feelings of depression. The depression was related to June's being overwhelmed at work and feeling financially stressed, in part because she was paying for her own surgery. During this phase, the therapist contacted the nutritionist about June's progress and wrote a letter to the bariatric surgeon about her readiness for gastric banding surgery.

In the postsurgical period, June's symptoms of depression remitted. She successfully altered her relationship with food by focusing intently on labeling her emotions, finding effective distractions, and using relaxation techniques. She had been divorced for some years and began dating. She was promoted to a new position at work and became far more satisfied with her career. Treatment ended after she lost more than 120 pounds, had no depressive relapses, and reported feeling much happier than she had in years. Her health was markedly improved. June's case illustrates that successful treatment of the obese cardiac patient requires a multidisciplinary effort and a long-term approach.

Many morbidly obese cardiac patients are depressed, demoralized, and unmotivated. The patient who has the more typical presentation of being moderately overweight and in reasonable psychological health is typically referred to cardiac rehabilitation, advised to join a gym or Weight Watchers, or recommended to follow one of the standard diets appropriate for the patient's medical condition. Behavioral cardiology clinicians are likely to get referrals of people who are morbidly obese with existing cardiovascular risk factors, and rightfully so, because effective treatment of psychiatric distress improves quality of life, motivation, and confidence, which in turn may positively affect weight reduction efforts.

PSYCHOLOGICAL ASSESSMENT

Weight and Diet History

There are many tools to measure eating disorders and specifically binge eating, and clinically oriented interviews such as the Weight and Lifestyle Inventory (Wadden et al., 2001) are very good but somewhat lengthy. Clinicians who need a more general assessment of eating patterns and weight history could obtain this information through clinical interview. The assessment would evaluate many domains, including the following:

- weight history (the patient's weight as a child, teen, young adult, after being married, after having children, etc.);
- weight of parents and parental influences on food;
- body image (how does the patient feel about his or her body generally and with reference to specific parts of the body that he or she likes or does not like);
- experiences of being teased about weight;
- diet history (what diets were tried, was weight lost, how long was it kept off);
- past treatment for eating disorders or untreated eating disorders;
- a "typical day" of eating (what is eaten, how much, at what time of day, percentage of calories eaten after evening meal);
- history of eating to self-soothe, out of habit, and in social situations; and
- history of waking up to eat at night.

Cumulatively, this information provides a portrait of the degree to which the cardiac patient is adversely affected by his or her weight and the level of difficulty posed by attempting to change eating patterns. Asking patients about their dietary patterns and weight history serves both an assessment and a therapeutic function in that these types of questions stimulate many thoughts and feelings. For many patients, this type of interview may be the first in which they make connections between psychological states and dietary consumption.

Assessment of Physical Activity

One easy way to screen for sedentary behavior is to use the following item from the Harvard Alumni Survey: "How many times a week do you engage in any regular activity, such as brisk walking, jogging, bicycling, etc., *long enough to work up a sweat?*" (italics added; Lee, Hsieh, & Paffenbarger, 1995). The indication that the level of exertion is "enough to work up a sweat" is an easy way to differentiate those people who exercise with sufficient intensity from those who do not. In clinical practice, a more thorough examination of physical activity could use the Baecke Questionnaire of Habitual Physical Activity (Baecke, Burema, & Frijters, 1982). This 16-item, self-report measure has been used in research studies and can discriminate between active and inactive people. The questionnaire is also easy for clinicians to use, with items about level of activity at work, at home, and during leisure time as well as engagement in sports. The degree to which the person believes his or her activity level is normative compared with others of the same age and the amount of time spent watching television are also measured. Test–retest reliability indices have ranged from .74 to .86 (Baecke et al., 1982). Although the Baecke Questionnaire has been designed for use in research studies, it is easy to incorporate into routine practice for those clinicians seeking a pre–post assessment of physical activity.

PSYCHOTHERAPEUTIC APPROACHES FOR CARDIAC PATIENTS WHO ARE MORBIDLY OBESE

The focus of most behavioral clinical trials with morbidly obese populations has emphasized the endpoints of body weight, dietary intake, and exercise habits rather than alleviation of psychological distress. Implied in this approach is the notion that body weight is the most important outcome when treating the morbidly obese patient. Mental health providers are limited in their ability to influence weight, because so many factors (e.g., hormonal influences on hunger and satiety) greatly influence outcome. A less commonly used psychotherapeutic approach for morbidly obese patients is to focus on the many psychosocial issues (depression, childhood maltreatment, body image, marital functioning, sexual functioning, societal discrimination) that are overrepresented in this population and respond well to psychotherapeutic intervention. Therapeutic approaches that address many of these issues were covered in previous chapters in this book. Accordingly, this section of the chapter focuses on techniques to improve body image and counseling for weight loss surgery candidates.

Strategies to Improve Body Image

Psychotherapy for people who are morbidly obese may focus on many psychological issues but almost always includes exploration of their feelings about their body. Morbidly obese patients are often very dissatisfied with their body and may feel a deep sense of shame with respect to their body, weight, or eating patterns. This suggests the need for psychotherapists to focus on techniques that reduce shame and promote positive feelings about the self and body. Some strategies to improve body image include providing support, helping to change dysfunctional thinking, and intervening to derail maladaptive emotions. Each is discussed briefly in the following sections.

Support

Some psychotherapeutic approaches to improve body image are primarily supportive in nature. Supportive psychotherapy is often dismissed in the psychotherapy literature but is the most widely practiced form of individual therapy today (Winston, 2004). People who are morbidly obese face a great many challenges in terms of their psychological, occupational, and relational functioning as well as their physical health. Many overweight patients understand the problems that they face and need additional support beyond what can be provided by their own network of friends, family, and health care team members. Supportive psychotherapy incorporates at least the following elements that are central to all forms of psychotherapy: positive regard for the patient, careful listening, encouragement of expression of feelings, exploration of the patient's problems, and psychoeducation. A psychotherapist who listens carefully and does not attempt to give recommendations on how to lose weight will be a welcome change to patients who have already received a great deal of advice in this regard.

Cognitions

Cognitive techniques are helpful in influencing body image. Cognitive therapy that does not focus directly on weight loss but instead focuses on nondieting, regular exercise, and alternative coping skills has been found to enhance psychological well-being in obese patients (Tanco, Linden, & Earle, 1998). Cognitive techniques were described earlier in this book for the treatment of depression. In this context, the therapist is more likely to focus on the recognition of dysfunctional thoughts about weight or body and to help the patient develop alternative interpretations. For example, patients can be asked to look at their reflection in the mirror, focusing on both the parts of the body that they like and those that they do not like. What might a nonjudgmental friend say about their body? A therapist who simply refutes illogical thoughts about the body may have less success than the clinician who stays focused on the outcome of the patient's maladaptive cognitions. For example, many cardiac patients enrolled in a rehabilitation program hate how they look in workout gear. Exploration of this thought (e.g., does the individual fear that other people will judge how she or he looks?) combined with examination of the potential consequence (e.g., how will weight loss be possible if the person refuses to exercise in front of other people?) can help promote body acceptance. Social rejection or embarrassment can be a theme that surfaces repeatedly when focusing on body image. Do the patients refuse social engagements because they dislike how they look or because they feel they cannot find flattering attire for the occasion? Is there a tendency to try to hide, for example, by sitting at the back of the room, trying to remain unobtrusive, or wearing overly baggy, shapeless clothes? What are the costs of such thoughts? Often patients will report that they have missed out on a lot of fun, for example, days at the beach missed for fear of wearing a bathing suit, a holiday party not attended resulting from feeling too fat in dressy clothes, or refusal to have sex with a loved partner because of fear of rejection or judgment. Cognitive approaches that focus only on how patients feel about their body can be extremely helpful in promoting better self-image as well as decreasing social avoidance strategies that often result from poor body image.

Emotions

The active involvement of the therapist can play a critical role in help-ing to attenuate feelings of shame and develop a more balanced perspective about the body. Use of the therapeutic relationship (McCullough et al., 2003) can be a critical aspect to explore the emotions blocking positive body im-age, as the following example illustrates:

Patient: There is nothing I like about my body. I can't even look in the mirror!

Therapist: Really, what do you imagine I feel toward you as you say that?

Patient: I have no idea.

Therapist: Try for a moment and see if you can imagine what I am feeling.

Patient: You are probably feeling like I'm too critical of myself. (Starts to cry)

Therapist: This brings up a lot of feeling.

Patient: Yes, I really feel so badly about myself.

Therapist: Perhaps we can try to face this together so you won't feel so overwhelmed with these negative feelings.

McCullough's model suggests that people become more self-accepting when they are able to reframe maladaptive cognitions and emotions about their bodies. This might be accomplished by role playing. For example, a patient who expresses a deep longing for her parent to provide validating support about her looks might be asked to imagine what that parent would say if the parent were in the room. This might be contrasted with how the patient would respond to her own children (if applicable) to build a sense of positive feeling about the body. As is probably evident, the underlying theme when addressing body dissatisfaction is to help the patient identify and ex-press positive feelings about the self that have been inhibited by shame or self-contempt.

Counseling for Weight Loss Surgery Patients

Some patients who plan to undertake weight loss surgery benefit from presurgical and postsurgical counseling. Of course, clinicians who work with this patient population need to familiarize themselves with the procedures, the pre- and postsurgical medical regimen, and typical results.

Presurgical Counseling

Some of the problems commonly encountered during the presurgical period include the following: ambivalence about whether to undergo the surgery, anxiety about the procedure and ability to cope with the necessarily lifestyle changes, lack of support from spouse or family, financial worries posed if patients are paying for the surgery themselves, and stress inherent in taking a great deal of time off from work to attend medical appointments. People who undergo bariatric surgery will have lifelong medical follow-up, and some patients underestimate the level of commitment required. It is easy when planning for bariatric surgery to minimize the degree of effort required to make lifestyle changes, and patients who appear to be overconfident may benefit from counseling that focuses on their perceptions of the postsurgery regimen and intentions to make behavioral change. Some patients may have unrealistic goals following surgery in terms of the amount of weight they will lose or the degree to which weight loss will affect their life. Psychotherapy that focuses on the individual's hopes for the postsurgery period can help to correct unrealistic expectations beforehand.

Insurance companies often initially deny weight loss surgery candidates, and patients may need to deal with insurance denials and appeals. Many patients pay for bariatric surgery out of pocket, which in turn can stimulate a great deal of emotion. Feelings of anger and frustration at the many factors outside of the individual's control are a natural result of the process. Counseling during the presurgical period can provide a patient with an advocate who helps to process negative emotions associated with this phase, provide psychoeducation about the procedure, and help the patient to work through ambivalence about whether to undergo the surgery and cope adaptively with setbacks.

Mental illness and current eating disorders (especially binge-eating disorder) are not always automatic rule-outs for weight loss surgery, but patients with such problems need help in exploring the potential untoward consequences of having the surgery without complete resolution of the psychiatric problem. A comprehensive review of 17 studies of how psychological factors affect outcome in weight loss surgery candidates suggests that the patients with the lowest levels of psychological functioning receive the greatest benefit from bariatric surgery (I. Greenberg, Perna, Kaplan, & Sullivan, 2005).

Postsurgical Counseling

After surgery, many patients experience an increase in psychological well-being, but a minority do not (van Hout, 2005; van Hout, Boekestein, Fortuin, Pelle, & van Heck, 2006). Patients whose expectations are unrealistic, who lack strong social support, who have low levels of confidence, who do not understand the amount of effort involved in weight loss, who have significant financial stress, or who lack good problem-solving skills face more obstacles to making change than patients without such difficulties. Once the patients have undergone the procedure, it is vital that they stay involved with a team of professionals to achieve the best possible outcome. It is at this point that poor psychological health places the patients at risk of drifting away from their medical care team. Psychotherapists who work with patients who are demoralized or nonadherent can use motivational techniques and supportive counseling to keep the patients engaged in their own treatment.

The restrictive dieting inherent after weight loss surgery can make people who were prone to binge eating beforehand more likely to binge under the stress of such a pronounced change (van Hout, van Oudheusden, & van Heck, 2004). Continuous vigilance for binging is important. Cognitive behavioral approaches can effectively stop binging behavior. Identification of the antecedents of the binge (often hunger or negative affect; Fairburn, Cooper, & Shafran, 2003) is an important first step in finding alternative behaviors to cope with the precipitant. Difficulty in coping with negative mood surfaces repeatedly as an obstacle to change in terms of weight (Fairburn et al., 2003). People with night-eating disorder have been shown to derive benefit from 20 minutes of progressive relaxation in terms of less depression, anger, fatigue, anxiety, stress, and, most importantly, fewer episodes of night eating (Pawlow & Jones, 2005; Pawlow, O'Neil, & Malcolm, 2003).

Other indicators of poor prognosis in terms of dieting success include eating in secret, feeling preoccupied with food or weight, and fear of losing control over eating (Fairburn, Cooper, Doll, & Davies, 2005). Exploration of these issues may reveal underlying emotional conflict or core maladaptive beliefs that can be modified with psychotherapy. For example, feeling defective or shamed about the self, viewing the self as lacking self-control, and perceiving the self as failing to achieve have all been identified as core maladaptive beliefs associated with greater severity of pathology among patients with eating disorders (Waller, Ohanian, Meyer, & Osman, 2000).

Even patients who are in robust psychological health will find the postsurgery regimen to be psychologically and behaviorally challenging. Once the weight is lost, many patients have very loose skin, and it is not uncommon to undergo additional plastic surgery to correct this. Family members and friends may relate to patients differently once they are thinner. Many patients are very receptive to postsurgical counseling and find the support and problem solving that can be offered through psychotherapy extremely helpful.

SUMMARY

As the prevalence of morbid obesity increases and the public becomes more aware of and familiar with weight loss surgery, there are likely to be more referrals of patients with morbid obesity to mental health professionals. Such patients may have existing cardiovascular disease or may be at high risk for a future cardiac event. Some therapists are generally opposed to weight loss surgery, and many clinicians do not have expertise in dietary and exercise change. Nonetheless, there is still a tremendous demand for general psychotherapy to address the emotional, cognitive, and interpersonal issues that can affect people who are morbidly obese, and behavioral cardiology practitioners are likely to see many referrals of such patients because there is considerable overlap in the cardiac and morbidly obese patient populations.

12

PSYCHOTROPIC MEDICATIONS

Medications to treat depression, anxiety, sleep problems, and smoking cessation are often prescribed to people with heart disease by their primary care physicians or cardiologists. These categories of medication are commonly encountered by therapists working with a cardiac population and are thus the focus of this chapter. The relative advantages of pharmacotherapy combined with psychotherapy have been demonstrated in many clinical trials (I. W. Miller & Keitner, 1996). A basic working knowledge of psychotropic medications commonly used in cardiac patients can be helpful to therapists. Patients often have a difficult time discriminating between somatic symptoms that may be caused by psychological distress, heart problems, a side effect of medication, or some combination of these factors. Pharmacological treatment for psychological problems in people with heart disease is complex and requires attention to the effect that the medication will have on cardiac function, potential to improve psychological well-being, severity of the psychological problem, and the patient's history of compliance with other medical regimens.

REMEMBERING PSYCHOLOGY 101

For those who have long since left the classroom, a quick refresher on the brain can help to refresh the memory about how drugs work. Signals in the brain are relayed between nerve cells through a synapse, a small gap between the cells. Psychiatrist Eric Chamberlin explains the process:

> Neurotransmitters are chemicals released by the presynaptic neuron. Common neurotransmitters include dopamine, serotonin, and norepinephrine. After being released by the presynaptic neuron, the neurotransmitter defuses across the synapse and binds to receptors on the postsynaptic neuron. This binding causes the neuron to fire (depolarization) and the signal is propogated. The neurotransmitter separates from the receptor and is transported back into the presynaptic neuron where it can be used again, a process called reuptake. If the reuptake process is blocked, the neurotransmitter will remain in the synapse and continue to trigger firing of the postsynaptic neuron. Most antidepressants work by blocking the reuptake of one or more neurotransmitters. (personal communication, March 4, 2007)

ANTIDEPRESSANTS

Antidepressants include tricyclic antidepressants (TCAs), monoamine oxidase (MAO) inhibitors, selective serotonin reuptake inhibitors (SSRIs), and nontricyclic antidepressants. TCAs and MAO inhibitors affect cardiac conduction, contractility, and rhythm and are associated with orthostatic hypotension. People who are using vasodilators or have heart failure are very susceptible to orthostatic hypotension when using TCAs. TCAs slow cardiac conduction; therefore, in people who have preexisting conduction dysfunction, TCAs can be lethal. For this reason, at the time of this writing, SSRIs are considered the first line of treatment for depression in people with heart disease (Roose & Miyazaki, 2005).

SSRIs

SSRIs are antidepressants that can also be used to treat anxiety problems and may even modify personality traits. SSRI drugs include the following (brand names in the United States listed in parentheses): citalopram (Celexa), escitalopram oxalate (Lexapro), fluoxetine (Prozac), fluvoxamine meleate (Luvox), paroxetine (Paxil), and sertraline (Zoloft). Serotonin dysregulation occurs when people are depressed. SSRIs work by increasing the level of serotonin, inhibiting its reuptake into the presynaptic cell and thus leaving more of it available in the synaptic cleft, between cells. The "selective" part of the name refers to the fact that this drug does not bind to noradrenaline and dopamine transporters. It can take up to 2 weeks before patients get relief from depression on SSRI medications. In the first few days, many people actually feel an increase in anxiety levels. Side effects of SSRIs include nausea, sleepiness, headaches, vivid dreams, dizziness, appetite change with resultant weight loss or gain, loss of libido, tremors, orthostatic hypertension, sweating, racing thoughts, feelings of depersonalization, or increased suicidality. Some SSRIs commonly used in the treatment of cardiac patients are discussed subsequently.

Sertraline

Sertraline hydrochloride (Zoloft) is an SSRI used to treat depression and anxiety. One major clinical trial testing the safety and efficacy of sertraline for people with heart disease has been completed. The Sertraline Antidepressant Heart Attack Randomized Trial (SADHART) study was a multicenter, randomized controlled trial of 369 people with depression and ischemic heart disease (Glassman et al., 2002). Sertraline was demonstrated to be more effective than placebo in reducing symptoms of depression in people with heart disease, even among people with severe and recurrent depression. Sertraline was also found to be safe, with no effect on left ventricular function, systolic or diastolic blood pressure, cardiac conduction, or heart rhythm. The placebo group in the SADHART study did have a nonsignificant trend toward worse cardiovascular outcomes in terms of cardiovascular morbidity and all-cause mortality, but this finding should be interpreted with caution, because the study was not powered to find an effect on these outcomes.

The Enhancing Recovery in Coronary Heart Disease (ENRICHD) trial, described in chapter 4, this volume, was designed as a clinical trial to evaluate the efficacy of cognitive behavioral therapy (CBT) for the treatment of depression in patients with acute coronary syndrome (Berkman et al., 2003), but the ENRICHD protocol offered a flexible approach in that it allowed depressed participants who did not initially respond to CBT to be treated with sertraline. In addition, some patients sought out antidepressant medication on their own during the course of the study. A post hoc analysis of the study participants who were treated with SSRIs showed that they had lower overall and cardiovascular-related mortality (Carney et al., 2004).

Citalopram

Citalopram (Celexa) is an SSRI that does not have significant cardiovascular side effects, is less toxic if overdosed, and is less likely to have drug interaction effects. In 2007, the results of a large-scale, randomized controlled trial of citalopram were published in the *Journal of the American Medical Association*. The Canadian Cardiac Randomized Evaluation of Antidepressant and Psychotherapy Efficacy (CREATE) trial randomized 284 patients with coronary heart disease (CHD) and major depression to an intervention lasting 12 weeks (Lesperance et al., 2007). The CREATE trial, also described in chapter 4 of this volume, was designed as a 2 × 2 factorial testing citalopram versus placebo and interpersonal therapy (IPT) versus clinical management. Thus the participants were randomized twice: to citalopram or placebo, and then to IPT or clinical management. Citalopram was superior to placebo in reducing depressive symptoms at 12 weeks postbaseline, with 35.9% of subjects who took citalopram attaining the goal of a score of ≤ 8 on the Hamilton Depression Inventory, whereas only 22% of patients taking placebo reached this goal. At the time of this writing, the long-term efficacy data are not yet available for this study.

Citalopram is also being tested in the Myocardial Infarction and Depression–Intervention Trial (MIND–IT), albeit as a secondary line of treatment (van den Brink et al., 2002). This trial is based in the Netherlands, enrolling 2,140 post-MI patients who are randomized to receive mirtazpine (Remeron) or placebo. Mirtazpine is a nontricyclic antidepressant that does not produce the anticholinergic effects that are associated with TCAs. With respect to the MIND–IT, in the case of refusal or nonresponse to mirtazpine, open treatment with citalopram is offered to patients. The results of this trial are not published at the time of this writing but will offer additional data on the effects of these antidepressants on cardiac prognosis. Analysis of baseline data from this study has indicated that the combined variables of younger age, severe left ventricular dysfunction, and a positive screen for depression using the Beck Depression Inventory (BDI) were strongly predictive of depression following MI (van Melle et al., 2006).

Paroxetine

Paroxetine (Paxil) is an SSRI used to treat depression and a spectrum of anxiety disorders. A randomized controlled trial comparing paroxetine with nortriptyline in depressed patients with heart disease showed that although both drugs were effective at treating depression, paroxetine normalized platelet activity and is thus thought to be safer for people with heart disease. By contrast, nortriptyline was associated with an increase in heart rate, decreased heart rate variability, and worse cardiovascular outcomes (Roose et al., 1998).

Fluoxetine

Fluoxetine (Prozac) was the first SSRI on the market in the United States and is used for treatment for multiple psychological disorders, including those commonly encountered by psychologists working with cardiac patients: depression, hypochondria, and panic disorder. A randomized controlled trial that evaluated the efficacy and safety of fluoxetine in patients ($n = 54$) with major depression after a first MI did not find a significant improvement in depressive symptoms in the treated group (Strik et al., 2000). However, the treatment group did have a better response rate compared with placebo, and in people with mild depression, fluoxetine was associated with greater improvements in symptom relief. Hostility scores were also favorably affected by treatment with fluoxetine, raising the possibility that this medication might be considered for patients with hostile affect. No decreases in cardiac function were associated with treatment using fluoxetine. Generally, fluoxetine has been associated with significantly fewer anticholinergic, antihistaminergic, and cardiotoxic side effects in the treatment of major depressive disorders, but isolated cases of dysrhythmia (atrial fibrillation and bradycardia) and syncope have been reported (Pacher, Ungvari, Kecskemeti, & Furst, 1998).

Clinical Example

Joe was a 58-year-old artist who had not suffered a heart attack but had CHD that was treated with coronary bypass surgery about 2 months before he was referred for therapy. Joe had a history of depression and had been treated once previously with antidepressants and psychotherapy, in his 30s after the breakup of a long-term relationship. When Joe entered the therapist's office, he looked very sad. However, his score on the BDI was just 8, generally below the threshold for screening depression. He was not tearful but described that in the month prior to his heart attack, he had become extremely fatigued, so much that he often collapsed after work at the end of the week and slept the weekend away. His mood seemed terribly sad, and he attributed this to a great deal of job stress and the death of a beloved brother during the previous year.

Joe came into the office quietly, appeared withdrawn, and never smiled. Despite this, he denied feeling depressed. Joe never became defensive, but over time, it became clear that he thought that all artists were prone to low mood and that what the therapist saw as depression was to him a melancholy, artistic personality trait. Joe and the therapist agreed that they would work together but that Joe would consult with a psychiatrist if he did not improve after 6 weeks. After 6 weeks, things were still not improved. Joe resisted being seen by a psychiatrist but did agree to let the therapist talk with his primary care physician, who prescribed fluoxetine. Within 2 weeks, Joe's affect was markedly improved, and he reported having greater energy and feeling in better spirits. He smiled and joked more in therapy sessions and, with the benefit of hindsight, agreed that he had been depressed. He did not like the resulting weight gain and loss of libido that the medication produced. His primary care physician asked him to stay on the medication for the year because of the high risk of relapse. He agreed but spent multiple sessions in therapy focused on the effect of Prozac on his personality. "Is it me," he wondered, "to feel this light and carefree, or is it just the drug?" Joe ruminated less and was more outgoing socially when he was on Prozac. At the same time, as an artist, he mourned the diminution of his angst and the loss of sexual passion. When the year was up, he was eager to stop taking the medication. His depression did not return. He agreed that, in the future, he would be better able to recognize a worsening of depressive symptoms and would be more receptive to taking medications from the outset if he became depressed.

This clinical example illustrates that some patients taking SSRI drugs report changes in characteristics that were traditionally thought to be personality traits (e.g., interpersonal sensitivity and social inhibition). Kramer (1993) wrote about this topic in the book *Listening to Prozac*, and underscored that human character traits have tremendous potential to be affected at the chemical level. Given that traits such as social inhibition are associated with dramatically increased predilection for negative affect and also for coronary artery disease (Denollet, Pedersen, Ong, et al., 2006), more trials of SSRI drugs in cardiac populations are needed. Cardiac patients who take SSRIs also have better outcomes in terms of their heart disease, as described in the next section.

Cardiac Benefit of SSRI Medications

Not only do SSRI medications have fewer cardiovascular side effects compared with TCAs and MAO inhibitors, but they are also generally associated with protection against MI in a depressed population. A study of 653 smokers with first MI found that the odds ratio for MI among current SSRI users compared with nonusers was .35 (Sauer, Berlin, & Kimmel, 2001). The protective effect of SSRIs against cardiovascular disease is thought to be caused by the attenuation of platelet activation caused by depleted serotonin storage. Platelets contain serotonergic receptors, and depression is associated with exaggerated platelet reactivity, an inflammatory response (Musselman et al., 1996, 2000). Inflammation is known to promote coronary artery disease progression by increasing macrophage and lipid deposition within coronary arteries and by instability and rupture of existing atherosclerotic lesions. A separate study by the same research group cited earlier compared 1,080 patients with first MI with 4,256 control cases and found that the odds ratio of MI associated with current SSRI use compared with nonuse was .59 (Sauer, Berlin, & Kimmel, 2003). After the SSRI group was compared with patients using tricyclic or atypical antidepressants, the data showed that only SSRIs were associated with reduced risk for MI (Sauer et al., 2003). In summary, the evidence to date suggests that SSRIs are safe for use with cardiac patients and have the potential to protect against MI in people treated for depression.

ANXIOLYTICS

Anxiolytics are drugs that reduce tension and relax muscles. Benzodiazepines represent the majority of anxiolytics prescribed. Benzodiazepines potentiate the effect of gamma-aminobutyric acid (usually referred to as GABA), an inhibitory neurotransmitter, by binding to benzodiazepine receptors, producing sedation of the central nervous system and thus making people feel more relaxed and less anxious. Benzodiazapines include lorazepam (Ativan), alprazolam (Xanax), and diazepam (Valium). Benzodiazepines can be recommended for short-term and long-term use depending on diagnosis, history of addiction, and other clinical variables, but they have significant potential for addiction. Side effects include sleepiness, forgetfulness, impaired coordination, and headache. No randomized trials have evaluated the efficacy or safety of benzodiazepines, specifically for cardiac patients. Benzodiazepine use can impair or facilitate psychotherapy, depending on the patient's level of anxiety. Although the majority of psychiatrists and primary care physicians who prescribe anxiolytic medications aim to titrate until the patient has eliminated symptoms of anxiety, benzodiazepine use can also facilitate psychotherapy. Eric Chamberlin explains this process:

> It is similar to learning and level of arousal, in that there is an optimal level. Too little or too much arousal and learning doesn't take place. Ideally, pharmacotherapy complements psychotherapy. When patients reach the optimal zone of anxiety pharmacologically with medication, they can progress more rapidly in psychotherapy. (personal communication, March 4, 2007)

Effective team partnerships between the psychotherapist, primary care physician, and psychiatrist are essential to the success of treatment.

As noted earlier in chapter 5 on anxiety and the heart, 15% to 20% of people who present to the emergency room with chest pain meet criteria for full-blown or subclinical panic disorder (Katon, Von Korff, & Lin, 1992; Yingling, Wulsin, Arnold, & Rouan, 1993). Therefore, it is not surprising that a number of cardiac patients seen in a psychotherapist's office will have been prescribed clonazepam (Klonopin), a highly potent medication for treatment of anxiety disorders. Clonazepam is a benzodiazepine derivative that is commonly prescribed for panic. The primary side effects of clonazepam are sleepiness, poor motor coordination, euphoria, dizziness, memory problems, and, important for cardiac patients, heart palpitations. When patients stop taking clonazepam, their symptoms of anxiety may recur. Thus, nearly one third of patients who use clonazepam for an extended period of time develop low-dose dependence in that they cannot stop taking the drug, but increased dosages are not needed to get the same effect, so they do not develop tolerance. At the time of this writing, there are no published studies about the use of clonazepam specifically in people with heart disease.

SLEEP MEDICATION

Many people with heart disease complain that they sleep poorly, and 13% of outpatients with CHD meet criteria for primary insomnia (Bankier, Januzzi, & Littman, 2004). When medication is prescribed, a nonbenzodiazepine hypnotic agent is often used. A commonly prescribed sleep medication is zolpidem tartrate (Ambien), which acts by potentiating GABA. Zolpidem works relatively quickly and has a half-life of just a few hours. It is approved for short-term use of less than 6 weeks. Side effects of zolpidem can include memory problems, hallucinations, delusions, poor motor coordination, euphoria or dysphoria, increased appetite, increased libido, impaired judgment, increased impulsivity, and, when the drug is stopped, re recurrence of insomnia. More recently, an extended release version of this medication was introduced in the United States. There are no studies on the safety of zolpidem for people with heart problem available in the literature at the time of this writing.

BETA-BLOCKERS

Beta-adrenergic blockers are commonly prescribed to treat high blood pressure and slow heart rate and to improve many types of cardiac problems. This class of medications blocks the stimulation of the beta-receptors in the body to reduce the overall workload of the ventricles. Beta-blockers are commonly prescribed for cardiac patients and are included in this chapter because they can reduce symptoms of anxiety and feelings of anger or irritability. Beta-blockers work by counteracting the effect of adrenaline and depressing sympathetic activity; thus it is not surprising that they reduce symptoms of anxiety (Mealy et al., 1996), although they are not approved by the Food and Drug Administration (FDA) for that purpose. Smokers have very high levels of anxiety when they present to the emergency room with MI and are 60% more likely to be prescribed beta-blockers (Sheahan et al., 2006). Beta-blockers can also be effective at reducing aggression and anger (Fava, 1997). As previously noted in chapter 6 on anger, hostility, and the heart, episodes of anger can trigger cardiac events (Mittleman et al., 1995). In a sample of 699 patients with MI, anger 1 hour or less beforehand increased risk for MI, but use of beta-blockers decreased that risk substantially (Moller et al., 1999). Most cardiac patients who are prescribed beta-blockers are not necessarily aware that they may have the added benefit of attenuating the cardiovascular response to feelings of anxiety and anger. Because so many cardiac patients are commonly prescribed this type of medication, therapists can benefit from this knowledge as well.

SMOKING CESSATION MEDICATIONS

The first medications approved by the FDA for smoking cessation were introduced to the market in the United States in 1984. The availability of such pharmaceutical aides has contributed to the decline in smoking rates over the past 40 years (Centers for Disease Control and Prevention, 2007), which in turn, has been associated with declines in coronary heart disease mortality (Ford & Capewell, 2007).

Nicotine Replacement

The general consensus from the literature is that nicotine replacement therapy (NRT) is not dangerous for the heart. It is tobacco rather than nicotine that has adverse cardiovascular side effects. Although it is true that nicotine does increase sympathetic activity, which results in increased heart rate and blood pressure as well as vasoconstriction, and can precipitate glucose intolerance and aggravate diabetes, the level of nicotine in NRT is typically far less than that created by cigarette smoking. Cigarette smoking poses most of its cardiac risk by increasing levels of carbon monoxide, risk for clot formation, and lipid problems (Benowitz & Gourlay, 1997). Studies of NRT have generally established the safety and efficacy of this class of medications for cardiac patients (Joseph & Fu, 2003a, 2003b). It is important to note that even cardiac patients who smoke while using the nicotine patch have not been shown to be at higher risk for adverse events (Joseph et al., 1996).

At the time of this writing, the FDA has approved five types of NRT for the treatment of smoking cessation: gum, patch, nasal spray, inhaler, and lozenge. Nicotine polacrilex gum increases the likelihood of stopping smoking by 50%, can be bought over the counter, comes in several flavors, and is self-titrating. People who have dentures or jaw problems often do not like the gum. The gum is less expensive than other types of NRT (Fiore et al., 2000). The nicotine transdermal patch increases the likelihood of quitting smoking by 90%, is available over the counter, and offers the highest dose of nicotine (up to 21 mg) in a continuous dosage. People like the patch because it is easy to use; the most common complaint about the patch is that it can cause skin irritation. Nicotine nasal spray provides a fast route for nicotine to reach the brain and increases the chance of stopping smoking by 170%. However, it is available only by prescription and effectively amounts to squirting nicotine up the nose, making it unappealing for some people. The nicotine inhaler closely mimics actual smoking because the nicotine is encased in a plastic cartridge shaped like a cigarette. Although it is called an inhaler, the nicotine is absorbed through the mouth tissues. The inhaler increases the likelihood of cessation by 180% (Fiore et al., 2000). The nicotine lozenge is available over the counter and is similar to the gum in that it is self-dosing, but it does not require chewing. It takes a long time for the lozenge to dissolve, which is a relative advantage to some patients and disadvantage to others. All NRT products can be combined with other non-nicotine treatments, such as bupropion, discussed subsequently.

Non-Nicotine Medications for Smoking Cessation

There are two non-nicotine medications approved by the FDA at the time of this writing for the treatment of smoking cessation: bupropion hydrochloride (Zyban) and varenicline (Chantix). Bupropion is an atypical anti-depressant that is effective for smoking cessation. One of the advantages of bupropion is that it reduces feelings of irritability and negative affect in the early stages of cessation. There is no evidence that bupropion causes an effect on heart rate, ejection fraction, cardiac conduction, or blood pressure. A study by Rigotti et al. (2006) established the safety of using bupropion for smoking cessation at the standard dose of 300 mg in patients with recent MI or unstable angina. A question that often arises from cardiologists is whether bupropion might effectively treat both smoking cessation and depression in a person with heart disease. Because bupropion is not considered a first-line treatment for depression in cardiac patients, a first episode of depression should be thoroughly evaluated, and if medication is prescribed, many factors beyond the potential benefit to smoking cessation should be considered (e.g., severity of the depression, potential side effects). Beyond this, acutely depressed patients are less likely to achieve long-term abstinence from smoking, and thus, a first effort to effectively treat the depression should improve the odds that the patient will successfully stop smoking.

Varenicline (Chantix) was approved by the FDA for the treatment of smoking cessation and is a partial agonist at the α4β2 nicotinic acetylcholine receptor. As a partial agonist, varenicline has a dual mechanism of action in that it reduces cravings and withdrawal symptoms while at the same time decreases the feelings of pleasure that accompany smoking.

A report showed that long-term abstinence rate for varenicline was 23% compared with 10% of subjects on placebo and 14.6% of subjects using bupropion (Jorenby et al., 2006). There are ongoing studies, but no data yet available at the time of this writing, on the safety of varenicline in people with established heart disease.

MEDICATIONS IN CONJUNCTION WITH PSYCHOTHERAPY

Cardiac patients who seek therapy often have no history of mental health treatment and may have very positive or negative expectations about the value of using pharmacologic treatment. Clinicians might weigh several considerations when deciding whether to recommend a consultation with a psychiatrist for medication. On the one hand, some people are highly anxious, prone to hypochondriasis, and seek medication to treat even slight levels of dysphoria. On the other hand, other patients are stoic by nature, prone to denying their distress, and are sufficiently shamed by psychological symptoms such that they would not resort to using medication. Systematic reviews of randomized controlled trials of combined psychotherapy and drug treatment have established that patients with depression who are receiving combined treatment improve significantly compared with those receiving drug treatment alone, particularly in treatments lasting longer than 12 weeks

(Pampallona, Bollini, Tibaldi, Kupelnick, & Munizza, 2004). In particular, sequenced or crossover treatments (adding one treatment once the response to the other has been inadequate) consistently seem to show benefit (Segal, Vincent, & Levitt, 2002). Many medical patients express a preference for psychotherapy over medication, as was shown in the IMPACT trial in which 51% of the sample of older adult patients recruited from primary care clinics stated a preference for psychotherapy for treatment of depression (Unutzer et al., 2002). A smaller study showed that patient preference for medication versus psychotherapy affects the therapeutic alliance (Iacoviello et al., 2007). This study reported on 75 depressed patients randomized to receive either supportive-expressive therapy or medication for depression. Those in the medication arm were randomized again to sertraline or placebo. Patients who preferred and received therapy had alliance scores that increased over time, whereas those who preferred therapy but received medication (active or placebo) experienced a decrease in alliance scores. For those who preferred medication, there was no change in alliance on the basis of patient preference in any of the groups (Iacoviello et al., 2007). Therapeutic alliance is one of the strongest predictors of mental health outcome according to a review by Horvath (2001) and also has tremendous influence in use of pharmacotherapy (Krupnick et al., 1996). So perhaps more important than the decision to refer a patient for pharmacotherapy is the need for a strong alliance, such that the patient will make good use of the referral.

SUMMARY

Clinicians who work with cardiac patients need to achieve some level of proficiency in understanding major classes of psychotropic medications that are commonly prescribed for this population. This chapter focused selectively on medications that are commonly used for people with heart disease and, where clinical trial data exist, summarized the results of those studies. Ideally, prescriptions for psychotropic medications would be written by psychiatrists. However, in practice, psychiatry is often inaccessible because many providers don't accept insurance, waiting times for appointments are often long, and many cardiac patients find such referrals to be stigmatizing. It therefore behooves the mental health professional who does not prescribe to have some familiarity with the major classes of psychotropic medications so that her or she can properly educate their patients as to the value of psychotropic medications when appropriate.

13

SEX DIFFERENCES

There are important differences between women and men in the risk for and presentation of heart disease. Some of these differences are rooted in biological and physiological characteristics of the sexes. However, with respect to psychological risks for heart disease, many of the male–female differences are complex and rooted in a social context. This chapter first reviews the concrete, biologically rooted contrasts in cardiac illness in women compared with men, followed by an exploration of the broader social context of psychological differences in risk for heart disease. The last part of this chapter outlines similarities and differences in conducting psychotherapy with female versus male cardiac patients.

On average, a first heart attack occurs for men at about age 65 and for women at about age 70 (American Heart Association, 2005). In both men and women, increasing age is associated with risk for heart disease. Less is known about heart disease in women than in men, primarily because for decades only men were enrolled in research studies to investigate and treat cardiac illness. Even today, only 25% of study participants in clinical trials are women. Although heart disease is the leading cause of death for men and women, the onset, presentation, risk factors, course of illness, and treatment outcomes are different. Heart disease in women under the age of 50 is less common (Wenger, Speroff, & Packard, 1993), and traditionally women have perceived themselves to be at risk for breast cancer rather than coronary heart disease (CHD). However, far more women die from heart disease than from breast cancer at all ages. One out of 29 deaths in women is caused by breast cancer compared with 1 out of 2.4 deaths caused by cardiovascular disease (Mosca, Ferris, Fabunmi, & Robertson, 2004).

A variety of interrelated factors account for gender differences in cardio-vascular disease, including biological, psychological, and sociocultural factors. The physical, biological distinctions between the sexes are addressed next.

BIOLOGICAL DIFFERENCES

Obviously, the biology of men and women is different. From a physical perspective, women have smaller hearts and arteries. Women are more likely to have microvascular (small vessel) disease, and the detection of symptoms of heart disease in women is not as straightforward as it is in men. Women are more likely to have plaque erosions, whereas men are more likely to have plaque rupture, which in turn affects the way that atherosclerosis is diagnosed and treated. The composition of the plaque itself can be different in women, with some evidence that women have less dense and calcified plaque compared with men (Rossi, Merlini, & Ardissino, 2001; Virmani, Burke, & Farb, 1999).

Women are more likely than men to have more chronic types of heart disease, such as heart failure, and women with heart disease have higher rates of diabetes, hypertension, high cholesterol, and thyroid dysfunction compared with men. Women diagnosed with coronary artery disease tend to be older, have greater severity of disease, and have more comorbid illnesses (Wenger et al., 1993). Probably as a consequence of being older, women have fewer forms of support in that they are more likely to be living alone, widowed, retired, or unemployed (Schuster & Waldron, 1991) and also less likely to have adequate medical insurance. So perhaps it is not a great surprise that many studies have shown that heart disease in women is not treated with the same level of aggression as it is in men. Women receive fewer angioplasties, stents, implantable defibrillators, and open-heart surgeries compared with men (American Heart Association, 2005). Only 22% of heart transplants (Harper & Rosendale, 1996) are done in women. Women are less likely to receive beta-blockers, ACE (angiotensin converting enzyme) inhibitors, or aspirin after heart attack and less likely to be referred to cardiac rehabilitation. They are twice as likely as men to die following bypass surgery (Sjoland, Caidahl, Karlson, Karlsson, & Herlitz, 1997). A woman is more likely than a man to die from cardiac arrest before reaching the hospital. Women's attitudes even seem different in that, compared with men, they tend to opt for conservative treatments and are more likely to refuse cardiac rehabilitation programs and aggressive treatments such as heart transplant

(Cupples, 1997; L. Young & Little, 2004). At the same time, studies on this topic have been mixed, with some researchers noting that the sex differences in treatment have been relatively small and in many cases insignificant when national databases are used for analysis (Gold & Krumholz, 2006).

Clinical Example

Susan was a trim, youthful-looking woman in her early 50s when she was referred for psychotherapy by one of the nurses in cardiac rehabilitation. She was married with one adult child and was the primary caretaker of her brother, who was mentally disabled. Her mother had also lived with her but had died 6 months ago from chronic obstructive pulmonary disease. "I have no risk factors for heart disease that I know of," she said, "except that I have extremely high levels of caregiver stress." She had suffered a heart attack in the late summer. She described the weeks prior to the event as "hell."

"My mother was failing and I could not leave her alone for a minute. My brother kept getting upset at the chaos in the house and we had to give him medication to calm him. One weekend, I was feeling really sick but I still kept pushing myself to take care of everyone else. That night, I had the heart attack and wound up in the hospital." Susan's stress was evident on her face as she told her story.

In her cardiologist's office, following discharge, Susan wept as she described what seemed to be a hopeless situation of endless caregiver burden. She questioned whether she would be able to take time to attend the cardiac rehabilitation program. To her surprise, her cardiologist did not try to impress on her the need for cardiac rehabilitation. In hindsight, she looked back at that moment as a crossroads. "I knew if I didn't put myself first, there might not be a next time for me. And I realized that my doctor is not infallible. All he heard was that I am too busy and he let it go. I'll bet if I were a 50-year-old man saying I was too busy for rehabilitation and wanted to go back to work, he would have argued with me."

As this clinical example demonstrates, an array of complex, interrelated factors influence cardiac care. Why is the onset and course of heart disease different for men and women? One reason that women develop heart disease later is because of hormonal differences, as described subsequently.

Once women reach the age of menopause and as their estrogen levels fall, their risk for heart disease escalates dramatically. Estrogen protects against the atherosclerotic plaque formation that characterizes coronary artery disease. Ironically, about 10 years after menopause, higher levels of estrogen are also associated with plaque rupture. The Heart and Estrogen/Progestin Replacement Study (HERS) trial showed that lipid reduction resulting from hormone replacement therapy was not associated with decreased risk for cardiac events (Grady et al., 2002). It has since been hypothesized that estrogen alters plaque instability using inflammatory mechanisms, thereby offsetting the potential benefit derived from lipid reduction that occurs during hormone replacement therapy (Nguyen & McLaughlin, 2002).

Estrogen and progesterone influence serotonin and norepinephrine, and so hormonal factors may also help to explain the dramatic differences in depression rates between men and women. The sex differences in depression rates are particularly pronounced in adolescence, when girls have a far greater risk for depression close to the age of menstruation compared with similar-age boys. Women's risk for depression is elevated during times that hormone levels fluctuate greatly, for example, onset of menstruation, during pregnancy, and after pregnancy. Similarly, women who have more perimenopausal symptoms and those with premenstrual syndrome have a greater vulnerability to depression. Thus, depression is an independent risk for heart disease, and both depression and heart disease are affected by hormonal factors. A discussion of sex-related differences in terms of psychological risk for heart disease is presented later in this chapter.

There are also differences in how men and women are treated by the medical system, on the job, and in our culture that exert direct and indirect influence on their heart health. A brief discussion of this follows.

SOCIOCULTURAL FACTORS

Health care takes place in a cultural and social context. Beliefs, attitudes, social structures, cultural norms, and medical systems are all related to sex differences in the diagnosis and treatment of risk factors for heart disease.

Physician Variables

Physicians are human and vary widely in their approach to identifying and treating psychological problems according to their training, age, gender, and cultural characteristics. More often than not, physicians miss the diagnosis of depression (Schwenk, Coyne, & Fechner-Bates, 1996) in both men and women, and cardiac patients are no exception. The tendency to refer cardiac patients less often for psychotherapy might be a result of age. In general, older patients are less likely to use or be referred for psychotherapy services. A survey of the beliefs and referral practices of general practitioners in Canada found that physicians were far less likely to treat and refer aging patients for mental health problems compared with younger patients and more likely to believe that psychotherapy alone or even combined with medication is less effective in older patients (Mackenzie, Gekoski, & Knox, 1999).

Beliefs, attitudes, and stereotypes influence the recognition and interpretation of cardiac symptoms. However, it is not overt bias but rather more subtle beliefs and attitudes that are manifested only in certain contexts, as demonstrated in a study by Chiaramonte and Friend (2006). Medical students and residents were recruited to participate in two studies that they believed were unrelated. The first study tested their memory about symptom presentation, and the second examined medical practitioner attitudes. The students and residents read vignettes about patients with cardiac symptoms and were asked to give a diagnosis, treatment, and interpretation of symptoms. Four possible vignettes of patients with symptoms of heart disease were presented, contrasting male and female patients and contextual differences with and without stress and anxiety. The vignettes with the stress and anxiety context indicated that the patients felt anxious after not receiving a promotion at work and was concerned about their health. The authors found that a woman presenting with cardiac symptoms, in the context of stressful life events, was less likely to be diagnosed with heart disease or referred to a cardiologist than a man with the identical presentation. Male and female residents and medical students did not differ in their interpretation. There is strong evidence that women's cardiac symptoms are often attributed to mental stressors (Eastwood & Doering, 2005). These findings underscore that it is difficult, if not impossible, for medical professionals to divest themselves of socially and culturally normative beliefs.

Employment and Social Class

Men and women are influenced differently by socioeconomic factors in terms of effect on risk factors for heart disease. Employment stress poses a risk to heart health for men and women. In particular, people who work at jobs that exert great stress but offer little control or jobs that are poorly rewarded relative to the demands are at disproportionately higher risk for heart disease (Theorell & Karasek, 1996). Both types of job stress are well captured by Barbara Ehrenreich, who went undercover to document the plight of the working poor in the United States in her book *Nickel and Dimed: On (Not) Getting By in America* (Ehrenreich, 2001). To determine whether a person can live on $6 to $7 an hour, Ehrenreich found employment working at various locations in states across the country, at Wal-Mart, a truck stop, washing dishes in a nursing home, and as a housecleaner. She demonstrated that even when people work two such jobs to survive, they must often subsist with barely enough money to pay for substandard housing and nutritionally poor meals, and they are not able to afford health or dental care. Women are disproportionately affected by poverty (U.S. Census Bureau, 2004). In 2003, the U.S. poverty standard was just over $9,000 for one person and $12,000 for a family of two. About 1 out of every 8 women is poor, compared with 1 out of every 11 men. Among people over age 65, women are 70% more likely to be poor than men (Legal Momentum: Advancing Women's Rights, 2004). It is not difficult for most people to imagine that the resentment, worry, and indignities suffered as a result of poverty might influence a person's ability to comply with treatment regimens, which in turn could confer risk for heart disease.

Clinical Example

Elena had been working since the age of 14 in a variety of jobs, gradually working her way up to the top. She was diagnosed with Marfan's syndrome (a genetically inherited cardiac disease) in her late 20s but continued to work two jobs to support her two children who lived with her, as well as her aging mother who lived in South America. Her primary day job was in a group home for residents with mental retardation, and her secondary job was cleaning houses at night. She described struggling to put food on the table, yet was creative and so thrifty that she had managed to save enough money to purchase a used car in cash. She often commented that she was so fortunate, that her job paid benefits, including 2 weeks of paid vacation a year. Secretly, the therapist thought that Elena's wages bordered on exploitive for a 10-year employee and the therapist could not begin to imagine how she managed to cope with her many stressors.

When her ailing mother began to fail, Elena made plans to travel to South America for 3 weeks with her children, to give herself one last time to say goodbye, and to give her children their first visit with their grandparent. The trip was also important because Elena had not told her sisters that she was diagnosed with Marfan's syndrome. Because the disease is genetic, she wanted to tell them in person, so that they could themselves be tested. Although she had earned the vacation, her supervisor would not allow her to take 2 consecutive weeks. He warned her that she would lose her job if she did not return on the 8th day. Elena was faced with the choice—to pay thousands of dollars (roughly 10% of her annual household income) for herself and her children, on a plane trip that would require a day of travel each way and spend only 5 days with her family, or leave for 3 weeks as originally planned and find a new job when she returned. She was troubled in therapy over this dilemma. She ultimately chose to find a new job, counting on her industrious work ethnic to carry her through her grief over the loss of her mother. Such choices are patently unfair, yet too often people who are marginalized often face decisions such as these.

Both men and women who are less empowered by virtue of their socioeconomic status are more likely to work in lower-paying, low-control jobs that pose high risk for heart disease. Women, in particular, traditionally faced fewer job options. However, as more women obtain a higher education, the wage gap continues to narrow. In 2005, women made 82 cents for every dollar earned by men, according to the Bureau of Labor and Statistics, and this represented a substantial increase from the 66.6 cents women made, relative to men, in 1983 (U.S. Department of Labor, 2007). Women have entered the labor force in high numbers. More than 7 out of 10 women ages 25 to 54 worked full time year round in 1998. Yet women spend about the same amount of time on child care in 2003 as they did in 1965 (Bianchi, 2000). This has occurred because the time that women devote to self-care and sleep has decreased, family size has decreased, more women have delayed child bearing, and simultaneously, the amount of time that fathers spend on child rearing has increased. Only time will tell what impact the transformation of women's participation and roles in the workforce will have on their heart health. As must seem evident, from a sociocultural perspective, it is difficult to untangle the complex mix of interrelated economic and social factors that contribute to risk for heart disease, let alone tease out the independent effects of sex differences on those factors.

BIASES IN THE COLLECTIVE PSYCHE?

The presumption that heart disease is less salient for women than for men is deeply embedded in the collective psyche. Women themselves buy into the unspoken presumption that heart disease is not as important for them to think about. Women tend to delay seeking treatment and are less likely to acknowledge the seriousness of their risk for heart disease (Hansen, 2003). Few people raise an eyebrow about the fact that virtually all of the medical equipment for cardiovascular surgery has traditionally been developed for use with men (Cupples, 1997). Ironically, even life-saving technologies that are relatively recent, such as left ventricular assist devices, have been developed to fit the male physique (Hansen, 2003), and the development of smaller devices to fit women is undertaken only after the device is developed for the prototype, a male cardiac patient. Physicians can be slow to adapt treatments specifically for women. For example, implantable cardioverter defibrillators (ICDs) and pacemakers are known to present a specific adjustment challenge for women. The spot where the ICD is placed is less comfortable, the weight of the breast is pulled down from the device, women's clothing often leaves the device exposed, and the scarring from the surgery is associated with body image concerns (Sowell, Kuhl, Sears, Klodell, & Conti, 2006). Surgical techniques are available that allow the pacemakers and ICDs to be implanted so that the device will not bulge out, create scarring, or be as visible (Giudici, 2001), but they are termed "cosmetic" and have not yet been widely adopted by electrophysiologists. Such techniques require extra time and effort, necessitate the presence of an additional surgeon during the procedure, and have the potential for additional cost. Perhaps gender bias accounts for the fact that female patients are rarely presented with multiple options for device placement, and industry appears unmotivated to design devices to meet the needs of women. Sex bias is normative and is influenced by psychological factors, which are discussed next.

PSYCHOLOGICAL FACTORS

Even when age and comorbid illnesses are accounted for, women still report greater levels of psychiatric symptomatic distress following a cardiac event. Psychological dysfunction, in turn, undoubtedly affects the treatment that women receive for heart disease. In general, women with heart disease are older and have more comorbid illness, greater severity of cardiovascular disease, fewer social supports, fewer financial resources, and worse medical insurance coverage, at least in the United States (Con, Linden, Thompson, & Ignaszewski, 1999; Linden, 2000). The literature supports that women are less likely to be referred to cardiac rehabilitation and also more likely to refuse or drop out when they are referred. When women are compared with men prior to entering cardiac rehabilitation, they report more functional impairment, somatic complaints, social inhibition, and exhaustion (Linden, 2000; Nolan & Nolan, 1998; Schuster & Waldron, 1991).

As is true in the general population, rates of depression are twice as high among female cardiac patients compared with male cardiac patients. The lifetime risk for depression in women is 20% to 26%, or put another way, more than one out of five women will become depressed in the course of their life (Szewczyk & Chennault, 1997). More often than not, women have a first onset of depression during their 20s. The child-bearing years between ages 18 and 44 represent the most vulnerable period over the life span. Some types of depression, by definition, can only affect women (e.g., postpartum depression). Across the spectrum of depressive disorders, women consistently show greater susceptibility compared with men (Szewczyk & Chennault, 1997).

Among people with cardiovascular disease, 50% of women, compared with 25% of men, meet criteria for mild to moderate depression following myocardial infarction (MI; Frasure-Smith, Lesperance, Juneau, Talajic, & Bourassa, 1999). Women with depression are at higher risk for death following MI (Carney, Freedland, Smith, Lustman, & Jaffe, 1991). This finding has led to the hypothesis that depression could partially account for the higher mortality rate associated with MI found for women (Carney et al., 1991).

At the same time, men are three to five times more likely than women to commit suicide (Moscicki, 1994). Addictive behaviors, particularly substance abuse and cigarette smoking, are all disproportionately more common in men compared with women. Men are more likely to smoke cigarettes, use cocaine, and abuse alcohol, leading many researchers to question whether men experience depression or anxiety that is masked and manifested through substance abuse and risk-taking behaviors (Addis & Cohane, 2005).

The literature on sex differences with respect to hostility seems to confirm that hostility is manifested differently in men than in women. A study of 101 men and 95 women who were administered the Structured Interview (SI; originally called the Type A Structured Interview) developed by Rosenman (1978). The SI uses an interviewing technique designed to elicit anger and hostility by asking questions in such a way as to provoke these emotions in the interviewee. The interviewee is rated on their competitiveness, impatience, and hostility/aggression. Participants were also administered the Cook–Medley Hostility Scale, and thallium stress testing showed that subtle and indirect antagonism predicted risk for CHD in women, whereas overt expressions of anger were associated with higher risk for men (Siegman, Townshend, Civelek, & Blumenthal, 2000).

The Coronary Artery Risk Development in Young Adults (CARDIA) study enrolled 3,308 Black and White young adults and followed them for 15 years (Yan et al., 2003). The baseline data showed that participants with high scores in time urgency and impatience were more likely to be women, and those with higher scores on achievement striving and competitiveness were more likely to be men. Time urgency and impatience were measured with four items from the Framingham Type A Questionnaire: (a) feeling pressured for time in general, (b) feeling pressured at the end of an average work or housework day, (c) eating too quickly, and (d) getting quite upset when having to wait for anything. Achievement striving and competitiveness was measured with four other items from the same questionnaire: (a) having a strong need to excel in most things, (b) being bossy or dominating, (c) being hard driving and competitive, and (d) thinking about work after working hours or all day long.

Of course, when these items are examined individually, it is clear that traditional sex role orientation could be confounded with the constructs of time urgency, impatience, achievement striving, and competitiveness. Indeed, studies that have examined sex role orientation and Type A behavior pattern have supported that both women and men with Type A tend to score higher on "masculinity" (Nix & Lohr, 1981). Nonetheless, there is evidence that men may be more responsive to treatments for hostility and time urgency. A small study of Swedish male and female primary care patients who participated in an intervention designed to positively affect hostility and time pressure showed that men improved on these measures to a greater degree than women (Karlberg, Krakau, & Unden, 1998). Unfortunately, there have been no large-scale studies testing the effect of treatment for time urgency or hostility, let alone examining sex differences.

GENDER-SPECIFIC PSYCHOTHERAPY TREATMENT EFFECTS

One would think that because there are dramatic gender-related differences in the prevalence, onset, and course of depression, there would be a rich literature on gender-specific effects on treatment. In fact, this literature is very sparse in noncardiac populations. Not much is known about whether men and women respond differently to therapeutic technique. A small study showed that women have more symptomatic relief and improvements in depression with supportive short-term therapy, whereas men have better outcomes in interpretative short-term therapy (Ogrodniczuk, Piper, Joyce, & McCallum, 2001). Overall, major clinical trials have not reported much in the way of sex differences in response to psychotherapy. Results from the National Institute of Mental Health Treatment of Depression Collaborative Research Program showed no differences in outcome between men and women for treatment of depression. In that study, participants were randomized to interpersonal therapy, cognitive behavioral therapy, imipramine plus clinical management, or placebo plus clinical management. The analysis of gender differences in response to treatment included 188 subjects, 134 of whom were women, and it investigated whether gender had a main effect or interacted with treatment modality, attitudes, life events, or social support on outcome at 6, 12, and 18 months after treatment. No evidence of main or interaction effects was demonstrated in that study, providing evidence that both men and women respond similarly to treatment for depression, even with different therapy modalities (Zlotnick, Shea, Pilkonis, Elkin, & Ryan, 1996).

However, with respect to cardiac patients, the picture is less clear. Two major clinical trials have shown that depressed, female cardiac patients respond poorly to psychosocial intervention. In the Montreal Heart Attack Readjustment Trial, nurses made telephone calls and home visits for counseling for male and female cardiac patients with depression. The treatment had no impact on cardiac mortality for men at 1 year. However, women who received the treatment were nearly twice as likely to die from cardiac and noncardiac causes compared with women who were in the usual-care control condition (Frasure-Smith et al., 1997). Women with depression enrolled in the ENRICHD trial who received cognitive behavioral therapy were more likely to die or have another heart attack compared with women enrolled in the usual-care group (Berkman et al., 2003; Schneiderman et al., 2004). Controlling for age and comorbid illness attenuated this effect, but the authors noted that future research is needed to determine whether effects of depression treatments differ by sex in cardiac patients. The message for clinicians is that it remains important to treat depression in cardiac patients, but there may be contextual differences that are not yet understood that influence how women respond to treatment compared with men. Although this issue is important, it rarely permeates the clinical practice setting. When discussion of gender arises in clinical practice, the question that is raised most frequently is not whether the treatment will work for women versus men but rather whether the therapist is a man or a woman.

When surveys are conducted, most people do not express a gender preference when seeking a therapist. Of those who do, the majority overwhelmingly prefer women. In a sample of 124 patients seeking psychotherapy, with a mean age of 36 years old and a sample with 54 men and 69 women, 37% had a gender preference in seeking a therapist, and women therapists were preferred by a 5 to 1 ratio by those who expressed a preference (M. Kaplan, 1996). Kaplan noted that more research should be devoted to understanding what patients believe they will experience with a female therapist.

In clinical practice, the help-seeking behavior of women also differs from men. Women are more likely to seek mental health treatment as compared with men, and once they are there, they are more likely to attend a greater number of counseling sessions on average than men (Hatchett & Park, 2004). So although female cardiac patients might have a greater vulnerability to mental health problems, the reluctance of men to seek help makes it equally important to create awareness and outreach efforts for both men and women.

PSYCHOTHERAPEUTIC APPROACHES INFORMED BY GENDER DIFFERENCES

Sometimes cardiac patients present with problems that reflect classic sex role differences, such as women with heavy child-rearing responsibilities or men in leadership positions at work with incredibly long work hours. Both men and women often have a deep sense of shame about seeking out mental health treatment, although there is some suggestion that this poses a greater barrier for men (Levant, 2001). Psychotherapy with male and female cardiac patients is more alike than different, and individual variables play a far greater role in influencing the therapeutic approach used compared with the sex of the patient. Many would argue that it is the degree of rigidity of sex role orientation that seems to be associated with poor mental health. Nonetheless, as this chapter has emphasized, there are important differences in the lived experience of men and women in our society and there are therapy models that focus on the development of gender-specific approaches to therapy. Two such models are described in this section, but first, in lieu of a clinical example, some of my personal reflections on this topic are noted.

Clinical Reflections

The gender differences that I am most aware of in my own work are reflected in the demographic composition of my practice. Compared with many of my psychotherapist colleagues, about 65% of my psychotherapy patients are men, and the remaining 35% are women under the age of 65. Many of my female patients are in their 40s and 50s. Most of my patients are referred from the nurses in our cardiac rehabilitation program, cardiologists affiliated with the hospital, or self-referred through word of mouth or through their own research. The age range of my female patients is skewed toward younger ages. These patients often reflect a greater sense of isolation because they often do not know other younger women who have heart disease. Although there is no shortage of female patients in their 70s and older with heart disease, older women do not present as often for treatment, perhaps because heart disease becomes more normative with the aging process. Thus my own experience also agrees with the literature in that fewer women with heart disease seem to seek out, be referred, or accept a referral for psychotherapy. By contrast, my male patients tend to have a wide age range from mid-30s to early 80s. Older male cardiac patients can benefit from an approach that keeps their socialization history in mind. This next section illustrates one such approach.

Psychotherapy With Men

Stereotypical perceptions of masculinity have valued emotional stoicism, self-sufficiency, and strength (Addis & Cohane, 2005), or the so-called "Dirty Harry persona" (Magnavita, 1997). The enduring icon created by actor Clint Eastwood is a man who successfully detaches from emotions and who handles overwhelming adversity by relying only on himself. This stereotype is powerfully embedded in U.S. culture and for some patients can pose a major barrier to seeking or accepting psychotherapeutic help. Psychologist Ronald Levant has named this *normative male alexithymia* (Levant, 2001), described as the inability to recognize emotions or put them into words that occurs as a result of socialization to traditional sex roles. Alexithymia refers to difficulty in experiencing, expressing, or describing emotional responses. The inability to be adept at emotional expression is a stereotypical masculine trait. Levant proposed that a subclinical alexithymia syndrome develops as a result of parenting practices and sociocultural norms. Traditional sex role socialization promotes an identification with masculinity that values the avoidance of things seen as feminine, restricted emotions, toughness and aggression, self-reliance, achievement and status, nonrelational attitudes toward sexuality, and fear and hatred of homosexuals. Research on early childhood development confirms that parents are more likely to discourage little boys from expressing fear and sadness and even to punish boys who are not able to restrict emotional expression (Levant & Pollack, 1995). In clinical practice, male cardiac patients often do present with a paucity of skill in understanding or expressing their own emotional states, as the following example illustrates.

Clinical Example

Fred's wife called the therapist to set up his appointment. She described him as being extremely depressed and anxious but very reluctant to seek help. Fred had a heart attack about 9 months ago and was not cleared by his physician to return to work. He had two episodes of chest pain that brought him to the emergency room but were deemed to be "stress related." His cardiologist recommended that he seek therapy. His wife complained that although he seemed distraught, he would not talk to her and sat by himself in his study for hours at a time. In his first session, Fred sat expressionless as he listed a number of stressful events that had occurred in the preceding 12 months, including his heart attack, the death of his father, and his inability to return to work. "I just don't really know how you are going to help me with any of these things, though," he said. "What is done, is done. I'm dealing with it fine."

This example demonstrates the challenge in working with patients who have little awareness of their own emotions, a fair amount of severity in terms of the problem, and considerable doubt about the value of psychotherapy. It can be hard to form a collaborative alliance, because that requires some comfort with the emotional states of intimacy and closeness. An active but respectful stance is needed to engage the patient, instill a sense of hope, and forge an emotional bond from the earliest point in therapy.

A structured psychoeducational approach to this conundrum is described by Levant (2001). Levant's treatment program for normative male alexithymia uses five steps aimed at helping male psychotherapy patients to become more aware of affect. Goals of treatment include the capacity to be better able to recognize and express emotions constructively. The steps are as follows:

1. Psychoeducation about normative alexithymia: This step consists of providing information on the patient's limitations on ability to express emotions and an understanding of the historical context of how those limitations developed.
2. Development of a vocabulary for emotion: In this step, the therapist assists the patient with naming emotions correctly in the session and between sessions (e.g., by recording words for feelings).
3. Understanding emotional states of other people: In this step, the therapist focuses on other people and encourages the patient to observe the verbal and nonverbal expressions of others and to imagine what their emotional responses are in any given situation.
4. Track emotional responses: In this step, Levant recommends that the patient keep a diary of emotional responses noting any sensations in the body, the relational or social context, and the predominant emotions that were experienced.
5. Practice: The final step involves the repetition through role play, videotape, or by observing others.

Levant noted that this approach is designed for men who are unaware of their emotional states but are motivated to follow a directive, homework-based psychotherapy program. This approach has some direct parallels with the movement toward greater focus on affect from other therapists (Fosha & Slowiaczek, 1997; L. S. Greenberg & Bolger, 2001; McCullough et al., 2003). The difference, however, is that this approach is more structured and directly involves the patient through exercises and homework, rather than relying only on therapist technique. There are many patients, both men and women, who have little ability to name their emotions, and this approach is a viable method for specifically instructing patients in how they might develop a language for emotion. However, the treatment program is designed for men and, accordingly, the explanation of how traditional male socialization leads to the development of subclinical alexithymia has face validity only for male patients. If this approach were used with women, psychoeducation would need to focus on the patient's early development and derive an explanation of how the patient is presumed to have developed deficits in the ability to recognize and express feeling.

Psychotherapy With Women

Feminist paradigms for psychotherapy have examined the power differential between men and women. Masculinity is associated with higher levels of political, social, and economic power across all cultures. Feminist psychotherapy is guided by an understanding of how power and oppression affect the mental health of women (L. S. Brown, 1994). The Stone Center model (discussed in chap. 7, this volume) was developed specifically for women and incorporates some features of feminist theory but emphasizes the importance of the quality of relationships to women's mental health (Jordan, 1997). This philosophy of therapy defines the centrality of relational connection, particularly in the development of women. From this perspective, traditional psychotherapeutic approaches that focus on the importance of autonomy and self-reliance are thought to be less important as a therapeutic goal, compared with the ability for relational connection. Relational psychotherapy assumes that women grow through growth-fostering relationships. Relational psychotherapy as described by the Stone Center emphasizes the importance of *mutuality*, which is characterized by a shared sense of purpose between patient and therapist, shared commitment and emotional investment in the therapeutic relationship as a mechanism for change, and responsiveness and openness on the part of the therapist to being changed by the patient. To this end, the therapist might be more likely to express feelings about the client, to admit uncertainty or error, or to validate accurate perceptions about him- or herself (Jordan, 2000).

This model for therapy also emphasizes *relational competence*, or the ability to acknowledge interdependence and to reach out for help. Stiver and Baker-Miller (1997) wrote a chapter called "From Depression to Sadness in Women's Psychotherapy" that sounds very similar to the flip side of Levant's argument. In this chapter, Stiver and Baker-Miller acknowledged that men are raised to be "less in touch with their feelings" (p. 235), and although they do not acknowledge the importance of relationships, they are surrounded by women who provide relationships for them. The authors made a case that in traditional marriages, men are better taken care of in terms of their emotional needs, and that as many of the studies in behavioral cardiology show, marriage has a protective effect for men. The authors noted that women are more likely to feel frustration and sadness when their needs for relational connection are continuously frustrated in the marital relationship. They questioned whether this might partially account for the higher rates of depression in women compared with men.

The Stone Center description of relational therapy has considerable overlap with therapeutic alliance research describing the salient features of the emotional bond between patient and therapist. Indeed, the writers from the Stone Center do not describe this as a psychotherapy model per se so much as a philosophical stance to therapeutic work, much the same way that motivational interviewing is described. The critical aspects of mutuality that have also been described in research on the emotional bond between patient and therapist include the following: the communication that the therapist is genuinely concerned for the patient's welfare, the therapist appreciates the patient as a person, the therapeutic relationship seems important to the therapist, and the patient is able to express feelings toward the therapist without fear of censure (Hatcher & Barends, 1996). Although research on the emotional bond between patient and therapist confirms the importance of the therapist's ability to demonstrate appreciation of, engagement with, and positive feeling toward the patient, there is little research that has described precisely how good therapists achieve this. Jordan (1997) and the other Stone Center theorists take the field a step further in suggesting that the therapist's ability to be emotionally affected by the patient and to effectively communicate that his or her own degree of engagement is a critical determinant of therapy outcome.

SUMMARY

This chapter has reviewed differences in the presentation and treatment of heart disease in men and women and described some features of the social context in which male and female cardiac patients seek psychotherapy. Both male and female writers make the point that men and women in our culture experience rigid sex role orientations. Robert Bly (1990) used mythological analogy in the book *Iron John* to make the point that child-rearing practices in the postindustrial age have created generations of distant fathers and disconnected sons. It is impossible to make any sweeping generalizations about the influence of rigid sex role orientation on the development or treatment of mental health problems in cardiac patients. However, it is certainly true that men and women who were born 6 to 8 decades ago were raised with far different cultural norms about the expression of emotion compared with those born in the last 3 to 4 decades. To the extent that the historical context of a patient's upbringing and ingrained values about male versus female roles are relevant to the cardiac patient's suffering, these must be addressed in therapy.

There are so many societal and cultural attitudes and beliefs that mediate sex differences that the topic could leave clinicians feeling overwhelmed.

Therapist attunement to the unique circumstances of each patient may be the best antidote to this. Some cardiac patients might benefit from a psychotherapeutic approach that incorporates specific emphasis on how the patient may have been affected by female or male socialization norms, whereas for other patients, this is a nonissue and not salient to their treatment.

A final note on this topic is that there are undeniable beliefs about power and male and female roles, and people can suffer powerful repercussions for stepping out of those roles. For example, the public seemed to have far greater difficulty with Hillary Clinton's role as First Lady compared with Laura Bush's role as First Lady, perhaps because Clinton had her own career aspirations. Author Anna Fels (2006) noted,

> I've often wondered how the media would have reacted if Chelsea Clinton, by all reports a lovely young woman, had been arrested multiple times for underage use of alcohol instead of the daffy Bush twins. I suspect that Hillary Clinton, lawyer and politician, would have been raked over the coals. Yet there has been nary a whisper about Laura Bush's mothering skills or failures. (p. 298)

This contemporary example underscores the point that perceptions heavily influence how people interpret events and situations. None of us are free from subjective bias, and so as therapists, the best we can do is to be as aware as possible of our own attitudes, beliefs, and stereotypes.

CONCLUSION:
THE PRACTICE OF
BEHAVIORAL CARDIOLOGY

Many overlapping and synonymous phrases describe the practice of providing psychotherapy to cardiac patients, including cardiac psychology, medical psychology, psychosomatic medicine, health psychology, behavioral medicine, and behavioral health. Each term has a slightly different meaning, but generally they all concern applying the principles and science of psychology to the prevention, treatment, and management of disease, with the larger goals of improving both mental and physical well-being. Some readers of this volume will already be engaged in providing psychotherapy to cardiac patients and may want to expand their scope of practice, whereas other readers may want to begin to develop this niche practice but feel stymied at how to begin. This chapter concludes the book with some ideas about how to become trained in behavioral cardiology, explores various models for practice (e.g., in a hospital vs. a private practice), and discusses some of the rewards and pitfalls of this field from a personal perspective. I also discuss the future of behavioral cardiology services and the implications of this for psychotherapists who want to market their services to people with heart disease.

TRAINING IN BEHAVIORAL CARDIOLOGY

How much education about heart disease should a clinician seek before working with cardiac patients? Ideally, therapists would have formal training in behavioral cardiology before working with cardiac patients. However, the reality is that many therapists already work with people who have cardiovascular disease, although often, in these instances, neither the patient nor the therapist conceptualizes the medical illness as pertinent to the presenting problem or treatment plan. The difference between a therapist who has training in the field versus one who does not is that the former is more likely to consider the patient from a behavioral cardiology perspective, whereas the latter might miss many opportunities for intervention.

Clinicians already have a challenging task in learning the general knowledge needed for adult psychotherapy, and there are obvious differences in emphasis between different disciplines. The goal of training in behavioral cardiology is to become an expert clinician with an understanding of heart disease as opposed to an expert in two fields. There is little advantage to specialization that occurs prior to the development of a solid fund of general knowledge in the clinician's own field of study (e.g., clinical psychology, psychiatry, social work, or counseling). Just as mastering psychotherapy is an ongoing process, knowledge of behavioral cardiology evolves over a period of many years. Some programs in clinical health psychology offer generic training in clinical psychology but also have a strong focus on the application of psychology to health promotion and prevention of illness. In these types of medically oriented educational programs, training sites are generally in hospitals, primary care clinics, and other medical sites rather than in the traditional settings of psychiatric hospitals and community mental health clinics.

Many physicians and psychologists have the opportunity to rotate through a behavioral medicine unit during their training. Training programs in the Veterans Affairs (VA) health care system, some hospitals, and many large academic medical centers have a cardiac rotation in behavioral medicine. In the United States, training in behavioral cardiology postings may be listed with national organizations such as the American Psychological Association, Society for Behavioral Medicine, American College of Cardiology, National Association of Social Workers, American Psychosomatic Society, and American Heart Association.

One of the core competencies that a clinician practicing in this area will develop is basic knowledge of the cardiovascular system. Although some formal training programs offer classes on this topic, most do not. Therefore, at the time of this writing, the interested clinician must be assertive in educating him- or herself. I have observed that students use a variety of ways to obtain an understanding about the anatomy, physiology, and function of the heart. One practical method to begin is with training in cardiopulmonary resuscitation (CPR). This type of training could one day save a life, and it provides some hands-on experience in understanding the heart. A class in CPR will teach risk factors for heart disease and stroke, information about normal heart and lung function, how to recognize a life-threatening emergency, and how to provide CPR. Beyond this, today's CPR classes will also teach how to use an automated external defibrillator to defibrillate a person who is in cardiac arrest. Such classes offer a starting point to assess interest in the field, have a societal benefit, and perhaps might be the most cost-effective training that a clinician might obtain in terms of the payoff of knowledge learned relative to the time and money invested.

Classes for laypeople on heart disease are sometimes offered as consumer education from hospitals and universities. Through the Preventive Cardiology Department at Hartford Hospital, we offer "Cardiology College," a consumer education class for the layperson to learn more about heart disease. There are also many DVDs and books that provide a great deal of information on the physiology of the heart. Many academic medical centers offer a "mini-medical school" consumer education course that can be helpful for those who want to investigate more about medicine before committing to a course of study that focuses on behavioral cardiology.

Postgraduate training under a talented mentor already working in the field is probably the best possible way to bring together formal coursework and personal interest in the field, with knowledge about how to apply the skills. Although there are many paths to the development of a great clinician, researcher, or educator, virtually all good professionals have served an apprenticeship with a talented mentor (Matarazzo, 1980). In behavioral cardiology, there may be a greater number of would-be apprentices than there are mentors to train them. There are extremely strong research-based training programs in this area that offer excellent mentoring opportunities with leaders in the field. There are also opportunities to work with clinicians who serve a predominantly cardiac population, although more often than not these folks are highly in demand from every discipline. Thus most clinicians often describe themselves as generalists in health psychology rather than specialists in behavioral cardiology.

PRACTICE SETTINGS

Prior to training, many mental health professionals have little appreciation of the wide variety of practice settings that exist in general, let alone the type of setting that is specific to a practitioner of behavioral cardiology. A survey of psychologists in 2001 by the American Psychological Association included more than 1,100 licensed clinical psychologists (American Psychological Association, 2003). The majority of respondents (65%) worked in independent practice, and 14% worked in a hospital setting, which includes both private and public general hospitals, psychiatric hospitals, and VA hospitals. In general, factors to weigh when considering each type of practice setting, relative to long-term occupational satisfaction, include the following: the appeal of the setting and type of work available, pay rates, opportunities for collaboration, flexibility of work hours, perceived status of the job, level of bureaucracy, and opportunity for balance between work and home life.

Sometimes perceptions about each setting should be tested out beforehand. For example, although VA hospitals have a mission to conduct research, a survey of time allocation of various types of mental health practitioners in several VA settings showed that the majority of time was allocated to clinical activities, followed by administrative activities, and that research accounted for only 2% of the time (Sullivan, Jinnett, Mukherjee, & Henderson, 2003). Even once on the job, the practitioners' expectations of their own role versus the perceptions of their colleagues are often different. A survey of 500 physicians, nurses, and social workers examined perceptions about the unique role of medical social workers. Results revealed that although medical social workers viewed counseling patients on psychological and emotional issues to be their exclusive role, nurses and physicians did not agree that this role was unique to medical social workers and instead focused on the exclusive role of the social worker as limited to working with families, resolving social–environmental problems, and providing referrals (Cowles & Lefcowitz, 1992, 1995). Although many clinicians will not know what setting they will ultimately practice in, the experience of pregraduate training offers many opportunities to examine each setting in some detail before making a long-term commitment.

Cardiology Inpatient Training

Programs that provide a rotation on the cardiology inpatient units and cardiac intensive care unit offer a great exposure to the world of the hospital-based provider. In this type of setting, trainees can get exposed to the fast pace of medical inpatient work. There is a need for psychotherapists on the inpatient side, and many opportunities exist for intervention. Patients awaiting cardiac catheterization, procedures, or surgeries are usually highly anxious, and mental health professionals can teach strategies to calm the body. Cardiac inpatients commonly have transient depression, sleep problems, delirium, and dementia after a cardiac event or surgery. Some patients lie in hospital beds for months at a time awaiting heart transplant, being supported by a ventricular assist device, in recovery from acute illness such as pregnancy-related cardiac conditions, or facing end-of-life issues. Such patients can derive great benefit from supportive counseling or medical family therapy. Comprehensive training in inpatient cardiology is found in the VA system in the United States, for which the system of care is closed (similar to health care systems such as Kaiser Permanente) and the training in behavioral medicine is well established.

Cardiac Rehabilitation

Cardiac rehabilitation is probably the most widely available training site for practitioners of behavioral cardiology. Accredited cardiac rehabilitation programs incorporate a mental health professional to deliver stress management education and classes into the curriculum. Patients referred from cardiac rehabilitation can have any of the types of heart disease described throughout this book. As outpatients, they are in an ideal phase to obtain benefit from psychotherapy because they have survived the most acute part of their illness, and every effort is made to rehabilitate them to their former level of functioning or better. Trainees can often sit in on or even provide stress management classes in cardiac rehabilitation. Most rehabilitation nurses, therapists, and exercise physiologists are only too willing to refer appropriate patients for psychotherapy. Because rehabilitation professionals typically conduct a lengthy assessment and see the patients three times a week for 12 weeks, they are in a good position to judge whether a patient will be receptive to such a referral.

Preventive Cardiology

When my hospital established a Department of Preventive Cardiology, I was able to join the multidisciplinary team from the beginning, and I have been fortunate to work closely with Paul D. Thompson, who is thought to be one of the nation's leading preventive cardiologists. Not all health care systems have a department dedicated to primary, secondary, and tertiary prevention of heart disease. Ours offers services in cholesterol management, smoking cessation, psychotherapy, stress management, exercise physiology, nutrition counseling, and treatment of heart disease in competitive athletes. The team includes a cardiologist specially trained in preventive cardiology, nurses, cardiology residents, exercise physiologists, a clinical psychologist, a counselor, a research psychologist, and predoctoral and postdoctoral psychology trainees. Institutions that offer similar programs can provide excellent training in outpatient behavioral cardiology.

There are admittedly few psychotherapists working in any of the areas described earlier. So how is a clinician to proceed, without a mentor already established?

Blazing a New Trail

If there is no mental health professional already affiliated with any of these programs, the would-be trainee is in the position of having to establish his or her course of training with little mentoring on the psychological side. Some clinicians who are particularly motivated to learn the field can pull together multiple mentors and have enough confidence to integrate the various perspectives. Most trainees prefer to follow the path of an established mentor already working in the field. There are advantages to either course. Training with an established mentor will not have the same steep learning curve or the abounding opportunities to make mistakes of ignorance! At the same time, there are many various specializations within the field of behavioral cardiology. The pioneering spirit that is required to "create" a mentoring experience from a diverse multidisciplinary group will serve the clinician well in his or her subsequent efforts to develop a career in this field.

COLLABORATIVE CARE WITH PHYSICIANS AND HEALTH CARE PRACTITIONERS

There are many models for collaborative care between mental health professionals and other health care practitioners (Seaburn, Lorenz, Gunn, Gawinski, & Mauksch, 2003). These include use of the mental health professional as a direct provider of service, a consultant to the patient, or a consultant to the treatment team. Over the past 3 decades, there have been many outstanding opportunities for clinicians to find jobs in VA hospitals, rehabilitation hospitals, or general hospitals that offer opportunities to treat cardiac patients. However, these postings are often for positions with broad duties devoted to the spectrum of medical patients. Clinicians who want to focus primarily on serving cardiac patients are often still left with unanswered questions, particularly about how to market themselves. Many clinicians want to set up outpatient practices alongside cardiologists or in a cardiology practice but have never encountered a real example of how this model works. Reading books on collaborative care, such as that by Seaburn and colleagues, can be an excellent starting point, because the philosophy of collaborative care can be as foreign to mental health practitioners as it is to physicians and other health care clinicians. Although a collaborative approach to the care of the medical patient is desirable, it can be most difficult to achieve during the earliest stages of setting up a new service, when paradoxically, the spirit of partnership is most important.

Perhaps the most important advice about practice in the field of behavioral cardiology is to take a long-term view. For reasons that are not completely clear, it has been more difficult to integrate mental health professionals into cardiology than into the fields of oncology or reproductive medicine, even though the empirical evidence that supports such integration exists. A long-term perspective requires acknowledging the learning deficits that exist in the early phases of career development. It can take a great deal of time to build collaborative partnerships, and these relationships will inevitably evolve as each professional learns more about how to work with the other. Flexibility is extremely important, particularly when the other party is unfamiliar with how to integrate the mental health professional into the medical environment. Cultural norms in medicine are different from those in traditional mental health fields. For example, psychotherapy practitioners may have been trained to designate appointment slots (e.g., 50 minutes on the same day of the week at the same time), a practice that may not work for many medical patients. Space is always at a premium in a medical setting, and many health care practitioners will not understand the needs of the mental health clinician, so the negotiation for adequate space can be a delicate process.

The spirit of collaboration extends not just to the other clinicians involved in the patient's care but to the support staff as well. My own practice is integrated with a large clinic of cardiac patients, and initially multiple members of the support team expressed concern about the influx of "mental health" patients into the waiting room—even though these patients also had heart disease! With a long-term view, the clinician will remember that mental health treatment is still stigmatized and the support staff in medicine may not appreciate increases in patient load, let alone the differences that may exist with respect to billing, charting, privacy, and space needs (e.g., examination rooms for physicians vs. counseling rooms for therapists).

SOLICITING REFERRALS

Clinicians need to consider the view of the health care team to envision how a nurse or physician might make a referral. Compared with cardiologists, other medical specialists (e.g., oncologists and family care practitioners) receive far more training in recognizing and referring patients with psychological distress. Health care professionals are extremely busy, and one of the more effective ways to increase referrals is through simple screening methods, for example, asking all patients to complete the Beck Depression Inventory (BDI) prior to cardiac rehabilitation, on entrance to the congestive heart disease program, or for treatment in an arrhythmia clinic. If a screening system is put in place and is sufficiently simple (e.g., refer all assenting patients with a BDI score greater than 10 for consultation), then it will not be difficult to generate a strong referral base. This type of system can work very well for clinicians who are employed in some type of hospital or clinic-based health care system that is affiliated with the cardiology program, because it is presumably part of their mission to identify treatment resources for all patients in their system of care. Conversely, it is usually not the mission of clinicians in private practice to provide consultation and psychotherapy services for patients who cannot pay for services or who are not appropriate. Private practice clinicians might need to identify the types of patients that they can treat and provide some different referral options for patients who cannot be treated within their practice.

Inpatient Referrals

Although many behavioral cardiology clinicians will gravitate to outpatient work, some can be successful at practicing in a cardiac inpatient setting. There is a tremendous need for therapists who can help to assess and treat mental health problems in inpatient cardiology. Traditionally, inpatient behavioral cardiology has been under the purview of consultation–liaison psychiatry and medical social work teams. There are some inherent challenges to cardiac inpatient work. Although the clinical need for service certainly exists, the clinician may face the dilemma of how to get paid for therapy services, provide privacy for counseling, document notes in the medical record, and deal with the many interruptions inherent in inpatient care. A cardiac patient has little privacy, and medical professionals tend to be in and out of the room constantly to deliver medications, check vital signs, take the patient for tests, and so on. In addition, patients are uniquely vulnerable in the inpatient setting—partially clothed, often catheterized, and feeling poorly. My own experience is that most patients are appreciative of a therapist who can help them process their emotions in the moment when they need the help; however, the inpatient provider role is uniquely stressful for the mental health provider and requires a great deal of flexibility, confidence, and clinical acumen. Providers who work in settings such as VA hospitals or closed health care settings (e.g., Kaiser Permanente hospitals) are in a somewhat better position to get paid for assessment and counseling of cardiac inpatients if they are already employees of the system. For the most part, patients can benefit from inpatient behavioral health services, and if such services are provided, the challenge remains to help patients connect to more traditional outpatient mental health settings following hospital discharge to provide continuity of care.

Soliciting Referrals to Independent Practice

Many cardiologists and cardiac nurses are only too happy to refer patients if the psychotherapist is a credible practitioner, thus obtaining some postdoctoral training in the field is a necessary first step. However, even after completing such training, clinicians will encounter many types of heart problems that are new to them, and it is important to simply learn from the patient about his or her illness. Equally important, the cardiologist or nurse who referred the patient is usually happy to provide a layperson's understanding of the patient's heart condition or prognosis. Often, mental health practitioners in their early experiences in medical settings try to overcompensate for their discomfort in a new situation in a variety of ways (Seaburn et al., 2003).

Some psychotherapists use psychological or medical jargon that is unintelligible and confusing to the medical provider. Others come across to members of the health care team as too arrogant. Enthusiasm for the field can be overexpressed to the point that the mental health clinician appears overly zealous in his or her efforts to address the mind–body connection. Physicians and nurses do not expect mental health professionals to have the same level of knowledge about medicine that they have. A little cross-disciplinary respect and thoughtful questioning will go a long way toward smoothing the path of collaboration and contributing to the clinician's fund of knowledge. Similarly, the spirit of partnership necessitates an appreciation of the health care practitioner's own knowledge about the psychosocial realm. It can be only too easy for mental health clinicians to consider the emotional and psychosocial needs of the patient as "their" territory and to dismiss the considerable knowledge and effect that the patient's physician or other health practitioner can have in this regard (Seaburn et al., 2003).

There are many creative ways for independent practitioners to solicit referrals. The first step is to identify the local hospital(s) or health care centers that are treating cardiac patients. The next step involves assessing what mental health professionals are already involved with the program. Inevitably, in U.S. hospitals, there is a beleaguered medical social worker or similar sort who is called on to deal with the psychiatric needs of every cardiac patient who is encountered. Usually, such a person is only too willing and delighted to have a community practitioner to whom he or she can refer. It is important to avoid alienating or competing with the mental health provider who is already involved in meeting the psychosocial needs of cardiac patients.

Ideally, the independent practitioner will then begin to visit local cardiac rehabilitation programs and might even consider offering a regular class (e.g., on stress management) to the patient population. Such relationship building can be time consuming and might take several meetings. Too often, in my experience, people unfamiliar with a health care system will attempt to save time by "going straight to the top" to influence a decision maker—usually an extremely busy physician with a heavy administrative load—to solicit referrals. Although this could work, I have learned it is more common that the providers on the front lines have the patient contact and are the true decision makers for referrals. These nurses and rehabilitation professionals are savvy clinicians in their own right, and referrals will likely depend on the quality of the relationship that the mental health professional is able to foster.

Questions that the clinician might consider asking include the following: (a) Would the cardiac rehabilitation program employ the mental health clinician for a set number of hours in a teaching capacity? (b) Might the program have a private office where patients could be seen for outpatient therapy? My own experience suggests that cardiac rehabilitation programs need to employ behavioral health specialists to teach traditional classes such as stress management. These would be considered bundled services that could not be billed separately. However, mental health providers who are able to be reimbursed from third-party payers under their own license can easily set up outpatient therapy services and can even facilitate additional groups using the cardiac rehabilitation patient population as the referral base.

Cardiologists in private practice, as well as the nurses and physician assistants who work with them, are also likely to need a competent psychotherapist to whom they can refer their patients. Pharmaceutical representatives typically call on providers in this type of setting frequently (at least, that has been my observation in the United States). Accordingly, it is vital that mental health clinicians differentiate themselves in their attempts to underscore the need for their services. Independent practitioners may gain more referrals by initially providing a grand rounds lecture on topics, such as "psychological factors associated with heart disease," than by attempting to cold call and visit each individual practice. Physicians and nurses typically need the continuing education credits provided in grand rounds lectures. Of course, the grand rounds lecture should be in cardiology, or at the minimum in medicine rather than psychiatry, lest the target audience comprise professionals who are not in a position to refer patients. Grand rounds lectures are often planned a year in advance, so it is wise to have a long-term view when using this approach. A few providers typically account for the majority of referrals. As such, it is helpful to cultivate these "behavior-friendly" medical professionals by providing them with prompt feedback on their patients and by reinforcing to their patients the high regard that you have for their doctors. Patients usually appreciate that they obtain better care when the members of their health care team work well together.

Community lectures and events also provide an opportunity to reach out directly to the lay public. Topics such as stress management, reducing time urgency, and caregiver stress are highly popular. For a different twist on the community lecture strategy, the mental health clinician might consider pairing his or her efforts with those of a nurse, cardiologist, or other professional to provide a more holistic perspective on the topic. Some clinicians are extremely media savvy and can consequently solicit a newspaper article or exposure by radio or television about their practice.

REWARDS AND PITFALLS OF A CAREER IN CLINICAL BEHAVIORAL CARDIOLOGY

There are significant contrasts in the provision of therapy to cardiac patients versus the general adult psychotherapy population. This practice niche is not well understood in medicine or mental health, let alone by the lay public, so it can be difficult for the clinician to feel confident and secure in his or her professional identity (Seaburn et al., 2003). Clinicians often have to explain what they do, again and again. Accordingly, it can be difficult to convey the scope of one's services or the role that the clinician would like to play in the delivery of the patient's care. However, most patients and providers are enthusiastic once they understand the function of the mental health clinician. People intuitively tend to grasp the importance of good psychological health in terms of its importance to overall physical well-being. It is typically mental health professionals, not cardiologists and nurses, who have the most difficulty in "getting out of the box," to consider a different paradigm for the delivery of service. It can be difficult to relax the perspective that years of training and practice in traditional psychiatric settings can cultivate. Many divisions of psychiatry and psychology are reluctant to relinquish control over the delivery of care. By housing such services in the traditional psychiatric setting, the provider has the advantage of a built-in network of mental health colleagues. However, the downside of this approach is that the stigma associated with mental health can make it less likely that patients will comply with a referral. Similarly, unless clinicians are employed in a particularly progressive department of psychology or psychiatry, they may set up services using anachronistic models rather than immersing themselves in the medical setting and setting up the service line accordingly. All this is to say that there are often certain tensions between disciplines. Even though there may be no one treating the patient population, it is wise to anticipate turf battles, particularly after the development of a successful practice. Talented clinicians have the know-how to stay "under the radar" in some circumstances and to promote their services appropriately in others.

THE FUTURE OF BEHAVIORAL CARDIOLOGY

The field of behavioral cardiology is abundant with opportunity, in part, because the field is so broad and the number of clinical practitioners is few. Therefore, the degree of unmet psychological need in this patient population is great. In the decades to come, there will be an increasing degree of specialization by clinicians who work in the field of behavioral cardiology. For example, the needs of patients with implantable cardioverter devices are far different from those who have had a heart attack or those living with heart failure. The future also brings a challenge for behavioral cardiology researchers to quickly disseminate their findings to clinicians through evidence-based practice guidelines. Training programs for health psychologists, medical social workers, and psychiatrists focused on psychosomatic medicine will need to include this field and may have to reach out to develop new connections with cardiologists. Above all, the successful advancement of this field will depend on the ability of researchers and clinicians to work productively together to integrate behavioral cardiology into the routine delivery of medical care.

Integrated Delivery of Service

Population demographics will soon force greater attention to the importance of preventive medicine. As the proportion of people over the age of 65 increases, the U.S. medical care system will either integrate more behavioral experts into the delivery of care to address the issues of preventable disease or face the risk of collapse under the weight of caring for a disproportionate number of older citizens with long-term chronic diseases. It takes a forward-thinking health care system to have a strong program for prevention. A sure path toward that end is through a model that integrates clinical behavioral cardiology into the delivery of cardiac care.

An integrated behavioral health service is more complicated to set up but ultimately rewarding in terms of the improvement in care that can come from a genuinely multidisciplinary health care team. Some larger medical and academic settings have a department of preventive cardiology. In my own setting, preventive cardiology encompasses a lipid clinic, an exercise physiology clinic, a program treating heart problems of elite athletes, nutritional counseling, cardiac research, and my own behavioral health programs that include both smoking cessation and outpatient psychotherapy. Other preventive cardiology services may also include clinics to provide specialized care for hypertension, congestive heart disease, or rare cardiac conditions. Mental health practitioners may find this type of setting very rewarding as well because the setup of the service implies that mental health is just one of many important cardiac risk factors, similar to sedentary behavior, poor nutrition, hypertension, or high cholesterol. This setting is not stigmatizing in that patients are not identified as mental health patients.

Similarly, mental health practitioners may consider a truly integrated cardiac private practice setting whereby they can lease an office in a cardiology private practice. Cardiology practices tend to be underused during certain hours (e.g., when the cardiologists are rounding in the hospital or during evening hours), and thus it can be very cost-effective for cardiologists to lease space to mental health practitioners on off hours or to include a consult room in the design of their office space dedicated to the delivery of counseling (e.g., behavioral, nutritional, stress management, smoking cessation) services. Cardiology practices that provide easy access to behavioral health specialists, nutritionists, and other health care professionals are at an advantage compared with other practice settings in that they offer ready access to a full spectrum of services.

Traditional Mental Health Settings

In the short term, independent mental health practitioners will probably develop more niche practices focused on behavioral cardiology because it will take time for the integrated practice model to gain acceptance. The difficulty with this model is that so many suffering patients are not treated. The medical practitioners will easily spot the patients with severe mental health pathology but will often miss the opportunity to refer patients with run-of-the-mill psychological issues. For example, difficult-to-treat patients with severe personality and somatization disorders will be easily identified and referred for therapy. Although the mental health setting is no doubt a far more appropriate setting, such patients are challenging for any practitioner, and few therapists want to build a practice with a disproportionate number of such challenging cases. At the same time, a multitude of higher functioning patients suffer in silence with problems that would respond well to psychosocial intervention. Those patients are often treated with antidepressant medication only or missed altogether. Consequently, in this type of setting, therapists who want to encourage referrals could also suggest routine screening for depression and anxiety, as was described in the section on cardiac rehabilitation, and offer to follow up with assenting patients who screen positively.

In summary, there are a multitude of settings in which clinicians can deliver behavioral cardiology services. Each setting provides its own rewards and risks. Personality characteristics of the clinician will help to determine the right choice of setting. Practitioners need to weigh some of the following factors:

- How much tolerance do I have for making mistakes? Inevitably, the less traveled the path, the more mistakes will be made. For example, it is difficult to appreciate how ingrained the level of hierarchy can be in some medical settings. Mental health clinicians can often be astounded to learn that many conservative and traditionally trained physicians do not consider them as peers in any sense of the word! It is easy to make the mistake of not communicating with enough deference, and this will undoubtedly occur repeatedly in the high turnover world of medicine.

- How important is it to get paid for my services? Some degree of investment is required to build up a practice, and remuneration for these services will depend on the type of client (e.g., self-pay vs. covered by insurance) that the mental health practitioner hopes to cultivate. The most challenging type of practice to cultivate will be a self-pay, independent practice that focuses exclusively on treating cardiac patients. Because most medical patients come with health insurance and little history of mental health treatment, they can be shocked to realize that psychotherapy is difficult to access through their plan, let alone psychotherapy with a clinician trained in cardiac psychology who is a provider on their insurance panel!

- How much do I enjoy working with older adults? Although heart disease can occur at any stage of life, the majority of heart disease is found in people over the age of 65. As people age and have health problems, they may need some accommodations in service, such as handicapped accessibility. That being said, younger cardiac patients are the ones at greatest risk for psychological problems such as depression and anxiety, so a practice devoted to this specialty is likely to have a wide spectrum of age ranges, although the distribution is likely to be skewed to the older age range.

- What strengths do I bring to this profession? As my child's kindergarten teacher once remarked, "Everyone is good at something. No one is good at everything." Every practitioner of behavioral cardiology will bring his or her own unique strengths to this field. A passion for advocacy can be translated into participation in the local chapter of the American Heart Association or a similar public health agency. A practitioner with strong quantitative research skills can help to collect the type of data that justify and validate the practice of behavioral cardiology. Specific training in relaxation methods, health promotion, exercise, and so forth can extend the breadth of service that the practitioner can provide. Personal experience with heart disease can yield greater empathy with the experience of patients.
- Can I work with severely ill medical patients and tolerate the high rate of mortality inherent in this work? Severe physical symptoms such as shortness of breath are distracting in therapy sessions. Patients who are severely ill often have difficulty in coming to sessions. Losing a patient with whom one has bonded to a sudden, unexpected cardiac death never becomes easier over time. Similar to psychooncology, some clinicians gravitate to the field, but it is not the right choice for many practitioners.

The best way to determine the right context for providing services is to try to gain some exposure to as many settings as possible and evaluate the goodness of fit from a personal perspective. There are many leaders in the field who might prefer to wait until such time as our field has reached a consensus on the core competencies needed to practice behavioral cardiology. Despite decades of research, we are a long way from agreeing on and disseminating evidence-based guidelines for treatment of this patient population. Coronary heart disease is the leading cause of death in the United States, and psychological factors are known to be an independent predictor of mortality and morbidity. We cannot afford to wait until our profession reaches consensus to increase our efforts to recognize and treat cardiac patient with comorbid psychological distress. Perhaps the most important aspect of developing a practice in behavioral cardiology concerns the need to remember that seeking help for mental health issues is still overwhelmingly difficult for most people. Just because you build it does not necessarily mean patients will come, unless you make your services as accessible and easy as possible.

OVERCOMING RELUCTANCE TO SEEK PSYCHOLOGICAL HELP

Few of the people who need psychotherapy actually seek treatment, presumably because they foresee so many disadvantages (Fischer & Turner, 1970). People worry about the costs, have negative beliefs about both psychotherapy and psychotherapists, do not believe that psychotherapy will help, and often see many other practical inconveniences. In addition, most people seek help through their primary care doctor and might anticipate that they will be stigmatized and judged by other people (e.g., family members) if they were to seek out a psychotherapist.

Cardiac patients often have little exposure to psychotherapy and often only seek mental health treatment as a last resort. Thus, when a request for appointment is finally made, it is more likely the patient will show up if the clinician can bring the patient in as soon as possible rather than waiting weeks for an appointment. Clinicians who talk with the patient over the phone rather than routing the call to a secretary can effectively quash negative perceptions of psychotherapists and engage the patient from the earliest point. In our setting, we label our services as "stress management and counseling services" rather than psychotherapy, because the word *stress* is ubiquitous, easy to endorse, and lacks the stigmatizing connotation associated with any word having the root *psych* (e.g., psychology, psychotherapy, psychiatry).

SUMMARY

Behavioral cardiology researchers have long been aware that a multitude of negative emotions affect patients with heart disease. Some researchers have urged for increased awareness and a call to action (Pickering, Clemow, Davidson, & Gerin, 2003). Others have defined the field and targeted the audience of cardiologists (Rozanski, Blumenthal, Davidson, Saab, & Kubzansky, 2005). Still others have compiled edited volumes with an academic and clinical audience in mind, incorporating chapters from experts in a variety of areas (Allan & Scheidt, 1996; Molinari, Compare, & Parati, 2006).

It would be exceedingly helpful if psychotherapists could turn to clinical practice guidelines for the treatment of distress in cardiac patients, but as of this writing, no such guidelines exist. Instead, the application of standard psychotherapeutic approaches adapted to the context of the cardiac patient and informed by clinical experience represents the best that the field has to offer. There are only a few psychotherapists who have formal training in behavioral cardiology and are employed in a clinical capacity primarily to work with people who have heart disease. The field is much in need of additional clinicians and expanded services, as well as talented leaders who can effectively communicate the value of psychosocial intervention for this patient population. Reimbursement for psychotherapy provided to cardiac patients is no more challenging than reimbursement for services provided to psychiatric patients. In general, there is tremendous potential for behavioral cardiology clinicians to align themselves with cardiologists and other health care practitioners with the goal of improved and comprehensive care of the patient with heart disease.

REFERENCES

Addis, M. E., & Cohane, G. H. (2005). Social scientific paradigms of masculinity and their implications for research and practice in men's mental health. *Journal of Clinical Psychology, 61*, 633–647.

Agard, A., Hermeren, G., & Herlitz, J. (2004). When is a patient with heart failure adequately informed? A study of patients' knowledge of and attitudes toward medical information. *Heart and Lung, 33*, 219–226.

Agency for Health Care Policy and Research. (1994). Heart failure: Management of patients with left-ventricular systolic dysfunction (AHCPR Publication No. 94-0613). *Quick Reference Guideline for Clinicians, 11*, 1–25.

Alexander, F. G. (1939). Emotional factors in essential hypertension. *Psychosomatic Medicine, 1*, 175–179.

Allan, R., & Scheidt, S. S. (1996). *Heart and mind: The practice of cardiac psychology.* Washington, DC: American Psychological Association.

Allen, J. K., & Blumenthal, R. S. (1998). Risk factors in the offspring of women with premature coronary heart disease. *American Heart Journal, 135*, 428–434.

Allison, K. C., Wadden, T. A., Sarwer, D. B., Fabricatore, A. N., Crerand, C. E., Gibbons, L. M., et al. (2006). Night eating syndrome and binge eating disorder among persons seeking bariatric surgery: Prevalence and related features. *Surgery for Obesity and Related Diseases, 2*, 153–158.

American Cancer Society. (2007). *Cancer facts and figures 2007.* Atlanta, GA: Author.

American Heart Association. (2001). *Sex and heart disease.* Dallas, TX: Author.

American Heart Association. (2005). *Heart disease and stroke statistics: 2005 update.* Dallas, TX: Author.

American Heart Association. (2006). *Heart and stroke encyclopedia.* Dallas, TX: Author.

American Psychiatric Association. (2000). *Diagnostic and statistical manual of mental disorders* (4th ed., text rev.). Washington, DC: Author.

American Psychological Association. (2003). *Salaries in psychology 2001: A report of the 2001 APA salary survey* Washington, DC: Author.

Amin, M., Gabelman, G., & Buttrick, P. (1991). Cocaine-induced myocardial infarction: A growing threat to men in their 30s. *Postgraduate Medicine, 90*, 50–55.

Anderson, H. V., Shaw, R. E., Brindis, R. G., Hewitt, K., Krone, R. J., Block, P. C., et al. (2002). A contemporary overview of percutaneous coronary interventions: The American College of Cardiology–National Cardiovascular Data Registry (ACC–NCDR). *Journal of the American College of Cardiology, 39*, 1096–1103.

Arafeh, J. M., & Baird, S. M. (2006). Cardiac disease in pregnancy. *Critical Care Nurse Quarterly, 29*, 32–52.

Aronson, D., & Rayfield, E. J. (2007). Diabetes. In E. J. Topol, R. Califf, E. N. Prystowsky, J. D. Thomas, & P. D. Thompson (Eds.), *Textbook of cardiovascular medicine* (3rd ed., pp. 36–54). Philadelphia: Lippincott, Williams & Wilkins.

Artinian, N. T. (2003). The psychosocial aspects of heart failure. *American Journal of Nursing, 103*, 32–42.

Asbury, E. A., & Collins, P. (2005). Cardiac syndrome X. *International Journal of Clinical Practice, 59*, 1063–1069.

Astin, F., Jones, K., & Thompson, D. R. (2005). Prevalence and patterns of anxiety and depression in patients undergoing elective percutaneous transluminal coronary angioplasty. *Heart and Lung, 34*, 393–401.

Attebring, M. F., Hartford, M., Hjalmarson, A., Caidahl, K., Karlsson, T., & Herlitz, J. (2004). Smoking habits and predictors of continued smoking in patients with acute coronary syndromes. *Journal of Advanced Nursing, 46*, 614–623.

Averbukh, Y., Heshka, S., El-Shoreya, H., Flancbaum, L., Geliebter, A., Kamel, S., et al. (2003). Depression score predicts weight loss following Roux-en-Y gastric bypass. *Obesity Surgery, 13*, 833–836.

Badgio, P. C., Halperin, G. S., & Barber, J. P. (1999). Acquisition of adaptive skills: Psychotherapeutic change in cognitive and dynamic therapies. *Clinical Psychology Review, 19*, 721–737.

Baecke, J. A., Burema, J., & Frijters, J. E. (1982). A short questionnaire for the measurement of habitual physical activity in epidemiological studies. *American Journal of Clinical Nutrition, 36*, 936–942.

Bankier, B., Januzzi, J. L., & Littman, A. B. (2004). The high prevalence of multiple psychiatric disorders in stable outpatients with coronary heart disease. *Psychosomatic Medicine, 66*, 645–650.

Barbato, A., & D'Avanzo, B. (2006). Marital therapy for depression. *Cochrane Database of Systematic Reviews, 2*, Article CD004188.

Barefoot, J. C. (1992). Developments in the measurement of hostility. In H. S. Friedman (Ed.), *Hostility, coping, and health* (pp. 13–31). Washington, DC: American Psychological Association.

Barefoot, J. C., Burg, M. M., Carney, R. M., Cornell, C. E., Czajkowski, S. M., Freedland, K. E., et al. (2003). Aspects of social support associated with depression at hospitalization and follow-up assessment among cardiac patients. *Journal of Cardiopulmonary Rehabilitation, 23*, 404–412.

Barefoot, J. C., Dodge, K. A., Peterson, B. L., Dahlstrom, W. G., & Williams, R. B., Jr. (1989). The Cook–Medley Hostility Scale: Item content and ability to predict survival. *Psychosomatic Medicine, 51*, 46–57.

Barefoot, J. C., Larsen, S., von der Lieth, L., & Schroll, M. (1995). Hostility, incidence of acute myocardial infarction, and mortality in a sample of older Danish men and women. *American Journal of Epidemiology, 142*, 477–484.

Barkham, M., & Hardy, G. E. (2001). Counselling and interpersonal therapies for depression: Towards securing an evidence base. *British Medical Bulletin, 57*, 115–132.

Barkham, M., Hardy, G. E., & Startup, M. (1994). The structure, validity and clinical relevance of the Inventory of Interpersonal Problems. *British Journal of Medical Psychology, 67*(Pt. 2), 171–185.

Barkham, M., Hardy, G. E., & Startup, M. (1996). The IIP–32: A short version of the Inventory of Interpersonal Problems. *British Journal of Clinical Psychology, 35*(Pt. 1), 21–35.

Batel, P., Pessione, F., Maitre, C., & Rueff, B. (1995). Relationship between alcohol and tobacco dependencies among alcoholics who smoke. *Addiction, 90,* 977–980.

Beck, A. T., Rush, A. J., Shaw, B. F., & Emery, G. (1979). *Cognitive therapy of depression.* New York: Guilford Press.

Beck, A. T., & Steer, R. A. (1984). Internal consistencies of the original and revised Beck Depression Inventory. *Journal of Clinical Psychology, 40,* 1365–1367.

Benowitz, N. L., & Gourlay, S. G. (1997). Cardiovascular toxicity of nicotine: Implications for nicotine replacement therapy. *Journal of the American College of Cardiology, 29,* 1422–1431.

Berkman, L. F. (1995). The role of social relations in health promotion. *Psychosomatic Medicine, 57,* 245–254.

Berkman, L. F., Blumenthal, J., Burg, M., Carney, R. M., Catellier, D., Cowan, M. J., et al. (2003). Effects of treating depression and low perceived social support on clinical events after myocardial infarction: The Enhancing Recovery in Coronary Heart Disease Patients (ENRICHD) Randomized Trial. *Journal of the American Medical Association, 289,* 3106–3116.

Bernstein, I. H., & Gesn, P. R. (1997). On the dimensionality of the Buss/Perry Aggression Questionnaire. *Behaviour Research and Therapy, 35,* 563–568.

Berry, D. S., & Pennebaker, J. W. (1993). Nonverbal and verbal emotional expression and health. *Psychotherapy and Psychosomatics, 59,* 11–19.

Bhattacharyya, M. R., Perkins-Porras, L., Whitehead, D. L., & Steptoe, A. (2007). Psychological and clinical predictors of return to work after acute coronary syndrome. *European Heart Journal, 28,* 160–165.

Bianchi, S. M. (2000). Maternal employment and time with children: Dramatic change or surprising continuity. *Demography, 37,* 401–414.

Birketvedt, G. S., Florholmen, J., Sundsfjord, J., Osterud, B., Dinges, D., Bilker, W., & Stunkard, A. (1999). Behavioral and neuroendocrine characteristics of the night-eating syndrome. *Journal of the American Medical Association, 282,* 657–663.

Birks, Y., Roebuck, A., & Thompson, D. R. (2004). A validation study of the Cardiac Depression Scale (CDS) in a UK population. *British Journal of Health Psychology, 9,* 15–24.

Bjerrum, L., Hamm, L. R. V., Toft, B., Munck, A. P., & Kragstrup, J. (2002). Cardiovascular risk factors: Different evaluations by physicians and patients. *Ugeskr Laeger, 164,* 5382–5386.

Blair, S. N., Kohl, H. W., III, Barlow, C. E., Paffenbarger, R. S., Jr., Gibbons, L. W., & Macera, C. A. (1995). Changes in physical fitness and all-cause mortality. A prospective study of healthy and unhealthy men. *Journal of the American Medical Association, 273,* 1093–1098.

Blom, M., Janszky, I., Balog, P., Orth-Gomer, K., & Wamala, S. P. (2003). Social relations in women with coronary heart disease: The effects of work and marital stress. *Journal of Cardiovascular Risk, 10,* 201–206.

Blum, D. (2002). *Love at Goon Park: Harry Harlow and the science of affection.* Cambridge, MA: Perseus.

Blumenthal, J. A., Babyak, M. A., Ironson, G., Thoresen, C., Powell, L., Czajkowski, S., et al. (2007). Spirituality, religion, and clinical outcomes in patients recovering from an acute myocardial infarction. *Psychosomatic Medicine, 69,* 501–508.

Blumenthal, J. A., Burg, M. M., Barefoot, J., Williams, R. B., Haney, T., & Zimet, G. (1987). Social support, Type A behavior, and coronary artery disease. *Psychosomatic Medicine, 49,* 331–340.

Bly, R. (1990). *Iron John: A book about men.* Reading, MA: Addison-Wesley.

Boltwood, M. D., Taylor, C. B., Burke, M. B., Grogin, H., & Giacomini, J. (1993). Anger report predicts coronary artery vasomotor response to mental stress in atherosclerotic segments. *American Journal of Cardiology, 72,* 1361–1365.

Botker, H. E., Frobert, O., Moller, N., Christiansen, E., Schmitz, O., & Bagger, J. P. (1997). Insulin resistance in cardiac syndrome X and variant angina: Influence of physical capacity and circulating lipids. *American Heart Journal, 134,* 229–237.

Bowen, M. (1966). The use of family theory in clinical practice. *Comprehensive Psychiatry, 7,* 345–374.

Bowen, M. (1974). Alcoholism as viewed through family systems theory and family psychotherapy. *Annals of the New York Academy of Sciences, 233,* 115–122.

Bowen, M. (1978). *Family therapy in clinical practice.* New York: Aronson.

Bradley, K. A., Boyd-Wickizer, J., Powell, S. H., & Burman, M. L. (1998). Alcohol screening questionnaires in women: A critical review. *Journal of the American Medical Association, 280,* 166–171.

Bramwell, L. (1990). Social support in cardiac rehabilitation. *Canadian Journal of Cardiovascular Nursing, 1,* 7–13.

Brecht, M. L., Dracup, K., Moser, D. K., & Riegel, B. (1994). The relationship of marital quality and psychosocial adjustment to heart disease. *Journal of Cardiovascular Nursing, 9,* 74–85.

Brown, B. B. (1978). Social and psychological correlates of help-seeking behavior among urban adults. *American Journal of Community Psychology, 6,* 425–439.

Brown, B. S., O'Grady, K. E., Farrell, E. V., Flechner, I. S., & Nurco, D. N. (2001). Factors associated with frequency of 12-step attendance by drug abuse clients. *American Journal of Drug and Alcohol Abuse, 27,* 147–160.

Brown, L. S. (1994). *Subversive dialogues: Theory in feminist therapy*. New York: Basic Books.

Brownson, R. C., Jones, D. A., Pratt, M., Blanton, C., & Heath, G. W. (2000). Measuring physical activity with the behavioral risk factor surveillance system. *Medicine and Science in Sports and Exercise, 32*, 1913–1918.

Brummett, B. H., Babyak, M. A., Barefoot, J. C., Bosworth, H. B., Clapp-Channing, N. E., Siegler, I. C., et al. (1998). Social support and hostility as predictors of depressive symptoms in cardiac patients one month after hospitalization: A prospective study. *Psychosomatic Medicine, 60*, 707–713.

Brummett, B. H., Babyak, M. A., Mark, D. C., Williams, R. B., Siegler, I. C., Clapp-Channing, N., et al. (2002). Predictors of smoking cessation in patients with a diagnosis of coronary artery disease. *Journal of Cardiopulmonary Rehabilitation, 22*, 143–147.

Brummett, B. H., Barefoot, J. C., Siegler, I. C., Clapp-Channing, N. E., Lytle, B. L., Bosworth, H. B., et al. (2001). Characteristics of socially isolated patients with coronary artery disease who are at elevated risk for mortality. *Psychosomatic Medicine, 63*, 267–272.

Brummett, B. H., Mark, D. B., Siegler, I. C., Williams, R. B., Babyak, M. A., Clapp-Channing, N. E., et al. (2005). Perceived social support as a predictor of mortality in coronary patients: Effects of smoking, sedentary behavior, and depressive symptoms. *Psychosomatic Medicine, 67*, 40–45.

Buchholz, S., & Rudan, G. (2007). Tako-Tsubo syndrome on the rise: A review of the current literature. *Postgraduate Medical Journal, 83*, 261–264.

Buchwald, H., Avidor, Y., Braunwald, E., Jensen, M. D., Pories, W., Fahrbach, K., et al. (2004). Bariatric surgery: A systematic review and meta-analysis. *Journal of the American Medical Association, 292*, 1724–1737.

Bugental, J. F. T. (1999). *Psychotherapy isn't what you think: Bringing the psychotherapeutic engagement into the living moment*. Phoenix, AZ: Zeig Tucker.

Bugental, J. F. T., & Sterling, M. M. (1995). Existential–humanistic psychotherapy: New perspectives. In A. S. Gurman & S. B. Messer (Eds.), *Essential psychotherapies: Theory and practice* (pp. 226–260). New York: Guilford Press.

Bunzel, B., Laederach-Hofmann, K., Wieselthaler, G. M., Roethy, W., & Drees, G. (2005). Posttraumatic stress disorder after implantation of a mechanical assist device followed by heart transplantation: Evaluation of patients and partners. *Transplantation Proceedings, 37*, 1365–1368.

Bunzel, B., Schmidl-Mohl, B., Grundbock, A., & Wollenek, G. (1992). Does changing the heart mean changing personality? A retrospective inquiry on 47 heart transplant patients. *Quality of Life Research, 1*, 251–256.

Burg, M. M., Benedetto, M. C., Rosenberg, R., & Soufer, R. (2003). Presurgical depression predicts medical morbidity 6 months after coronary artery bypass graft surgery. *Psychosomatic Medicine, 65*, 111–118.

Burg, M. M., Benedetto, M. C., & Soufer, R. (2003). Depressive symptoms and mortality two years after coronary artery bypass graft surgery (CABG) in men. *Psychosomatic Medicine, 65*, 508–510.

Burns, J. L., Serber, E. R., Keim, S., & Sears, S. F. (2005). Measuring patient acceptance of implantable cardiac device therapy: Initial psychometric investigation of the Florida Patient Acceptance Survey. *Journal of Cardiovascular Electrophysiology, 16,* 384–390.

Burns, M., Bird, D., Leach, C., & Higgins, K. (2003). Anger management training: The effects of a structured programme on the self-reported anger experience of forensic inpatients with learning disability. *Journal of Psychiatric and Mental Health Nursing, 10,* 569–577.

Bushman, B. J., Bonacci, A. M., Pedersen, W. C., Vasquez, E. A., & Miller, N. (2005). Chewing on it can chew you up: Effects of rumination on triggered displaced aggression. *Journal of Personality and Social Psychology, 88,* 969–983.

Buss, A. H., & Perry, M. (1992). The Aggression Questionnaire. *Journal of Personality and Social Psychology, 63,* 452–459.

Buss, K. A., Goldsmith, H. H., & Davidson, R. J. (2005). Cardiac reactivity is associated with changes in negative emotion in 24-month-olds. *Developmental Psychobiology, 46,* 118–132.

Cai, J., & Terasaki, P. I. (2004). Heart transplantation in the United States 2004. In J. M. Cecka & P. I. Terasaki (Eds.), *Clinical transplants 2004* (pp. 331–344). Los Angeles: UCLA Tissue Typing Laboratory.

Camps, M. A., Zervos, E., Goode, S., & Rosemurgy, A. S. (1996). Impact of bariatric surgery on body image perception and sexuality in morbidly obese patients and their partners. *Obesity Surgery, 6,* 356–360.

Cannon, W. B. (1929). *Bodily changes in pain, hunger, fear and rage.* New York: Appleton.

Carels, R. A., Szczepanski, R., Blumenthal, J. A., & Sherwood, A. (1998). Blood pressure reactivity and marital distress in employed women. *Psychosomatic Medicine, 60,* 639–643.

Cargill, B. R., Clark, M. M., Pera, V., Niaura, R. S., & Abrams, D. B. (1999). Binge eating, body image, depression, and self-efficacy in an obese clinical population. *Obesity Research, 7,* 379–386.

Carney, R. M., Blumenthal, J. A., Freedland, K. E., Youngblood, M., Veith, R. C., Burg, M. M., et al. (2004). Depression and late mortality after myocardial infarction in the Enhancing Recovery in Coronary Heart Disease (ENRICHD) study. *Psychosomatic Medicine, 66,* 466–474.

Carney, R. M., Fitzsimons, D., & Dempster, M. (2002). Why people experiencing acute myocardial infarction delay seeking medical assistance. *European Journal of Cardiovascular Nursing, 1,* 237–242.

Carney, R. M., Freedland, K. E., Rich, M. W., Smith, L. J., & Jaffe, A. S. (1993). Ventricular tachycardia and psychiatric depression in patients with coronary artery disease. *American Journal of Medicine, 95,* 23–28.

Carney, R. M., Freedland, K. E., Smith, L., Lustman, P. J., & Jaffe, A. S. (1991). Relation of depression and mortality after myocardial infarction in women. *Circulation, 84,* 1876–1877.

Carney, R. M., Freedland, K. E., Stein, P. K., Miller, G. E., Steinmeyer, B., Rich, M. W., et al. (2007). Heart rate variability and markers of inflammation and coagulation in depressed patients with coronary heart disease. *Journal of Psychosomatic Research, 62,* 463–467.

Carney, R. M., Freedland, K. E., Stein, P. K., Watkins, L. L., Catellier, D., Jaffe, A. S., et al. (2003). Effects of depression on QT interval variability after myocardial infarction. *Psychosomatic Medicine, 65,* 177–180.

Carney, R. M., Freedland, K. E., & Veith, R. C. (2005). Depression, the autonomic nervous system, and coronary heart disease. *Psychosomatic Medicine, 67*(Suppl. 1), S29–S33.

Carney, R. M., Rich, M. W., teVelde, A., Saini, J., Clark, K., & Freedland, K. E. (1988). The relationship between heart rate, heart rate variability and depression in patients with coronary artery disease. *Journal of Psychosomatic Research, 32,* 159–164.

Carney, R. M., Rich, M. W., teVelde, A., Saini, J., Clark, K., & Jaffe, A. S. (1987). Major depressive disorder in coronary artery disease. *American Journal of Cardiology, 60,* 1273–1275.

Carr, D., & Friedman, M. A. (2005). Is obesity stigmatizing? Body weight, perceived discrimination, and psychological well-being in the United States. *Journal of Health and Social Behavior, 46,* 244–259.

Carroll, K. M., Ball, S. A., Nich, C., Martino, S., Frankforter, T. L., Farentinos, C., et al. (2006). Motivational interviewing to improve treatment engagement and outcome in individuals seeking treatment for substance abuse: A multisite effectiveness study. *Drug and Alcohol Dependence, 81,* 301–312.

Case, R. B., Moss, A. J., Case, N., McDermott, M., & Eberly, S. (1992). Living alone after myocardial infarction: Impact on prognosis. *Journal of the American Medical Association, 267,* 515–519.

Cay, E. L., & Walker, D. D. (1988). Psychological factors and return to work. *European Heart Journal, 9*(Suppl. L), 74–81.

Centers for Disease Control and Prevention. (2002, April 12). Annual smoking-attributable mortality, years of potential life lost, and economic costs—United States, 1995–1999. *Morbidity and Mortality Weekly Report, 51*(14), 300–303. Retrieved from http://www.cdc.gov/MMWR/preview/mmwrhtml/mm5114a2.htm

Centers for Disease Control and Prevention. (2007). [Percentage of adults who were current, former, or never smokers, overall and by sex, race, Hispanic origin, age, education, and poverty status]. *National Health Interview Surveys, Selected Years— United States, 1965–2004.* Retrieved from http://www.cdc.gov/tobacco/data_statistics/tables/adult/table_2.htm

Chaput, L. A., Adams, S. H., Simon, J. A., Blumenthal, R. S., Vittinghoff, E., Lin, F., et al. (2002). Hostility predicts recurrent events among postmenopausal women with coronary heart disease. *American Journal of Epidemiology, 156,* 1092–1099.

Chiaramonte, G. R., & Friend, R. (2006). Medical students' and residents' gender bias in the diagnosis, treatment, and interpretation of coronary heart disease symptoms. *Health Psychology, 25,* 255–266.

Clemente, M. (2005, August 8). *The face of ABC news: "World News Tonight" anchor for 22 years* [Electronic version of transcript]. Retrieved December 14, 2007, from http://www.washingtonpost.com/wp-dyn/content/discussion/2005/08/08/DI2005080800431.html

Cobb, N. K., & Graham, A. L. (2006). Characterizing Internet searchers of smoking cessation information. *Journal of Medical Internet Research, 8,* e17.

Cobb, N. K., Graham, A. L., Bock, B. C., Papandonatos, G., & Abrams, D. B. (2005). Initial evaluation of a real-world Internet smoking cessation system. *Nicotine and Tobacco Research, 7,* 207–216.

Cohen, J. B., & Reed, D. (1985). The Type A behavior pattern and coronary heart disease among Japanese men in Hawaii. *Journal of Behavioral Medicine, 8,* 343–352.

Compare, A., Manzoni, G. M., & Molinari, E. (2006). Type A, type D, anger-prone behavior and risk of relapse in CHD patients. In E. Molinari, A. Compare, & G. Parati (Eds.), *Clinical psychology and heart disease* (pp. 187–215). Milan: Springer-Verlag.

Con, A. H., Linden, W., Thompson, J. M., & Ignaszewski, A. (1999). The psychology of men and women recovering from coronary artery bypass surgery. *Journal of Cardiopulmonary Rehabilitation, 19,* 152–161.

Cook, W., & Medley, D. (1954). Proposed hostility and pharisaic-virtue scales for the MMPI. *Journal of Applied Psychology, 38,* 414–418.

Cooper, A. F., Jackson, G., Weinman, J., & Horne, R. (2002). Factors associated with cardiac rehabilitation attendance: A systematic review of the literature. *Clinical Rehabilitation, 16,* 541–552.

Copeland, J., & Martin, G. (2004). Web-based interventions for substance use disorders: A qualitative review. *Journal of Substance Abuse Treatment, 26,* 109–116.

Cowles, L. A., & Lefcowitz, M. J. (1992). Interdisciplinary expectations of the medical social worker in the hospital setting. *Health and Social Work, 17,* 57–65.

Cowles, L. A., & Lefcowitz, M. J. (1995). Interdisciplinary expectations of the medical social worker in the hospital setting: Part 2. *Health and Social Work, 20,* 279–286.

Coyne, J. C., Rohrbaugh, M. J., Shoham, V., Sonnega, J. S., Nicklas, J. M., & Cranford, J. A. (2001). Prognostic importance of marital quality for survival of congestive heart failure. *American Journal of Cardiology, 88,* 526–529.

Critchley, J., & Capewell, S. (2003). Smoking cessation for the secondary prevention of coronary heart disease. *Cochrane Database of Systematic Reviews, 4,* Article CD003041.

Crits-Christoph, P. (1992). The efficacy of brief dynamic psychotherapy: A meta-analysis. *American Journal of Psychiatry, 149,* 151–158.

Cupples, S. A. (1997). Cardiac transplantation in women. *Critical Care Nursing Clinics of North America, 9,* 521–533.

Dalton, K. M., Kalin, N. H., Grist, T. M., & Davidson, R. J. (2005). Neural-cardiac coupling in threat-evoked anxiety. *Journal of Cognitive Neuroscience, 17,* 969–980.

Damasio, A. (2001, October 25). Fundamental feelings. *Nature, 413*, 781.

Das, S., & O'Keefe, J. H. (2006). Behavioral cardiology: Recognizing and addressing the profound impact of psychosocial stress on cardiovascular health. *Current Atherosclerosis Report, 8*, 111–118.

Davanloo, H. (1978). Evaluation and criteria for selection of patients for short-term dynamic psychotherapy. *Psychotherapy and Psychosomatics, 29*, 307–308.

Davanloo, H. (1980). *Short-term dynamic psychotherapy.* Northvale, NJ: Jason Aronson.

Davidson, K. W., Kupfer, D. J., Bigger, J. T., Califf, R. M., Carney, R. M., Coyne, J. C., et al. (2006). Assessment and treatment of depression in patients with cardiovascular disease: National Heart, Lung, and Blood Institute working group report. *Psychosomatic Medicine, 68*, 645–650.

Davidson, R. J. (2003a). Affective neuroscience and psychophysiology: Toward a synthesis. *Psychophysiology, 40*, 655–665.

Davidson, R. J. (2003b). Darwin and the neural bases of emotion and affective style. *Annals of the New York Academy of Sciences, 1000*, 316–336.

Davidson, R. J. (2003c). Seven sins in the study of emotion: Correctives from affective neuroscience. *Brain and Cognition, 52*, 129–132.

Davidson, R. J. (2004a). Well-being and affective style: Neural substrates and biobehavioural correlates. *Philosophical Transactions of the Royal Society B: Biological Sciences, 359*, 1395–1411.

Davidson, R. J. (2004b). What does the prefrontal cortex "do" in affect: Perspectives on frontal EEG asymmetry research. *Biological Psychology, 67*, 219–233.

Davidson, R. J., Coe, C. C., Dolski, I., & Donzella, B. (1999). Individual differences in prefrontal activation asymmetry predict natural killer cell activity at rest and in response to challenge. *Brain, Behavior and Immunity, 13*, 93–108.

Davidson, R. J., & Fox, N. A. (1989). Frontal brain asymmetry predicts infants' response to maternal separation. *Journal of Abnormal Psychology, 98*, 127–131.

Davidson, R. J., & Irwin, W. (1999). The functional neuroanatomy of emotion and affective style. *Trends in Cognitive Sciences, 3*, 11–21.

Davidson, R. J., Kabat-Zinn, J., Schumacher, J., Rosenkranz, M., Muller, D., Santorelli, S. F., et al. (2003). Alterations in brain and immune function produced by mindfulness meditation. *Psychosomatic Medicine, 65*, 564–570.

Davidson, R. J., Marshall, J. R., Tomarken, A. J., & Henriques, J. B. (2000). While a phobic waits: Regional brain electrical and autonomic activity in social phobics during anticipation of public speaking. *Biological Psychiatry, 47*, 85–95.

Day, R. C., Freedland, K. E., & Carney, R. M. (2005). Effects of anxiety and depression on heart disease attributions. *International Journal of Behavioral Medicine, 12*, 24–29.

DeBusk, R., Drory, Y., Goldstein, I., Jackson, G., Kaul, S., Kimmel, S. E., et al. (2000). Management of sexual dysfunction in patients with cardiovascular disease: Recommendations of the Princeton Consensus Panel. *American Journal of Cardiology, 86*, 175–181.

De Jong, M. J., Moser, D. K., An, K., & Chung, M. L. (2004). Anxiety is not manifested by elevated heart rate and blood pressure in acutely ill cardiac patients. *European Journal of Cardiovascular Nursing, 3,* 247–253.

Denollet, J. (1998). Personality and coronary heart disease: The Type-D Scale–16 (DS16). *Annals of Behavioral Medicine, 20,* 209–215.

Denollet, J. (2005). DS14: Standard assessment of negative affectivity, social inhibition, and type D personality. *Psychosomatic Medicine, 67,* 89–97.

Denollet, J., Pedersen, S. S., Ong, A. T., Erdman, R. A., Serruys, P. W., & van Domburg, R. T. (2006). Social inhibition modulates the effect of negative emotions on cardiac prognosis following percutaneous coronary intervention in the drug-eluting stent era. *European Heart Journal, 27,* 171–177.

Denollet, J., Pedersen, S. S., Vrints, C. J., & Conraads, V. M. (2006). Usefulness of Type D personality in predicting five-year cardiac events above and beyond concurrent symptoms of stress in patients with coronary heart disease. *American Journal of Cardiology, 97,* 970–973.

Derogatis, L. R., & Melisaratos, N. (1983). The Brief Symptom Inventory: An introductory report. *Psychological Medicine, 13,* 595–605.

Dew, M. A., Kormos, R. L., DiMartini, A. F., Switzer, G. E., Schulberg, H. C., Roth, L. H., et al. (2001). Prevalence and risk of depression and anxiety-related disorders during the first three years after heart transplantation. *Psychosomatics, 42,* 300–313.

Diamond, P. M., & Magaletta, P. R. (2006). The short-form Buss–Perry Aggression Questionnaire (BPAQ–SF): A validation study with federal offenders. *Assessment, 13,* 227–240.

Di Benedetto, M., Lindner, H., Hare, D. L., & Kent, S. (2006). Depression following acute coronary syndromes: A comparison between the Cardiac Depression Scale and the Beck Depression Inventory II. *Journal of Psychosomatic Research, 60,* 13–20.

DiClemente, C. C., Prochaska, J. O., Fairhurst, S. K., Velicer, W. F., Velasquez, M. M., & Rossi, J. S. (1991). The process of smoking cessation: An analysis of precontemplation, contemplation, and preparation stages of change. *Journal of Consulting and Clinical Psychology, 59,* 295–304.

DiGiuseppe, R., & Tafrate, R. C. (2007). *Understanding anger disorders.* New York: Oxford University Press.

DiLorenzo, T. A., Schnur, J., Montgomery, G. H., Erblich, J., Winkel, G., & Bovbjerg, D. H. (2006). A model of disease-specific worry in heritable disease: The influence of family history, perceived risk and worry about other illnesses. *Journal of Behavioral Medicine, 29,* 37–49.

Dolcos, F., LaBar, K. S., & Cabeza, R. (2004). Interaction between the amygdala and the medial temporal lobe memory system predicts better memory for emotional events. *Neuron, 42,* 855–863.

Dolcos, F., LaBar, K. S., & Cabeza, R. (2005). Remembering one year later: Role of the amygdala and the medial temporal lobe memory system in retrieving emotional memories. *Proceedings of the National Academy of Sciences, 102,* 2626–2631.

Domar, A. D., & Dreher, H. (1996). *Healing mind, healthy woman: Using the mind–body connection to manage stress and take control of your life.* New York: Henry Holt.

Dopp, J. M., Miller, G. E., Myers, H. F., & Fahey, J. L. (2000). Increased natural killer-cell mobilization and cytotoxicity during marital conflict. *Brain, Behavior and Immunity, 14,* 10–26.

Dornelas, E. A., & Magnavita, J. J. (2001). High-impact therapy for smoking cessation. *Journal of Clinical Psychology, 57,* 1311–1322.

Dornelas, E. A., Sampson, R. A., Gray, J. F., Waters, D., & Thompson, P. D. (2000). A randomized controlled trial of smoking cessation counseling after myocardial infarction. *Preventive Medicine, 30,* 261–268.

Dornelas, E. A., Swencionis, C., & Wylie-Rosett, J. (1994). Predictors of walking by sedentary older women. *Journal of Women's Health, 3,* 283–290.

Dornelas, E. A., & Thompson, P. D. (2007). Smoking cessation for cardiac patients. *Preventive Cardiology, 10,* 31–33.

Downey, G., Freitas, A. L., Michaelis, B., & Khouri, H. (1998). The self-fulfilling prophecy in close relationships: Rejection sensitivity and rejection by romantic partners. *Journal of Personality and Social Psychology, 75,* 545–560.

Dracup, K., Evangelista, L. S., Doering, L., Tullman, D., Moser, D. K., & Hamilton, M. (2004). Emotional well-being in spouses of patients with advanced heart failure. *Heart and Lung, 33,* 354–361.

Dreher, H. (2001). Counseling for type A and recurrent heart disease: Friedman et al. (1986). *Advances in Mind–Body Medicine, 17,* 10–15.

Dreher, H. (2004). Psychosocial factors in heart disease: A process model. *Advances in Mind–Body Medicine, 20,* 20–31.

Eastwood, J. A., & Doering, L. V. (2005). Gender differences in coronary artery disease. *Journal of Cardiovascular Nursing, 20,* 340–351.

Ehrenreich, B. (2001). *Nickel and dimed: On (not) getting by in America.* New York: Henry Holt.

Ekman, P., & Davidson, R. J. (1994). *The nature of emotion: Fundamental questions.* New York: Oxford University Press.

Elkin, I., Shea, M. T., Watkins, J. T., Imber, S. D., Sotsky, S. M., Collins, J. F., et al. (1989). National Institute of Mental Health Treatment of Depression Collaborative Research Program: General effectiveness of treatments. *Archives of General Psychiatry, 46,* 971–982.

Elliot, A. J. (2006). The hierarchical model of approach–avoidance motivation. *Motivation & Emotion 30,* 111–116.

Emery, S., Gilpin, E. A., Ake, C., Farkas, A. J., & Pierce, J. P. (2000). Characterizing and identifying "hard-core" smokers: Implications for further reducing smoking prevalence. *American Journal of Public Health, 90,* 387–394.

Eng, P. M., Fitzmaurice, G., Kubzansky, L. D., Rimm, E. B., & Kawachi, I. (2003). Anger expression and risk of stroke and coronary heart disease among male health professionals. *Psychosomatic Medicine, 65,* 100–110.

Eng, W., Heimberg, R. G., Hart, T. A., Schneier, F. R., & Liebowitz, M. R. (2001). Attachment in individuals with social anxiety disorder: The relationship among adult attachment styles, social anxiety, and depression. *Emotion, 1,* 365–380.

Eslick, G. D. (2004). Noncardiac chest pain: Epidemiology, natural history, health care seeking, and quality of life. *Gastroenterology Clinics of North America, 33,* 1–23.

Evangelista, L. S., Doering, L., & Dracup, K. (2003). Meaning and life purpose: The perspectives of post-transplant women. *Heart and Lung, 32,* 250–257.

Evangelista, L. S., Dracup, K., Doering, L., Westlake, C., Fonarow, G. C., & Hamilton, M. (2002). Emotional well-being of heart failure patients and their caregivers. *Journal of Cardiac Failure, 8,* 300–305.

Ewing, J. A. (1998). CAGE Questionnaire allows doctors to avoid focusing on specifics of drinking. *British Medical Journal, 316,* 1827.

Fabricatore, A. N., Wadden, T. A., Sarwer, D. B., Crerand, C. E., Kuehnel, R. H., Lipschutz, P. E., et al. (2006). Self-reported eating behaviors of extremely obese persons seeking bariatric surgery: A factor analytic approach. *Obesity, 14*(Suppl. 2), 83S–89S.

Fagerstrom, K. O., & Schneider, N. G. (1989). Measuring nicotine dependence: A review of the Fagerstrom Tolerance Questionnaire. *Journal of Behavioral Medicine, 12,* 159–182.

Fairburn, C. G., Cooper, Z., Doll, H. A., & Davies, B. A. (2005). Identifying dieters who will develop an eating disorder: A prospective, population-based study. *American Journal of Psychiatry, 162,* 2249–2255.

Fairburn, C. G., Cooper, Z., & Shafran, R. (2003). Cognitive behaviour therapy for eating disorders: A "transdiagnostic" theory and treatment. *Behaviour Research and Therapy, 41,* 509–528.

Fava, M. (1997). Psychopharmacologic treatment of pathologic aggression. *Psychiatric Clinics of North America, 20,* 427–451.

Fels, A. (2006). Julia. In L. M. Steiner (Ed.), *The mommy wars* (pp. 296–305). New York: Random House.

Ferri, M., Amato, L., & Davoli, M. (2006). Alcoholics Anonymous and other 12-step programmes for alcohol dependence. *Cochrane Database of Systematic Reviews, 3,* Article CD005032.

Finch, J. (1993). Prescription drug abuse. *Primary Care, 20,* 231–239.

Fiore, M. C., Bailey, W. C., Cohen, S. J., Dorfman, S. F., Goldstein, M. G., Gritz, E. R., et al. (2000). *Treating tobacco use and dependence: Clinical practice guideline.* Rockville, MD: U.S. Department of Health and Human Services.

Fiorentine, R. (1999). After drug treatment: Are 12-step programs effective in maintaining abstinence? *American Journal of Drug and Alcohol Abuse, 25,* 93–116.

Fischer, E. H., & Cohen, S. L. (1972). Demographic correlates of attitude toward seeking professional psychological help. *Journal of Consulting and Clinical Psychology, 39*, 70–74.

Fischer, E. H., & Turner, J. L. (1970). Orientations to seeking professional help: Development and research utility of an attitude scale. *Journal of Consulting and Clinical Psychology, 35*, 79–90.

Fleet, R. P., Dupuis, G., Marchand, A., Burelle, D., & Beitman, B. D. (1994). Panic disorder, chest pain and coronary artery disease: Literature review. *Canadian Journal of Cardiology, 10*, 827–834.

Ford, E. S., & Capewell, S. (2007). Coronary heart disease mortality among young adults in the U.S. from 1980 through 2002: Concealed leveling of mortality rates. *Journal of the American College of Cardiology, 50*, 2128–2132.

Fosha, D., & Slowiaczek, M. L. (1997). Techniques to accelerate dynamic psychotherapy. *American Journal of Psychotherapy, 51*, 229–251.

Francis, G. S. (2007). Pathophysiology of the heart failure clinical syndrome. In E. J. Topol, R. Califf, E. N. Prystowsky, J. D. Thomas, & P. D. Thompson (Eds.), *Textbook of cardiovascular medicine* (3rd ed., pp. 1339–1351). Philadelphia: Lippincott, Williams & Wilkins.

Frasure-Smith, N., & Lesperance, F. (2000). Coronary artery disease, depression and social support only the beginning. *European Heart Journal, 21*, 1043–1045.

Frasure-Smith, N., Lesperance, F., Gravel, G., Masson, A., Juneau, M., & Bourassa, M. G. (2002). Long-term survival differences among low-anxious, high-anxious and repressive copers enrolled in the Montreal Heart Attack Readjustment Trial. *Psychosomatic Medicine, 64*, 571–579.

Frasure-Smith, N., Lesperance, F., Gravel, G., Masson, A., Juneau, M., Talajic, M., & Bourassa, M. G. (2000). Depression and health-care costs during the first year following myocardial infarction. *Journal of Psychosomatic Research, 48*, 471–478.

Frasure-Smith, N., Lesperance, F., Juneau, M., Talajic, M., & Bourassa, M. G. (1999). Gender, depression, and one-year prognosis after myocardial infarction. *Psychosomatic Medicine, 61*, 26–37.

Frasure-Smith, N., Lesperance, F., Prince, R. H., Verrier, P., Garber, R. A., Juneau, M., et al. (1997). Randomised trial of home-based psychosocial nursing intervention for patients recovering from myocardial infarction. *Lancet, 350*, 473–479.

Frasure-Smith, N., Lesperance, F., & Talajic, M. (1995a). Depression and 18-month prognosis after myocardial infarction. *Circulation, 91*, 999–1005.

Frasure-Smith, N., Lesperance, F., & Talajic, M. (1995b). The impact of negative emotions on prognosis following myocardial infarction: Is it more than depression? *Health Psychology, 14*, 388–398.

Freedland, K. E., Carney, R. M., & Skala, J. A. (2005). Depression and smoking in coronary heart disease. *Psychosomatic Medicine, 67*(Suppl. 1), S42–S46.

Freedland, K. E., Rich, M. W., Skala, J. A., Carney, R. M., Davila-Roman, V. G., & Jaffe, A. S. (2003). Prevalence of depression in hospitalized patients with congestive heart failure. *Psychosomatic Medicine, 65,* 119–128.

French, T. M. (1964). Franz Alexander, M.D. 1891–1964. *Psychosomatic Medicine, 26,* 203–206.

Friedman, M., Thoresen, C. E., Gill, J. J., Ulmer, D., Powell, L. H., Price, V. A., et al. (1986). Alteration of Type A behavior and its effect on cardiac recurrences in post myocardial infarction patients: Summary results of the Recurrent Coronary Prevention Project. *American Heart Journal, 112,* 653–665.

Furlanetto, L. M., Mendlowicz, M. V., & Romildo, B. J. (2005). The validity of the Beck Depression Inventory—Short Form as a screening and diagnostic instrument for moderate and severe depression in medical inpatients. *Journal of Affective Disorders, 86,* 87–91.

Gallo, L. C., & Smith, T. W. (1998). Construct validation of health-relevant personality traits: Interpersonal circumplex and five-factor model analyses of the Aggression Questionnaire. *International Journal of Behavioral Medicine, 5,* 129–147.

Gami, A. S., Witt, B. J., Howard, D. E., Erwin, P. J., Gami, L. A., Somers, V. K., et al. (2007). Metabolic syndrome and risk of incident cardiovascular events and death: A systematic review and meta-analysis of longitudinal studies. *Journal of the American College of Cardiology, 49,* 403–414.

Gehi, A., Haas, D., Pipkin, S., & Whooley, M. A. (2005). Depression and medication adherence in outpatients with coronary heart disease: Findings from the Heart and Soul Study. *Archives of Internal Medicine, 165,* 2508–2513.

Gerin, W., Davidson, K. W., Christenfeld, N. J., Goyal, T., & Schwartz, J. E. (2006). The role of angry rumination and distraction in blood pressure recovery from emotional arousal. *Psychosomatic Medicine, 68,* 64–72.

Gidron, Y., Kupper, N., Kwaijtaal, M., Winter, J., & Denollet, J. (2007). Vagus-brain communication in atherosclerosis-related inflammation: A neuroimmunomodulation perspective of CAD. *Atherosclerosis, 195,* e1–e9.

Gillath, O., Bunge, S. A., Shaver, P. R., Wendelken, C., & Mikulincer, M. (2005). Attachment-style differences in the ability to suppress negative thoughts: Exploring the neural correlates. *Neuroimage, 28,* 835–847.

Giudici, M. C. (2001). Experience with a cosmetic approach to device implantation. *Pacing and Clinical Electrophysiology, 24,* 1679–1680.

Glassman, A. H., O'Connor, C. M., Califf, R. M., Swedberg, K., Schwartz, P., Bigger, J. T., Jr., et al. (2002). Sertraline treatment of major depression in patients with acute MI or unstable angina. *Journal of the American Medical Association, 288,* 701–709.

Glazer, K. M., Emery, C. F., Frid, D. J., & Banyasz, R. E. (2002). Psychological predictors of adherence and outcomes among patients in cardiac rehabilitation. *Journal of Cardiopulmonary Rehabilitation, 22,* 40–46.

Godemann, F., Ahrens, B., Behrens, S., Berthold, R., Gandor, C., Lampe, F., et al. (2001). Classic conditioning and dysfunctional cognitions in patients with panic disorder and agoraphobia treated with an implantable cardioverter/defibrillator. *Psychosomatic Medicine, 63*, 231–238.

Godemann, F., Butter, C., Lampe, F., Linden, M., Schlegl, M., Schultheiss, H. P., et al. (2004a). Panic disorders and agoraphobia: Side effects of treatment with an implantable cardioverter/defibrillator. *Clinical Cardiology, 27*, 321–326.

Godemann, F., Butter, C., Lampe, F., Linden, M., Werner, S., & Behrens, S. (2004b). Determinants of the quality of life (QoL) in patients with an implantable cardioverter/defibrillator (ICD). *Quality of Life Research, 13*, 411–416.

Gold, L. D., & Krumholz, H. M. (2006). Gender differences in treatment of heart failure and acute myocardial infarction: A question of quality or epidemiology? *Cardiology in Review, 14*, 180–186.

Golden, J., Conroy, R. M., & O'Dwyer, A. M. (2007). Reliability and validity of the Hospital Anxiety and Depression Scale and the Beck Depression Inventory (Full and FastScreen scales) in detecting depression in persons with hepatitis C. *Journal of Affective Disorders, 100*, 265–269.

Goldstein, N. E., Lampert, R., Bradley, E., Lynn, J., & Krumholz, H. M. (2004). Management of implantable cardioverter defibrillators in end-of-life care. *Annals of Internal Medicine, 141*, 835–838.

Goodman, M., Quigley, J., Moran, G., Meilman, H., & Sherman, M. (1996). Hostility predicts restenosis after percutaneous transluminal coronary angioplasty. *Mayo Clinic Proceedings, 71*, 729–734.

Gottman, J. M., & Levenson, R. W. (2002). A two-factor model for predicting when a couple will divorce: Exploratory analyses using 14-year longitudinal data. *Family Process, 41*, 83–96.

Gottman, J. M., & Notarius, C. I. (2002). Marital research in the 20th century and a research agenda for the 21st century. *Family Process, 41*, 159–197.

Grady, D., Herrington, D., Bittner, V., Blumenthal, R., Davidson, M., Hlatky, M., et al. (2002). Cardiovascular disease outcomes during 6.8 years of hormone therapy: Heart and Estrogen/Progestin Replacement Study follow-up (HERS II). *Journal of the American Medical Association, 288*, 49–57.

Grant, A. O., & Durrani, S. (2007). Mechanisms of cardiac arrhythmias. In E. J. Topol, R. Califf, E. N. Prystowsky, J. D. Thomas, & P. D. Thompson (Eds.), *Textbook of cardiovascular medicine* (3rd ed., pp. 950–963). Philadelphia: Lippincott, Williams & Wilkins.

Greenberg, I., Perna, F., Kaplan, M., & Sullivan, M. A. (2005). Behavioral and psychological factors in the assessment and treatment of obesity surgery patients. *Obesity Research, 13*, 244–249.

Greenberg, L. S., & Bolger, E. (2001). An emotion-focused approach to the over-regulation of emotion and emotional pain. *Journal of Clinical Psychology, 57*, 197–211.

Greenberg, L. S., & Johnson, S. M. (1988). *Emotionally focused psychotherapy for couples.* New York: Guilford Press.

Greenberg, L. S., & Pascual-Leone, A. (2006). Emotion in psychotherapy: A practice-friendly research review. *Journal of Clinical Psychology, 62*, 611–630.

Grewen, K. M., Anderson, B. J., Girdler, S. S., & Light, K. C. (2003). Warm partner contact is related to lower cardiovascular reactivity. *Behavioral Medicine, 29*, 123–130.

Grewen, K. M., Girdler, S. S., Amico, J., & Light, K. C. (2005). Effects of partner support on resting oxytocin, cortisol, norepinephrine, and blood pressure before and after warm partner contact. *Psychosomatic Medicine, 67*, 531–538.

Grewen, K. M., Girdler, S. S., & Light, K. C. (2005). Relationship quality: Effects on ambulatory blood pressure and negative affect in a biracial sample of men and women. *Blood Pressure Monitoring, 10*, 117–124.

Gudmundsdottir, H., Johnston, M., Johnston, D., & Foulkes, J. (2001). Spontaneous, elicited and cued causal attributions in the year following a first myocardial infarction. *British Journal of Health Psychology, 6*, 81–96.

Hall, S. M., Munoz, R. F., Reus, V. I., & Sees, K. L. (1993). Nicotine, negative affect, and depression. *Journal of Consulting and Clinical Psychology, 61*, 761–767.

Hansen, S. (2003). Mental health issues associated with cardiovascular disease in women. *Psychiatric Clinics of North America, 26*, 693–712.

Hare, D. L., & Davis, C. R. (1996). Cardiac Depression Scale: Validation of a new depression scale for cardiac patients. *Journal of Psychosomatic Research, 40*, 379–386.

Hariri, A. R., Drabant, E. M., Munoz, K. E., Kolachana, B. S., Mattay, V. S., Egan, M. F., et al. (2005). A susceptibility gene for affective disorders and the response of the human amygdala. *Archives of General Psychiatry, 62*, 146–152.

Harlow, H. F., & Suomi, S. J. (1974). Induced depression in monkeys. *Behavioral Biology, 12*, 273–296.

Harmon-Jones, E. (2003). Clarifying the emotive functions of asymmetrical frontal cortical activity. *Psychophysiology, 40*, 838–848.

Harmon-Jones, E. (2007). Trait anger predicts relative left frontal cortical activation to anger-inducing stimuli. *International Journal of Psychophysiology, 66*, 154–160.

Harper, A. M., & Rosendale, J. D. (1996). The UNOS OPTN waiting list and donor registry: 1988–1996. *Clinical Transplants*, 69–90.

Harris, J. A. (1997). A further evaluation of the Aggression Questionnaire: Issues of validity and reliability. *Behaviour Research and Therapy, 35*, 1047–1053.

Harrison, R. (2005). Psychological assessment during cardiac rehabilitation. *Nursing Standard, 19*, 33–36.

Hatcher, R. L., & Barends, A. W. (1996). Patients' view of the alliance of psychotherapy: Exploratory factor analysis of three alliance measures. *Journal of Consulting and Clinical Psychology, 64*, 1326–1336.

Hatchett, G. T., & Park, H. L. (2004). Revisiting relationships between sex-related variables and continuation in counseling. *Psychological Reports, 94*, 381–386.

Haworth, J. E., Moniz-Cook, E., Clark, A. L., Wang, M., Waddington, R., & Cleland, J. G. (2005). Prevalence and predictors of anxiety and depression in a sample of chronic heart failure patients with left ventricular systolic dysfunction. *European Journal of Heart Failure, 7*, 803–808.

Haynes, S. G., Feinleib, M., & Kannel, W. B. (1980). The relationship of psychosocial factors to coronary heart disease in the Framingham Study: III. Eight-year incidence of coronary heart disease. *American Journal of Epidemiology, 111*, 37–58.

Hays, R. D., & Revetto, J. P. (1992). Old and new MMPI-derived scales and the short-MAST as screening tools for alcohol disorder. *Alcohol and Alcoholism, 27*, 685–695.

Hebl, M. R., & Mannix, L. M. (2003). The weight of obesity in evaluating others: A mere proximity effect. *Personality and Social Psychology Bulletin, 29*, 28–38.

Hecker, M. H., Chesney, M. A., Black, G. W., & Frautschi, N. (1988). Coronary-prone behaviors in the Western Collaborative Group Study. *Psychosomatic Medicine, 50*, 153–164.

Hedley, A. A., Ogden, C. L., Johnson, C. L., Carroll, M. D., Curtin, L. R., & Flegal, K. M. (2004). Prevalence of overweight and obesity among US children, adolescents, and adults, 1999–2002. *Journal of the American Medical Association, 291*, 2847–2850.

Henri, H. C., & Rudd, P. (2007). Hypertension: Context and management. In E. J. Topol, R. Califf, E. N. Prystowsky, J. D. Thomas, & P. D. Thompson (Eds.), *Textbook of cardiovascular medicine* (3rd ed., pp. 88–108). Philadelphia: Lippincott, Williams & Wilkins.

Hensley, P. L. (2006). Treatment of bereavement-related depression and traumatic grief. *Journal of Affective Disorders, 92*, 117–124.

Heo, S., Moser, D. K., Lennie, T. A., Zambroski, C. H., & Chung, M. L. (2007). A comparison of health-related quality of life between older adults with heart failure and healthy older adults. *Heart and Lung, 36*, 16–24.

Heo, S., Moser, D. K., Riegel, B., Hall, L. A., & Christman, N. (2005). Testing a published model of health-related quality of life in heart failure. *Journal of Cardiac Failure, 11*, 372–379.

Hillbrand, M., Waite, B. M., Rosenstein, M., Harackiewicz, D., Lingswiler, V. M., & Stehney, M. (2005). Serum cholesterol concentrations and non-physical aggression in healthy adults. *Journal of Behavioral Medicine, 28*, 295–299.

Horvath A. O. (2001). The alliance. *Psychotherapy, 38*, 365–372.

Horvath, A. O., & Luborsky, L. (1993). The role of the therapeutic alliance in psychotherapy. *Journal of Consulting and Clinical Psychology, 61*, 561–573.

Houston, B. K., Chesney, M. A., Black, G. W., Cates, D. S., & Hecker, M. H. (1992). Behavioral clusters and coronary heart disease risk. *Psychosomatic Medicine, 54*, 447–461.

Hurst, J. W., Morris, D. C., & Alexander, R. W. (1999). The use of the New York Heart Association's classification of cardiovascular disease as part of the patient's complete problem list. *Clinical Cardiology, 22*, 385–390.

Hurst, T., Olson, T. H., Olson, L. E., & Appleton, C. P. (2006). Cardiac syndrome X and endothelial dysfunction: New concepts in prognosis and treatment. *American Journal of Medicine, 119*, 560–566.

Iacoviello, B. M., McCarthy, K. S., Barrett, M. S., Rynn, M., Gallop, R., & Barber, J. P. (2007). Treatment preferences affect the therapeutic alliance: Implications for randomized controlled trials. *Journal of Consulting and Clinical Psychology, 75*, 194–198.

Insel, T. R., Gingrich, B. S., & Young, L. J. (2001). Oxytocin: Who needs it? *Progress in Brain Research, 133*, 59–66.

Insel, T. R., & Young, L. J. (2001). The neurobiology of attachment. *Nature Reviews Neuroscience, 2*, 129–136.

Ironson, G., Taylor, C. B., Boltwood, M., Bartzokis, T., Dennis, C., Chesney, M., et al. (1992). Effects of anger on left ventricular ejection fraction in coronary artery disease. *American Journal of Cardiology, 70*, 281–285.

Jaarsma, T. (2002). Sexual problems in heart failure patients. *European Journal of Cardiovascular Nursing, 1*, 61–67.

Jackson, G., Betteridge, J., Dean, J., Hall, R., Holdright, D., Holmes, S., et al. (1999). A systematic approach to erectile dysfunction in the cardiovascular patient: A consensus statement. *International Journal of Clinical Practice, 53*, 445–451.

Jambekar, S. A., Masheb, R. M., & Grilo, C. M. (2003). Gender differences in shame in patients with binge-eating disorder. *Obesity Research, 11*, 571–577.

Janicki, D. L., Kamarck, T. W., Shiffman, S., Sutton-Tyrrell, K., & Gwaltney, C. J. (2005). Frequency of spousal interaction and 3-year progression of carotid artery intima medial thickness: The Pittsburgh Healthy Heart Project. *Psychosomatic Medicine, 67*, 889–896.

Jarvik, R. K. (1981). The total artificial heart. *Scientific American, 244*, 74–80.

Jenkins, C. D., Rosenman, R. H., & Zyzanski, S. J. (1974). Prediction of clinical coronary heart disease by a test for the coronary-prone behavior pattern. *New England Journal of Medicine, 290*, 1271–1275.

Jiang, W., Kuchibhatla, M., Cuffe, M. S., Christopher, E. J., Alexander, J. D., Clary, G. L., et al. (2004). Prognostic value of anxiety and depression in patients with chronic heart failure. *Circulation, 110*, 3452–3456.

Johnson, S. M., & Greenman, P. S. (2006). The path to a secure bond: Emotionally focused couple therapy. *Journal of Clinical Psychology, 62*, 597–609.

Johnson, S. M., & Williams-Keeler, L. (1998). Creating healing relationships for couples dealing with trauma: The use of emotionally focused marital therapy. *Journal of Marital and Family Therapy, 24*, 25–40.

Johnston, M., Foulkes, J., Johnston, D. W., Pollard, B., & Gudmundsdottir, H. (1999). Impact on patients and partners of inpatient and extended cardiac counseling and rehabilitation: A controlled trial. *Psychosomatic Medicine, 61*, 225–233.

Jones, L. W., Farrell, J. M., Jamieson, J., & Dorsch, K. D. (2003). Factors influencing enrollment in a cardiac rehabilitation exercise program. *Canadian Journal of Cardiovascular Nursing, 13*, 11–15.

Jordan, J. V. (1997). A relational perspective for understanding women's development. In J. V. Jordon (Ed.), *Women's growth in diversity* (pp. 9–24). New York: Guilford Press.

Jordan, J. V. (2000). The role of mutual empathy in relational/cultural therapy. *Journal of Clinical Psychology, 56,* 1005–1016.

Jorenby, D. E., Hays, J. T., Rigotti, N. A., Azoulay, S., Watsky, E. J., Williams, K. E., et al. (2006). Efficacy of varenicline, an alpha4beta2 nicotinic acetylcholine receptor partial agonist, vs placebo or sustained-release bupropion for smoking cessation: A randomized controlled trial. *Journal of the American Medical Association, 296,* 56–63.

Joseph, A. M., & Fu, S. S. (2003a). Safety issues in pharmacotherapy for smoking in patients with cardiovascular disease. *Progress in Cardiovascular Diseases, 45,* 429–441.

Joseph, A. M., & Fu, S. S. (2003b). Smoking cessation for patients with cardiovascular disease: What is the best approach? *American Journal of Cardiovascular Drugs, 3,* 339–349.

Joseph, A. M., Norman, S. M., Ferry, L. H., Prochazka, A. V., Westman, E. C., Steele, B. G., et al. (1996). The safety of transdermal nicotine as an aid to smoking cessation in patients with cardiac disease. *New England Journal of Medicine, 335,* 1792–1798.

Kaba, E., & Shanley, E. (1997). Identification of coping strategies used by heart transplant recipients. *British Journal of Nursing, 6,* 858–862.

Kaba, E., Thompson, D. R., & Burnard, P. (2000). Coping after heart transplantation: A descriptive study of heart transplant recipients' methods of coping. *Journal of Advanced Nursing, 32,* 930–936.

Kaba, E., Thompson, D. R., Burnard, P., Edwards, D., & Theodosopoulou, E. (2005). Somebody else's heart inside me: A descriptive study of psychological problems after a heart transplantation. *Issues in Mental Health Nursing, 26,* 611–625.

Kabat-Zinn, J. (1991). *Full catastrophe living: Using the wisdom of your body and mind to face stress, pain and illness.* New York: Delacorte.

Kabat-Zinn, J., Massion, A. O., Kristeller, J., Peterson, L. G., Fletcher, K. E., Pbert, L., et al. (1992). Effectiveness of a meditation-based stress reduction program in the treatment of anxiety disorders. *American Journal of Psychiatry, 149,* 936–943.

Kalarchian, M. A., Marcus, M. D., Levine, M. D., Courcoulas, A. P., Pilkonis, P. A., Ringham, R. M., et al. (2007). Psychiatric disorders among bariatric surgery candidates: Relationship to obesity and functional health status. *American Journal of Psychiatry, 164,* 328–334.

Kaplan, J. R., & Manuck, S. B. (1999). Status, stress, and atherosclerosis: The role of environment and individual behavior. *Annals of the New York Academy of Sciences, 896,* 145–161.

Kaplan, J. R., & Manuck, S. B. (2004). Ovarian dysfunction, stress, and disease: A primate continuum. *Institute of Laboratory Animal Resources Journal, 45,* 89–115.

Kaplan, M. (1996). Patients' preferences for sex of therapist. *American Journal of Psychiatry, 153,* 136–137.

Karlberg, L., Krakau, I., & Unden, A. L. (1998). Type A behavior intervention in primary health care reduces hostility and time pressure: A study in Sweden. *Social Science & Medicine, 46*, 397–402.

Katon, W. J., Von Korff, M., & Lin, E. (1992). Panic disorder: Relationship to high medical utilization. *American Journal of Medicine, 92*, 7S–11S.

Kayser-Jones, J. (2002). The experience of dying: An ethnographic nursing home study. *Gerontologist, 42*(3), 11–19.

Kendler, K. S., Heath, A. C., Neale, M. C., Kessler, R. C., & Eaves, L. J. (1993). Alcoholism and major depression in women: A twin study of the causes of comorbidity. *Archives of General Psychiatry, 50*, 690–698.

Keren, R., Aarons, D., & Veltri, E. P. (1991). Anxiety and depression in patients with life-threatening ventricular arrhythmias: Impact of the implantable cardioverter-defibrillator. *Pacing and Clinical Electrophysiology, 14*, 181–187.

Kessler, R. C., McGonagle, K. A., Zhao, S., Nelson, C. B., Hughes, M., Eshleman, S., et al. (1994). Lifetime and 12-month prevalence of *DSM–III–R* psychiatric disorders in the United States: Results from the National Comorbidity Survey. *Archives of General Psychiatry, 51*, 8–19.

Kessler, R. C., Zhao, S., Blazer, D. G., & Swartz, M. (1997). Prevalence, correlates, and course of minor depression and major depression in the National Comorbidity Survey. *Journal of Affective Disorders, 45*, 19–30.

Ketterer, M. W., Denollet, J., Goldberg, A. D., McCullough, P. A., John, S., Farha, A. J., et al. (2002). The big mush: Psychometric measures are confounded and non-independent in their association with age at initial diagnosis of Ischaemic Coronary Heart Disease. *Journal of Cardiovascular Risk, 9*, 41–48.

Kiecolt-Glaser, J. K., & Newton, T. L. (2001). Marriage and health: His and hers. *Psychological Bulletin, 127*, 472–503.

Kim, C. K., McGorray, S. P., Bartholomew, B. A., Marsh, M., Dicken, T., Wassertheil-Smoller, S., et al. (2005). Depressive symptoms and heart rate variability in postmenopausal women. *Archives of Internal Medicine, 165*, 1239–1244.

Kim, W. S., Yoon, Y. R., Kim, K. H., Jho, M. J., & Lee, S. T. (2003). Asymmetric activation in the prefrontal cortex by sound-induced affect. *Perceptual and Motor Skills, 97*, 847–854.

Klein, S. (2002). *The science of happiness: How our brains make us happy—and what we can do to get happier.* New York: Marlowe.

Klerman, G., Weissman, M., & Rounsaville, B. (1984). *Interpersonal psychotherapy of depression.* New York: Basic Books.

Koenig, H. G. (2002). A commentary: The role of religion and spirituality at the end of life. *Gerontologist, 42*(3), 20–23.

Koskenvuo, M., Kaprio, J., Rose, R. J., Kesaniemi, A., Sarna, S., Heikkila, K., et al. (1988). Hostility as a risk factor for mortality and ischemic heart disease in men. *Psychosomatic Medicine, 50*, 330–340.

Koszycki, D., Lafontaine, S., Frasure-Smith, N., Swenson, R., & Lesperance, F. (2004). An open-label trial of interpersonal psychotherapy in depressed patients with coronary disease. *Psychosomatics, 45*, 319–324.

Kowal, J., Johnson, S. M., & Lee, A. (2003). Chronic illness in couples: A case for emotionally focused therapy. *Journal of Marital and Family Therapy, 29*, 299–310.

Kramer, P. (1993). *Listening to Prozac*. New York: Penguin Books.

Krupnick, J. L., Sotsky, S. M., Simmens, S., Moyer, J., Elkin, I., Watkins, J., et al. (1996). The role of the therapeutic alliance in psychotherapy and pharmacotherapy outcome: Findings in the National Institute of Mental Health Treatment of Depression Collaborative Research Program. *Journal of Consulting and Clinical Psychology, 64*, 532–539.

Kubzansky, L. D., Davidson, K. W., & Rozanski, A. (2005). The clinical impact of negative psychological states: Expanding the spectrum of risk for coronary artery disease. *Psychosomatic Medicine, 67*(Suppl. 1), S10–S14.

Kubzansky, L. D., & Kawachi, I. (2000). Going to the heart of the matter: Do negative emotions cause coronary heart disease? *Journal of Psychosomatic Research, 48*, 323–337.

Kubzansky, L. D., Kawachi, I., Spiro, A., III, Weiss, S. T., Vokonas, P. S., & Sparrow, D. (1997). Is worrying bad for your heart? A prospective study of worry and coronary heart disease in the Normative Aging Study. *Circulation, 95*, 818–824.

Kubzansky, L. D., Koenen, K. C., Spiro, A., III, Vokonas, P. S., & Sparrow, D. (2007). Prospective study of posttraumatic stress disorder symptoms and coronary heart disease in the Normative Aging Study. *Archives of General Psychiatry, 64*, 109–116.

Kuhl, E. A., Dixit, N. K., Walker, R. L., Conti, J. B., & Sears, S. F. (2006). Measurement of patient fears about implantable cardioverter defibrillator shock: An initial evaluation of the Florida Shock Anxiety Scale. *Pacing and Clinical Electrophysiology, 29*, 614–618.

Kuhn, W. F., Davis, M. H., & Lippmann, S. B. (1988). Emotional adjustment to cardiac transplantation. *General Hospital Psychiatry, 10*, 108–113.

Kurita, A., Takase, B., & Ishizuka, T. (2001). Disaster and cardiac disease. *Anatolian Journal of Cardiology, 1*, 101–106.

Lackner, J. M., & Gurtman, M. B. (2005). Patterns of interpersonal problems in irritable bowel syndrome patients: A circumplex analysis. *Journal of Psychosomatic Research, 58*, 523–532.

Lampert, R., Joska, T., Burg, M. M., Batsford, W. P., McPherson, C. A., & Jain, D. (2002). Emotional and physical precipitants of ventricular arrhythmia. *Circulation, 106*, 1800–1805.

Lane, D., Carroll, D., & Lip, G. Y. (1999). Psychology in coronary care. *Quarterly Journal of Medicine, 92*, 425–431.

Lane, D., Carroll, D., Ring, C., Beevers, D. G., & Lip, G. Y. (2001a). Mortality and quality of life 12 months after myocardial infarction: Effects of depression and anxiety. *Psychosomatic Medicine, 63*, 221–230.

Lane, D., Carroll, D., Ring, C., Beevers, D. G., & Lip, G. Y. (2001b). Predictors of attendance at cardiac rehabilitation after myocardial infarction. *Journal of Psychosomatic Research, 51,* 497–501.

Lane, D. A., Chong, A. Y., & Lip, G. Y. (2005). Psychological interventions for depression in heart failure. *Cochrane Database of Systematic Reviews, 1,* Article CD003329.

Lane, R. D., Reiman, E. M., Ahern, G. L., Schwartz, G. E., & Davidson, R. J. (1997). Neuroanatomical correlates of happiness, sadness, and disgust. *American Journal of Psychiatry, 154,* 926–933.

Lang, T., Hauser, R., Schlumpf, R., Klaghofer, R., & Buddeberg, C. (2000). Psychological comorbidity and quality of life of patients with morbid obesity and requesting gastric banding. *Schweizerische Medizinische Wochenschrift, 130,* 739–748.

Larson, D. B., Larson, S. S., & Koenig, H. G. (2002). Mortality and religion/spirituality: A brief review of the research. *Annals of Pharmacotherapy, 36,* 1090–1098.

Latzer, Y., & Tzchisinki, O. (2003). Binge eating disorder (BED): New diagnostic category. *Harefuah, 142,* 544–549, 564.

Leary, T. (1957). *Interpersonal diagnosis of personality.* New York: Ronald.

Lee, I. M., Hsieh, C. C., & Paffenbarger, R. S., Jr. (1995). Exercise intensity and longevity in men: The Harvard Alumni Health Study. *Journal of the American Medical Association, 273,* 1179–1184.

Legal Momentum: Advancing Women's Rights. (2004). *Reading between the lines: Women's poverty in the United States, 2003.* New York: Author.

Leon, A. S., Franklin, B. A., Costa, F., Balady, G. J., Berra, K. A., Stewart, K. J., et al. (2005). Cardiac rehabilitation and secondary prevention of coronary heart disease: An American Heart Association scientific statement from the Council on Clinical Cardiology (Subcommittee on Exercise, Cardiac Rehabilitation, and Prevention) and the Council on Nutrition, Physical Activity, and Metabolism (Subcommittee on Physical Activity), in collaboration with the American Association of Cardiovascular and Pulmonary Rehabilitation. *Circulation, 111,* 369–376.

Lesperance, F., & Frasure-Smith, N. (2000). Depression in patients with cardiac disease: A practical review. *Journal of Psychosomatic Research, 48,* 379–391.

Lesperance, F., Frasure-Smith, N., Koszycki, D., Laliberte, M. A., van Zyl, L. T., Baker, B., et al. (2007). Effects of citalopram and interpersonal psychotherapy on depression in patients with coronary artery disease: The Canadian Cardiac Randomized Evaluation of Antidepressant and Psychotherapy Efficacy (CREATE) trial. *Journal of the American Medical Association, 297,* 367–379.

Lesperance, F., Frasure-Smith, N., & Talajic, M. (1996). Major depression before and after myocardial infarction: Its nature and consequences. *Psychosomatic Medicine, 58,* 99–110.

Lesperance, F., Frasure-Smith, N., Talajic, M., & Bourassa, M. G. (2002). Five-year risk of cardiac mortality in relation to initial severity and one-year changes in depression symptoms after myocardial infarction. *Circulation, 105,* 1049–1053.

Lett, H. S., Blumenthal, J. A., Babyak, M. A., Strauman, T. J., Robins, C., & Sherwood, A. (2005). Social support and coronary heart disease: Epidemiologic evidence and implications for treatment. *Psychosomatic Medicine, 67*, 869–878.

Levant, R. F. (2001). Desperately seeking language: Understanding, assessing, and treating normative male alexithymia. In G. R. Brooks & G. E. Glenn (Eds.), *The new handbook of psychotherapy and counseling with men: A comprehensive guide to settings, problems and treatment approaches* (pp. 424–443). San Francisco: Jossey-Bass.

Levant, R. F., & Pollack, W. S. (1995). *A new psychology of men.* New York: Basic Books.

Lichtenstein, E., Glasgow, R. E., Lando, H. A., Ossip-Klein, D. J., & Boles, S. M. (1996). Telephone counseling for smoking cessation: Rationales and meta-analytic review of evidence. *Health Education Research, 11*, 243–257.

Light, K. C., Grewen, K. M., & Amico, J. A. (2005). More frequent partner hugs and higher oxytocin levels are linked to lower blood pressure and heart rate in premenopausal women. *Biological Psychology, 69*, 5–21.

Light, K. C., Grewen, K. M., Amico, J. A., Brownley, K. A., West, S. G., Hinderliter, A. L., et al. (2005). Oxytocinergic activity is linked to lower blood pressure and vascular resistance during stress in postmenopausal women on estrogen replacement. *Hormones and Behavior, 47*, 540–548.

Linden, W. (2000). Psychological treatments in cardiac rehabilitation: Review of rationales and outcomes. *Journal of Psychosomatic Research, 48*, 443–454.

Lynn, J., Harrell, F., Jr., Cohn, F., Wagner, D., & Connors, A. F., Jr. (1997). Prognoses of seriously ill hospitalized patients on the days before death: Implications for patient care and public policy. *New Horizons, 5*, 56–61.

Lynn, J., Teno, J. M., & Harrell, F. E., Jr. (1995). Accurate prognostications of death: Opportunities and challenges for clinicians. *Western Journal of Medicine, 163*, 250–257.

MacIntosh, H. B., Johnson, S. M., & Lee, A. (2006). Hanging onto a heartbeat: Emotionally focused therapy. In E. Molinari, A. Compare, & G. Parati (Eds.), *Clinical psychology and heart disease* (pp. 391–412). Milan: Springer-Verlag.

Mackenzie, C. S., Gekoski, W. L., & Knox, V. J. (1999). Do family physicians treat older patients with mental disorders differently from younger patients? *Canadian Family Physician, 45*, 1219–1224.

Maes, M. (1999). Major depression and activation of the inflammatory response system. *Advances in Experimental Medicine and Biology, 461*, 25–46.

Magnavita, J. J. (1997). *Restructuring personality disorders: A short-term dynamic approach.* New York: Guilford Press.

Magnavita, J. J. (2005). *Personality-guided relational psychotherapy: A unified approach.* Washington, DC: American Psychological Association.

Magnavita, J. J. (2006). The centrality of emotion in unifying and accelerating psychotherapy. *Journal of Clinical Psychology, 62*, 585–596.

Mak, Y. M., Chan, W. K., & Yue, C. S. (2005). Barriers to participation in a Phase II cardiac rehabilitation programme. *Hong Kong Medical Journal, 11*, 472–475.

Martino, S., Carroll, K. M., Nich, C., & Rounsaville, B. J. (2006). A randomized controlled pilot study of motivational interviewing for patients with psychotic and drug use disorders. *Addiction, 101,* 1479–1492.

Matarazzo, J. D. (1980). Behavioral health and behavioral medicine: Frontiers for a new health psychology. *American Psychologist, 35,* 807–817.

Matthews, K. A., Glass, D. C., Rosenman, R. H., & Bortner, R. W. (1977). Competitive drive, Pattern A, and coronary heart disease: A further analysis of some data from the Western Collaborative Group Study. *Journal of Chronic Diseases, 30,* 489–498.

May, R. (1983). *The discovery of being: Writings in existential psychology.* New York: Norton.

McClelland, D. C., Floor, E., Davidson, R. J., & Saron, C. (1980). Stressed power motivation, sympathetic activation, immune function, and illness. *Journal of Human Stress, 6,* 11–19.

McCraty, R., & Tomasino, D. (2006). Coherence-building techniques and heart rhythm coherence feedback: New tools for stress reduction, disease prevention and rehabilitation. In E. Molinari, A. Compare, & G. Parati (Eds.), *Clinical psychology and heart disease* (pp. 487–509). Milan: Springer-Verlag.

McCullough, L., Kuhn, N., Andrews, S., Kaplan, A., Wolf, J., & Hurley, C. L. (2003). *Treating affect phobia: A manual for short-term dynamic psychotherapy.* New York: Guilford Press.

McDaniel, S. H., Hepworth, J., & Doherty, W. J. (1992). *Medical family therapy: A biopsychosoical approach to families and health problems.* New York: Basic Books.

Mealy, K., Ngeh, N., Gillen, P., Fitzpatrick, G., Keane, F. B., & Tanner, A. (1996). Propranolol reduces the anxiety associated with day case surgery. *European Journal of Surgery, 162,* 11–14.

Mental health: Does therapy help? (1995, November). *Consumer Reports,* 734–739.

Middel, B., Bouma, J., de Jongste, M., van Sonderen, E., Niemeijer, M. G., Crijns, H., et al. (2001). Psychometric properties of the Minnesota Living With Heart Failure Questionnaire (MLHF–Q). *Clinical Rehabilitation, 15,* 489–500.

Miller, I. W., & Keitner, G. I. (1996). Combined medication and psychotherapy in the treatment of chronic mood disorders. *Psychiatric Clinics of North America, 19,* 151–171.

Miller, K., Myers, T. J., Robertson, K., Shah, N., Delgado, R. M., III, & Gregoric, I. D. (2004). Quality of life in bridge-to-transplant patients with chronic heart failure after implantation of an axial flow ventricular assist device. *Congestive Heart Failure, 10,* 226–229.

Miller, W. R., & Rollnick, S. (1991). *Motivational interviewing: Preparing people to change addictive behavior.* New York: Guilford Press.

Miller, W. R., & Rollnick, S. (2002). *Motivational interviewing: Preparing people for change* (2nd ed.). New York: Guilford Press.

Mitchell, P. H., Powell, L., Blumenthal, J., Norten, J., Ironson, G., Pitula, C. R., et al. (2003). A short social support measure for patients recovering from myocardial infarction: The ENRICHD Social Support Inventory. *Journal of Cardiopulmonary Rehabilitation, 23,* 398–403.

Mitchell, R., Muggli, M., & Sato, A. (1999). Cardiac rehabilitation: Participating in an exercise program in a quest to survive. *Rehabilitation Nursing, 24,* 236–239.

Mittleman, M. A., Maclure, M., Sherwood, J. B., Mulry, R. P., Tofler, G. H., Jacobs, S. C., et al. (1995). Triggering of acute myocardial infarction onset by episodes of anger: Determinants of Myocardial Infarction Onset Study Investigators. *Circulation, 92,* 1720–1725.

Mittleman, M. A., Mintzer, D., Maclure, M., Tofler, G. H., Sherwood, J. B., & Muller, J. E. (1999). Triggering of myocardial infarction by cocaine. *Circulation, 99,* 2737–2741.

Molinari, E., Compare, A., & Parati, G. (2006). *Clinical psychology and heart disease.* Milan: Springer-Verlag.

Moller, J., Hallqvist, J., Diderichsen, F., Theorell, T., Reuterwall, C., & Ahlbom, A. (1999). Do episodes of anger trigger myocardial infarction? A case-crossover analysis in the Stockholm Heart Epidemiology Program (SHEEP). *Psychosomatic Medicine, 61,* 842–849.

Momtahan, K., Berkman, J., Sellick, J., Kearns, S. A., & Lauzon, N. (2004). Patients' understanding of cardiac risk factors: a point-prevalence study. *Journal of Cardiovascular Nursing, 19,* 13–20.

Monsen, K., & Havik, O. E. (2001). Psychological functioning and bodily conditions in patients with pain disorder associated with psychological factors. *British Journal of Medical Psychology, 74*(Pt. 2), 183–195.

Montoya, P., Campos, J. J., & Schandry, R. (2005). See red? Turn pale? Unveiling emotions through cardiovascular and hemodynamic changes. *Spanish Journal of Psychology, 8,* 79–85.

Montgomery, G. H., Erblich, J., DiLorenzo, T., & Bovbjerg, D. H. (2003). Family and friends with disease: Their impact on perceived risk. *Preventive Medicine, 37,* 242–249.

Morrow, L. (2004, September 20). Advice from a bypass buddy: A heart-surgery veteran offers Bill Clinton a sneak preview of his new life. *Time,* 84.

Mosca, L., Ferris, A., Fabunmi, R., & Robertson, R. M. (2004). Tracking women's awareness of heart disease: An American Heart Association national study. *Circulation, 109,* 573–579.

Moscicki, E. K. (1994). Gender differences in completed and attempted suicides. *Annals of Epidemiology, 4,* 152–158.

Moser, D. K., & Dracup, K. (1996). Is anxiety early after myocardial infarction associated with subsequent ischemic and arrhythmic events? *Psychosomatic Medicine, 58,* 395–401.

Moser, D. K., & Dracup, K. (2004). Role of spousal anxiety and depression in patients' psychosocial recovery after a cardiac event. *Psychosomatic Medicine, 66,* 527–532.

Muller, J. E., Mittleman, M. A., Maclure, M., Sherwood, J. B., & Tofler, G. H. (1996). Triggering myocardial infarction by sexual activity: Low absolute risk and prevention by regular physical exertion: Determinants of Myocardial Infarction Onset Study investigators. *Journal of the American Medical Association, 275,* 1405–1409.

Musselman, D. L., Evans, D. L., & Nemeroff, C. B. (1998). The relationship of depression to cardiovascular disease: Epidemiology, biology, and treatment. *Archives of General Psychiatry, 55,* 580–592.

Musselman, D. L., Marzec, U. M., Manatunga, A., Penna, S., Reemsnyder, A., Knight, B. T., et al. (2000). Platelet reactivity in depressed patients treated with paroxetine: Preliminary findings. *Archives of General Psychiatry, 57,* 875–882.

Musselman, D. L., Tomer, A., Manatunga, A. K., Knight, B. T., Porter, M. R., Kasey, S., et al. (1996). Exaggerated platelet reactivity in major depression. *American Journal of Psychiatry, 153,* 1313–1317.

Nakatani, D., Sato, H., Sakata, Y., Shiotani, I., Kinjo, K., Mizuno, H., et al. (2005). Influence of serotonin transporter gene polymorphism on depressive symptoms and new cardiac events after acute myocardial infarction. *American Heart Journal, 150,* 652–658.

National Cancer Institute. (2007). *National network of tobacco cessation quitlines.* Retrieved from http://cancercontrol.cancer.gov/tcrb/national_quitlines.html

National Register of Health Service Providers in Psychology. (2007). *National register of 13,000 psychologists database.* Washington, DC: Author.

Nemeroff, C. B., Musselman, D. L., & Evans, D. L. (1998). Depression and cardiac disease. *Depression and Anxiety, 8*(Suppl. 1), 71–79.

Neven, K., Dymek, M., leGrange, D., Maasdam, H., Boogerd, A. C., & Alverdy, J. (2002). The effects of Roux-en-Y gastric bypass surgery on body image. *Obesity Surgery, 12,* 265–269.

New York Organ Donor Network. (2007). *First time organ donor family and recipient meeting at the New York Organ Donor Network.* New York: Author.

Newcombe, D. A., Humeniuk, R. E., & Ali, R. (2005). Validation of the World Health Organization Alcohol, Smoking and Substance Involvement Screening Test (ASSIST): Report of results from the Australian site. *Drug and Alcohol Review, 24,* 217–226.

Newton, T. L., & Sanford, J. M. (2003). Conflict structure moderates associations between cardiovascular reactivity and negative marital interaction. *Health Psychology, 22,* 270–278.

Nguyen, V. H., & McLaughlin, M. A. (2002). Coronary artery disease in women: A review of emerging cardiovascular risk factors. *Mount Sinai Journal of Medicine, 69,* 338–349.

Nix, J., & Lohr, J. M. (1981). Relationship between sex, sex-role characteristics and coronary-prone behavior in college students. *Psychological Reports, 48,* 739–744.

Nolan, M., & Nolan, J. (1998). Cardiac rehabilitation following myocardial infarction. *British Journal of Nursing, 7,* 219–225.

Nolen-Hoeksema, S. (2000). The role of rumination in depressive disorders and mixed anxiety/depressive symptoms. *Journal of Abnormal Psychology, 109,* 504–511.

Noriuchi, M., Kikuchi, Y., & Senoo, A. (2008). The functional neuroanatomy of maternal love: Mother's response to infant's attachment behaviors. *Biological Psychiatry, 63,* 415–423.

Norvell, N., Conti, R., & Hecker, J. (1987). Contribution of psychology to the assessment of candidates for heart transplantation. *Primary Cardiology, 13,* 20–28.

O'Carroll, R. E., Smith, K. B., Grubb, N. R., Fox, K. A., & Masterton, G. (2001). Psychological factors associated with delay in attending hospital following a myocardial infarction. *Journal of Psychosomatic Research, 51,* 611–614.

Ockene, J., Kristeller, J. L., Goldberg, R., Ockene, I., Merriam, P., Barrett, S., et al. (1992). Smoking cessation and severity of disease: The Coronary Artery Smoking Intervention Study. *Health Psychology, 11,* 119–126.

O'Farrell, P., Murray, J., & Hotz, S. B. (2000). Psychologic distress among spouses of patients undergoing cardiac rehabilitation. *Heart and Lung, 29,* 97–104.

Ogrodniczuk, J. S., Piper, W. E., Joyce, A. S., & McCallum, M. (2001). Effect of patient gender on outcome in two forms of short-term individual psychotherapy. *Journal of Psychotherapy Practice and Research, 10,* 69–78.

Orth-Gomer, K., Wamala, S. P., Horsten, M., Schenck-Gustafsson, K., Schneiderman, N., & Mittleman, M. A. (2000). Marital stress worsens prognosis in women with coronary heart disease: The Stockholm Female Coronary Risk Study. *Journal of the American Medical Association, 284,* 3008–3014.

Owen, J. E., Bonds, C. L., & Wellisch, D. K. (2006). Psychiatric evaluations of heart transplant candidates: Predicting post-transplant hospitalizations, rejection episodes, and survival. *Psychosomatics, 47,* 213–222.

Pacher, P., Ungvari, Z., Kecskemeti, V., & Furst, S. (1998). Review of cardiovascular effects of fluoxetine, a selective serotonin reuptake inhibitor, compared to tricyclic antidepressants. *Current Medicinal Chemistry, 5,* 381–390.

Pampallona, S., Bollini, P., Tibaldi, G., Kupelnick, B., & Munizza, C. (2004). Combined pharmacotherapy and psychological treatment for depression: A systematic review. *Archives of General Psychiatry, 61,* 714–719.

Pate, R. R., Pratt, M., Blair, S. N., Haskell, W. L., Macera, C. A., Bouchard, C., et al. (1995). Physical activity and public health: A recommendation from the Centers for Disease Control and Prevention and the American College of Sports Medicine. *Journal of the American Medical Association, 273,* 402–407.

Paul, S., & Sneed, N. V. (2004). Strategies for behavior change in patients with heart failure. *American Journal of Critical Care, 13,* 305–313.

Pawlow, L. A., & Jones, G. E. (2005). The impact of abbreviated progressive muscle relaxation on salivary cortisol and salivary immunoglobulin A (sIgA). *Applied Psychophysiology and Biofeedback, 30,* 375–387.

Pawlow, L. A., O'Neil, P. M., & Malcolm, R. J. (2003). Night eating syndrome: Effects of brief relaxation training on stress, mood, hunger, and eating patterns. *International Journal of Obesity and Related Metabolic Disorders, 27,* 970–978.

Pearsall, P., Schwartz, G. E., & Russek, L. G. (2000). Changes in heart transplant recipients that parallel the personalities of their donors. *Integrative Medicine: Integrating Conventional and Alternative Medicine, 2,* 65–72.

Pedersen, S. S., & Denollet, J. (2003). Type D personality, cardiac events, and impaired quality of life: A review. *European Journal of Cardiovascular Prevention and Rehabilitation, 10,* 241–248.

Pedersen, S. S., & Denollet, J. (2004). Validity of the Type D personality construct in Danish post-MI patients and healthy controls. *Journal of Psychosomatic Research, 57,* 265–272.

Peeters, A., Barendregt, J. J., Willekens, F., Mackenbach, J. P., Al Mamun, A., & Bonneux, L. (2003). Obesity in adulthood and its consequences for life expectancy: A life-table analysis. *Annals of Internal Medicine, 138,* 24–32.

Pennebaker, J. W., & Seagal, J. D. (1999). Forming a story: The health benefits of narrative. *Journal of Clinical Psychology, 55,* 1243–1254.

Pfiffner, D., & Hoffmann, A. (2004). Psychosocial predictors of death for low-risk patients after a first myocardial infarction: A 7-year follow-up study. *Journal of Cardiopulmonary Rehabilitation and Prevention, 24,* 87–93.

Pickering, T., Clemow, L., Davidson, K., & Gerin, W. (2003). Behavioral cardiology: Has its time finally arrived? *Mount Sinai Journal of Medicine, 70,* 101–112.

Powell, L. H. (1996). The hook: A metaphor for gaining control of emotional reactivity. In R. Allan & S. S. Scheidt (Eds.), *Heart and mind: The practice of cardiac psychology* (pp. 313–327). Washington, DC: American Psychological Association.

Prochaska, J. O., & DiClemente, C. C. (1983). Stages and processes of self-change of smoking: Toward an integrative model of change. *Journal of Consulting and Clinical Psychology, 51,* 390–395.

Prochaska, J. O., & DiClemente, C. C. (1984). Self-change processes, self efficacy and decisional balance across five stages of smoking cessation. *Progress in Clinical and Biological Research, 156,* 131–140.

Prochaska, J. O., DiClemente, C. C., & Norcross, J. C. (1992). In search of how people change: Applications to addictive behaviors. *American Psychologist, 47,* 1102–1114.

Rader, D. J. (2007). Lipid disorders. In E. J. Topol, R. Califf, E. N. Prystowsky, J. D. Thomas, & P. D. Thompson (Eds.), *Textbook of cardiovascular medicine* (3rd ed., pp. 55–75). Philadelphia: Lippincott, Williams & Wilkins.

Rafanelli, C., Pancaldi, L. G., Ferranti, G., Roncuzzi, R., Tomba, E., Milaneschi, Y., et al. (2005). Stressful life events and depressive disorders as risk factors for acute coronary heart disease. *Italian Heart Journal, 6*(Suppl.), 105–110.

Rainville, P., Bechara, A., Naqvi, N., & Damasio, A. R. (2006). Basic emotions are associated with distinct patterns of cardiorespiratory activity. *International Journal of Psychophysiology, 61,* 5–18.

Rankin, S. H. (1992). Psychosocial adjustments of coronary artery disease patients and their spouses: Nursing implications. *Nursing Clinics of North America, 27,* 271–284.

Rankin-Esquer, L. A., Deeter, A., & Taylor, C. B. (2000). Coronary heart disease and couples. In K. B. Schmaling & T. Goldman Sher (Eds.), *The psychology of couples and illness: Theory, research, and practice* (pp. 43–70). Washington, DC: American Psychological Association.

Ray, R. D., Ochsner, K. N., Cooper, J. C., Robertson, E. R., Gabrieli, J. D., & Gross, J. J. (2005). Individual differences in trait rumination and the neural systems supporting cognitive reappraisal. *Cognitive, Affective & Biological Neuroscience, 5,* 156–168.

Rector, T. S., Kubo, S. H., & Cohn, J. N. (1993). Validity of the Minnesota Living With Heart Failure Questionnaire as a measure of therapeutic response to enalapril or placebo. *American Journal of Cardiology, 71,* 1106–1107.

Rector, T. S., Tschumperlin, L. K., Kubo, S. H., Bank, A. J., Francis, G. S., McDonald, K. M., et al. (1995). Use of the Living With Heart Failure Questionnaire to ascertain patients' perspectives on improvement in quality of life versus risk of drug-induced death. *Journal of Cardiac Failure, 1,* 201–206.

Rees, G., Fry, A., & Cull, A. (2001). A family history of breast cancer: Women's experiences from a theoretical perspective. *Social Science & Medicine, 52,* 1433–1440.

Rhodes, D. L., & Bowles, C. L. (2002). Heart failure and its impact on older women's lives. *Journal of Advanced Nursing, 39,* 441–449.

Rigotti, N. A., McKool, K. M., & Shiffman, S. (1994). Predictors of smoking cessation after coronary artery bypass graft surgery: Results of a randomized trial with 5-year follow-up. *Annals of Internal Medicine, 120,* 287–293.

Rigotti, N. A., Thorndike, A. N., Regan, S., McKool, K., Pasternak, R. C., Chang, Y., et al. (2006). Bupropion for smokers hospitalized with acute cardiovascular disease. *American Journal of Medicine, 119,* 1080–1087.

Roberts, B. (2004). *How to keep from breaking your heart: What every woman needs to know about cardiovascular disease.* Sudbury, MN: Jones & Bartlett.

Robinson, B. C. (1983). Validation of a caregiver strain index. *Journal of Gerontology, 38,* 344–348.

Robinson, L. A., Berman, J. S., & Neimeyer, R. A. (1990). Psychotherapy for the treatment of depression: A comprehensive review of controlled outcome research. *Psychological Bulletin, 108,* 30–49.

Rohrbaugh, M. J., Shoham, V., & Coyne, J. C. (2006). Effect of marital quality on eight-year survival of patients with heart failure. *American Journal of Cardiology, 98,* 1069–1072.

Rollnick, S., Butler, C. C., & Stott, N. (1997). Helping smokers make decisions: The enhancement of brief intervention for general medical practice. *Patient Education and Counseling, 31,* 191–203.

Rollnick, S., Heather, N., & Bell, A. (1992). Negotiating behaviour change in medical settings: The development of brief motivational interviewing. *Journal of Mental Health, 1,* 25–37.

Romanoff, B. D., & Terenzio, M. (1998). Rituals and the grieving process. *Death Studies, 22,* 697–711.

Roose, S. P., Laghrissi-Thode, F., Kennedy, J. S., Nelson, J. C., Bigger, J. T., Jr., Pollock, B. G., et al. (1998). Comparison of paroxetine and nortriptyline in depressed patients with ischemic heart disease. *Journal of the American Medical Association, 279,* 287–291.

Roose, S. P. & Miyazaki, M. (2005). Pharmacologic treatment of depression in patients with heart disease. *Psychosomatic Medicine, 67*(Suppl. 1), S54–S57.

Rosengren, A., Hawken, S., Ounpuu, S., Sliwa, K., Zubaid, M., Almahmeed, W. A., et al. (2004). Association of psychosocial risk factors with risk of acute myocardial infarction in 11119 cases and 13648 controls from 52 countries (the INTERHEART study): Case-control study. *Lancet, 364*, 953–962.

Rosenman, R. H. (1978). The interview method of assessment of the coronary-prone behavior pattern. In T. M. Dembroski, S. M. Weiss, J. L. Shields, S. G. Haynes, & M. Feinleib (Eds.), *Coronary-prone behavior* (pp. 55–70). New York: Springer-Verlag.

Rosenman, R. H., Brand, R. J., Jenkins, D., Friedman, M., Straus, R., & Wurm, M. (1975). Coronary heart disease in Western Collaborative Group Study: Final follow-up experience of 8 1/2 years. *Journal of the American Medical Association, 233*, 872–877.

Rosenman, R. H., Brand, R. J., Sholtz, R. I., & Friedman, M. (1976). Multivariate prediction of coronary heart disease during 8.5 year follow-up in the Western Collaborative Group Study. *American Journal of Cardiology, 37*, 903–910.

Rosik, C. H. (2005). Psychiatric symptoms among prospective bariatric surgery patients: Rates of prevalence and their relation to social desirability, pursuit of surgery, and follow-up attendance. *Obesity Surgery, 15*, 677–683.

Rossi, M. L., Merlini, P. A., & Ardissino, D. (2001). Percutaneous coronary revascularisation in women. *Thrombosis Research, 103*(Suppl. 1), S105–S111.

Roviaro, S., Holmes, D. S., & Holmsten, R. D. (1984). Influence of a cardiac rehabilitation program on the cardiovascular, psychological, and social functioning of cardiac patients. *Journal of Behavioral Medicine, 7*, 61–81.

Roy, P., & Waksman, R. (2006). How to approach drug-eluting stent restenosis. *Minerva Cardioangiologica, 54*, 571–576.

Rozanski, A., Blumenthal, J. A., Davidson, K. W., Saab, P. G., & Kubzansky, L. (2005). The epidemiology, pathophysiology, and management of psychosocial risk factors in cardiac practice: The emerging field of behavioral cardiology. *Journal of the American College of Cardiology, 45*, 637–651.

Rozanski, A., Krantz, D. S., & Bairey, C. N. (1991). Ventricular responses to mental stress testing in patients with coronary artery disease: Pathophysiological implications. *Circulation, 83*, II137–II144.

Rozensky, R. H., Sweet, J. J., & Tovian, S. M. (1997). *Psychological assessment in medical settings.* New York: Plenum Press.

Ruiz, J. M., Hamann, H. A., Coyne, J. C., & Compare, A. (2006). In sickness and in health: Interpersonal risk and resilience in cardiovascular disease. In E. Molinari, A. Compare, & G. Parati (Eds.), *Clinical psychology and heart disease* (pp. 233–272). Milan: Springer-Verlag.

Rymaszewska, J., Kiejna, A., & Hadrys, T. (2003). Depression and anxiety in coronary artery bypass grafting patients. *European Psychiatry, 18*, 155–160.

Sapolsky, R. M. (2004). *Why zebras don't get ulcers: An updated guide to stress, stress-related diseases and coping* (3rd ed.). New York: Henry Holt.

Sauer, W. H., Berlin, J. A., & Kimmel, S. E. (2001). Selective serotonin reuptake inhibitors and myocardial infarction. *Circulation, 104,* 1894–1898.

Sauer, W. H., Berlin, J. A., & Kimmel, S. E. (2003). Effect of antidepressants and their relative affinity for the serotonin transporter on the risk of myocardial infarction. *Circulation, 108,* 32–36.

Schiffer, A. A., Pedersen, S. S., Widdershoven, J. W., Hendriks, E. H., Winter, J. B., & Denollet, J. (2005). The distressed (Type D) personality is independently associated with impaired health status and increased depressive symptoms in chronic heart failure. *European Journal of Cardiovascular Rehabilitation and Prevention, 12,* 341–346.

Schneiderman, N., Saab, P. G., Catellier, D. J., Powell, L. H., DeBusk, R. F., Williams, R. B., et al. (2004). Psychosocial treatment within sex by ethnicity subgroups in the Enhancing Recovery in Coronary Heart Disease clinical trial. *Psychosomatic Medicine, 66,* 475–483.

Schulberg, H. C., Pilkonis, P. A., & Houck, P. (1998). The severity of major depression and choice of treatment in primary care practice. *Journal of Consulting and Clinical Psychology, 66,* 932–938.

Schulberg, H. C., Post, E. P., Raue, P. J., Have, T. T., Miller, M., & Bruce, M. L. (2007). Treating late-life depression with interpersonal psychotherapy in the primary care sector. *International Journal of Geriatric Psychiatry, 22,* 106–114.

Schum, J. L., Lyness, J. M., & King, D. A. (2005). Bereavement in late life: Risk factors for complicated bereavement. *Geriatrics, 60,* 18–20, 24.

Schuster, P. M., & Waldron, J. (1991). Gender differences in cardiac rehabilitation patients. *Rehabilitation Nursing, 16,* 248–253.

Schwartz, G. E., Weinberger, D. A., & Singer, J. A. (1981). Cardiovascular differentiation of happiness, sadness, anger, and fear following imagery and exercise. *Psychosomatic Medicine, 43,* 343–364.

Schwarz, E. R., Kapur, V., Bionat, S., Rastogi, S., Gupta, R., & Rosanio, S. (2008). The prevalence and clinical relevance of sexual dysfunction in women and men with chronic heart failure. *International Journal of Impotence Research, 20,* 85–91.

Schwenk, T. L., Coyne, J. C., & Fechner-Bates, S. (1996). Differences between detected and undetected patients in primary care and depressed psychiatric patients. *General Hospital Psychiatry, 18,* 407–415.

Seaburn, D. B., Lorenz, A. D., Gunn, W. B., Jr., Gawinski, B. A., & Mauksch, L. B. (2003). *Models of collaboration: A guide for mental health professionals working with health care practitioners.* New York: Basic Books.

Sears, S. F., & Conti, J. B. (2003). Understanding implantable cardioverter defibrillator shocks and storms: Medical and psychosocial considerations for research and clinical care. *Clinical Cardiology, 26,* 107–111.

Sears, S. F., Lewis, T. S., Kuhl, E. A., & Conti, J. B. (2005). Predictors of quality of life in patients with implantable cardioverter defibrillators. *Psychosomatics, 46,* 451–457.

Sears, S. F., Sowell, L. V., Kuhl, E. A., Handberg, E. M., Kron, J., Aranda, J. M., Jr., et al. (2006). Quality of death: Implantable cardioverter defibrillators and pro-active care. *Pacing and Clinical Electrophysiology, 29,* 637–642.

Sears, S. F., Todaro, J. F., Lewis, T. S., Sotile, W., & Conti, J. B. (1999). Examining the psychosocial impact of implantable cardioverter defibrillators: A literature review. *Clinical Cardiology, 22,* 481–489.

Sears, S. F., Todaro, J. F., Urizar, G., Lewis, T. S., Sirois, B., Wallace, R., et al. (2000). Assessing the psychosocial impact of the ICD: A national survey of implantable cardioverter defibrillator health care providers. *Pacing and Clinical Electrophysiology, 23,* 939–945.

Segal, Z., Vincent, P., & Levitt, A. (2002). Efficacy of combined, sequential and crossover psychotherapy and pharmacotherapy in improving outcomes in depression. *Journal of Psychiatry and Neuroscience, 27,* 281–290.

Seligman, M. E. (1995). The effectiveness of psychotherapy: The Consumer Reports study. *American Psychologist, 50,* 965–974.

Selye, H. (1956). *The stress of life.* New York: McGraw Hill.

Selye, H. (1974). *Stress without distress.* Philadelphia: Lippincott, Williams & Wilkins.

Sheahan, S. L., Rayens, M. K., An, K., Riegel, B., McKinley, S., Doering, L., et al. (2006). Comparison of anxiety between smokers and nonsmokers with acute myocardial infarction. *American Journal of Critical Care, 15,* 617–625.

Shedd, O. L., Sears, S. F., Jr., Harvill, J. L., Arshad, A., Conti, J. B., Steinberg, J. S., et al. (2004). The World Trade Center attack: Increased frequency of defibrillator shocks for ventricular arrhythmias in patients living remotely from New York City. *Journal of the American College of Cardiology, 44,* 1265–1267.

Shekelle, R. B., Hulley, S. B., Neaton, J. D., Billings, J. H., Borhani, N. O., Gerace, T. A., et al. (1985). The MRFIT behavior pattern study: II. Type A behavior and incidence of coronary heart disease. *American Journal of Epidemiology, 122,* 559–570.

Sher, L. (2005). Type D personality: The heart, stress, and cortisol. *Quarterly Journal of Medicine, 98,* 323–329.

Sherbourne, C. D., Hays, R. D., Wells, K. B., Rogers, W., & Burnam, M. A. (1993). Prevalence of comorbid alcohol disorder and consumption in medically ill and depressed patients. *Archives of Family Medicine, 2,* 1142–1150.

Siegman, A. W., Kubzansky, L. D., Kawachi, I., Boyle, S., Vokonas, P. S., & Sparrow, D. (2000). A prospective study of dominance and coronary heart disease in the Normative Aging Study. *American Journal of Cardiology, 86,* 145–149.

Siegman, A. W., Townsend, S. T., Blumenthal, R. S., Sorkin, J. D., & Civelek, A. C. (1998). Dimensions of anger and CHD in men and women: Self-ratings versus spouse ratings. *Journal of Behavioral Medicine, 21,* 315–336.

Siegman, A. W., Townsend, S. T., Civelek, A. C., & Blumenthal, R. S. (2000). Antagonistic behavior, dominance, hostility, and coronary heart disease. *Psychosomatic Medicine, 62,* 248–257.

Sifneos, P. E. (1981). Short-term dynamic psychotherapy: Its history, its impact and its future. *Psychotherapy and Psychosomatics, 35,* 224–229.

Sigfússon, N., Sigurdsson, G., Aspelund, T., & Gudnason, V. (2006). The health risk associated with smoking has been seriously underestimated: The Reykjavik Study. *Laeknabladid, 92*, 263–269.

Simpson, S., Corney, R., Fitzgerald, P., & Beecham, J. (2003). A randomised controlled trial to evaluate the effectiveness and cost-effectiveness of psychodynamic counselling for general practice patients with chronic depression. *Psychological Medicine, 33*, 229–239.

Sinha, R., Lovallo, W. R., & Parsons, O. A. (1992). Cardiovascular differentiation of emotions. *Psychosomatic Medicine, 54*, 422–435.

Sjoland, H., Caidahl, K., Karlson, B. W., Karlsson, T., & Herlitz, J. (1997). Limitation of physical activity, dyspnea and chest pain before and two years after coronary artery bypass grafting in relation to sex. *International Journal of Cardiology, 61*, 123–133.

Skala, J., Freedland, K. E., & Carney, R. (2005). *Heart disease.* Cambridge, MA: Hogrefe & Huber.

Smith, T. W., Glazer, K., Ruiz, J. M., & Gallo, L. C. (2004). Hostility, anger, aggressiveness, and coronary heart disease: An interpersonal perspective on personality, emotion, and health. *Journal of Personality, 72*, 1217–1270.

Sniehotta, F. F., Scholz, U., & Schwarzer, R. (2006). Action plans and coping plans for physical exercise: A longitudinal intervention study in cardiac rehabilitation. *British Journal of Health Psychology, 11*, 23–37.

Sotile, W. M. (1996). *Psychosocial interventions for cardiopulmonary patients: A guide for health care professionals.* Champaign, IL: Human Kinetics.

Sotile, W. M., & Cantor-Cooke, R. (2003). Reclaim your sex life and physical intimacy. In W. M. Sotile & R. Cantor-Cooke (Eds.), *Thriving with heart disease: A unique program for you and your family* (pp. 156–183). New York: Free Press.

Sowell, L. V., Kuhl, E. A., Sears, S. F., Klodell, C. T., & Conti, J. B. (2006). Device implant technique and consideration of body image: Specific procedures for implantable cardioverter defibrillators in female patients. *Journal of Women's Health, 15*, 830–835.

Spiegel, D., Bloom, J. R., Kraemer, H. C., & Gottheil, E. (1989). Effect of psychosocial treatment on survival of patients with metastatic breast cancer. *Lancet, 2*, 888–891.

Spielberger, C. D. (1999). *State–Trait Anger Expression Inventory—2.* Lutz, FL: Psychological Assessment Resources.

Spielberger, C. D., Gorsuch, R. L., & Lushene, R. (1968). *State–Trait Anxiety Inventory.* Palo Alto, CA: Consulting Psychologists Press.

Spielberger, C. D., Reheiser, E. C., & Sydeman, S. J. (1995). Measuring the experience, expression, and control of anger. *Issues in Comprehensive Pediatric Nursing, 18*, 207–232.

Spies, C. D., Sander, M., Stangl, K., Fernandez-Sola, J., Preedy, V. R., Rubin, E., et al. (2001). Effects of alcohol on the heart. *Current Opinion in Critical Care, 7*, 337–343.

Steer, R. A., Cavalieri, T. A., Leonard, D. M., & Beck, A. T. (1999). Use of the Beck Depression Inventory for Primary Care to screen for major depression disorders. *General Hospital Psychiatry, 21*, 106–111.

Stein, R. (2006, December 17). Devices can interfere with peaceful death: Implants repeatedly shock hearts of patients who cannot be saved. *Washington Post*, p. A01.

Steinmark, A., Dornelas, E. A., & Fischer, E. H. (2006). Determinants and barriers to participation in an Internet-based recovery program for cardiac patients. *Journal of Clinical Psychology in Medical Settings, 13*, 353–357.

Stiver, I., & Baker-Miller, J. (1997). From depression to sadness in women's psychotherapy. In J. V. Jordan (Ed.), *Women's growth in diversity* (pp. 217–238). New York: Guilford Press.

Striegel-Moore, R. H., & Franko, D. L. (2003). Epidemiology of binge eating disorder. *International Journal of Eating Disorders, 34*(Suppl.), S19–S29.

Striegel-Moore, R. H., Franko, D. L., May, A., Ach, E., Thompson, D., & Hook, J. M. (2006). Should night eating syndrome be included in the DSM? *International Journal of Eating Disorders, 39*, 544–549.

Strik, J. J., Denollet, J., Lousberg, R., & Honig, A. (2003). Comparing symptoms of depression and anxiety as predictors of cardiac events and increased health care consumption after myocardial infarction. *Journal of the American College of Cardiology, 42*, 1801–1807.

Strik, J. J., Honig, A., Lousberg, R., Lousberg, A. H., Cheriex, E. C., Tuynman-Qua, H. G., et al. (2000). Efficacy and safety of fluoxetine in the treatment of patients with major depression after first myocardial infarction: Findings from a double-blind, placebo-controlled trial. *Psychosomatic Medicine, 62*, 783–789.

Stunkard, A. J., Allison, K. C., & O'Reardon, J. P. (2005). The night eating syndrome: A progress report. *Appetite, 45*, 182–186.

Stunkard, A. J., Grace, W. J., & Wolff, H. G. (1955). The night-eating syndrome: A pattern of food intake among certain obese patients. *American Journal of Medicine, 19*, 78–86.

Sturm, R. (2007). Increases in morbid obesity in the USA: 2000–2005. *Public Health, 121*, 492–496.

Suarez, E. C. (2004). C-reactive protein is associated with psychological risk factors of cardiovascular disease in apparently healthy adults. *Psychosomatic Medicine, 66*, 684–691.

Suarez, E. C., Lewis, J. G., & Kuhn, C. (2002). The relation of aggression, hostility, and anger to lipopolysaccharide-stimulated tumor necrosis factor (TNF)-alpha by blood monocytes from normal men. *Brain, Behavior and Immunity, 16*, 675–684.

Sukhodolsky, D. G., Golub, A., & Cromwell, E. N. (2001). Development and validation of the Anger Rumination Scale. *Personality and Individual Differences, 31*, 689–700.

Sullivan, G., Jinnett, K. J., Mukherjee, S., & Henderson, K. L. (2003). How mental health providers spend their time: A survey of 10 Veterans Health Administration mental health services. *Journal of Mental Health Policy and Economics, 6,* 89–97.

Sullivan, M. T. (2002). Caregiver Strain Index. *Journal of Gerontological Nursing, 28,* 4–5.

Sullivan, M. T. (2003). Caregiver Strain Index (CSI). *Home Healthcare Nurse, 21,* 197–198.

Svartberg, M., Seltzer, M. H., & Stiles, T. C. (1998). The effects of common and specific factors in short-term anxiety-provoking psychotherapy: A pilot process-outcome study. *Journal of Nervous and Mental Disease, 186,* 691–696.

Svartberg, M., Stiles, T. C., & Seltzer, M. H. (2004). Randomized, controlled trial of the effectiveness of short-term dynamic psychotherapy and cognitive therapy for cluster C personality disorders. *American Journal of Psychiatry, 161,* 810–817.

Sykes, D. H., Arveiler, D., Salters, C. P., Ferrieres, J., McCrum, E., Amouyel, P., et al. (2002). Psychosocial risk factors for heart disease in France and Northern Ireland: The Prospective Epidemiological Study of Myocardial Infarction (PRIME). *International Journal of Epidemiology, 31,* 1227–1234.

Szewczyk, M., & Chennault, S. A. (1997). Women's health: Depression and related disorders. *Primary Care, 24,* 83–101.

Tamura, M., & Kawata, C. (1997). A survey of cognitive probability structure of risk of death by cause. *Nippon Koshu Eisei Zasshi, 44,* 558–567.

Tanco, S., Linden, W., & Earle, T. (1998). Well-being and morbid obesity in women: A controlled therapy evaluation. *International Journal of Eating Disorders, 23,* 325–339.

Taylor, H. A., Jr. (1999). Sexual activity and the cardiovascular patient: Guidelines. *American Journal of Cardiology, 84,* 6N–10N.

Taylor, S. E., Klein, L. C., Lewis, B. P., Gruenewald, T. L., Gurung, R. A., & Updegraff, J. A. (2000). Biobehavioral responses to stress in females: Tend-and-befriend, not fight-or-flight. *Psychological Review, 107,* 411–429.

Theorell, T., & Karasek, R. A. (1996). Current issues relating to psychosocial job strain and cardiovascular disease research. *Journal of Occupational Health Psychology, 1,* 9–26.

Thompson, P. D. (2005). Exercise prescription and proscription for patients with coronary artery disease. *Circulation, 112,* 2354–2363.

Thornton, M., & Travis, S. S. (2003). Analysis of the reliability of the modified caregiver strain index. *Journals of Gerontology Series B: Psychological Sciences and Social Sciences, 58,* S127–S132.

Titone, N. J., Cross, R., Sileo, M., & Martin, G. (2004). Taking family-centered care to a higher level on the heart and kidney unit. *Pediatric Nursing, 30,* 495–497.

Toll, B. A., Sobell, L. C., D'Arienzo, J., Sobell, M. B., Eickleberry-Goldsmith, L., & Toll, H. J. (2003). What do Internet-based alcohol treatment websites offer? *Cyberpsychology and Behavior, 6,* 581–584.

Tomkins, S. S. (1984). Affect theory. In K. R. Scherer & P. Ekman (Eds.), *Approaches to emotion* (pp. 163–196). Hillsdale, NJ: Erlbaum.

Topol, E. J. (2007). *Textbook of cardiovascular medicine* (3rd ed.). Philadelphia: Lippincott, Williams & Wilkins.

Tung, R., Kaul, S., Diamond, G. A., & Shah, P. K. (2006). Narrative review: Drug-eluting stents for the management of restenosis: A critical appraisal of the evidence. *Annals of Internal Medicine, 144,* 913–919.

U.S. Census Bureau. (2004). *Income, poverty and health insurance coverage in the United States: 2003* (Rep. No. P60-226). Washington, DC: Author.

U.S. Department of Labor. (2007). *Bureau of Labor Statistics.* Available from U.S. Bureau of Labor Statistics Web site: http://www.bls.gov/

United Network for Organ Sharing. (2007). *U.S. transplantation data: Heart transplant.* Richmond, VA: Author.

Unutzer, J., Katon, W., Callahan, C. M., Williams, J. W., Jr., Hunkeler, E., Harpole, L., et al. (2002). Collaborative care management of late-life depression in the primary care setting: A randomized controlled trial. *Journal of the American Medical Association, 288,* 2836–2845.

Urry, H. L., Nitschke, J. B., Dolski, I., Jackson, D. C., Dalton, K. M., Mueller, C. J., et al. (2004). Making a life worth living: Neural correlates of well-being. *Psychological Science, 15,* 367–372.

van den Brink, R. H., van Melle, J. P., Honig, A., Schene, A. H., Crijns, H. J., Lambert, F. P., et al. (2002). Treatment of depression after myocardial infarction and the effects on cardiac prognosis and quality of life: Rationale and outline of the Myocardial Infarction and Depression—Intervention Trial (MIND–IT). *American Heart Journal, 144,* 219–225.

van den Heuvel, E. T., de Witte, L. P., Schure, L. M., Sanderman, R., & Meyboom-de Jong, B. (2001). Risk factors for burn-out in caregivers of stroke patients, and possibilities for intervention. *Clinical Rehabilitation, 15,* 669–677.

van der Wal, M. H., Jaarsma, T., Moser, D. K., Veeger, N. J., van Gilst, W. H., & van Veldhuisen, D. J. (2006). Compliance in heart failure patients: The importance of knowledge and beliefs. *European Heart Journal, 27,* 434–440.

van Dijk, D., Jansen, E. W., Hijman, R., Nierich, A. P., Diephuis, J. C., Moons, K. G., et al. (2002). Cognitive outcome after off-pump and on-pump coronary artery bypass graft surgery: A randomized trial. *Journal of the American Medical Association, 287,* 1405–1412.

van Hout, G. (2005). Psychosocial effects of bariatric surgery. *Acta Chirurgica Belgica, 105,* 40–43.

van Hout, G. C., Boekestein, P., Fortuin, F. A., Pelle, A. J., & van Heck, G. L. (2006). Psychosocial functioning following bariatric surgery. *Obesity Surgery, 16,* 787–794.

van Hout, G. C. M., van Oudheusden, I., & van Heck, G. L. (2004). Psychological profile of the morbidly disease. *Obesity Surgery, 14,* 579–588.

van Melle, J. P., de Jonge, P., Kuyper, A. M., Honig, A., Schene, A. H., Crijns, H. J., et al. (2006). Prediction of depressive disorder following myocardial infarction data from the Myocardial Infarction and Depression—Intervention Trial (MIND–IT). *International Journal of Cardiology, 109,* 88–94.

van Melle, J. P., de Jonge, P., Spijkerman, T. A., Tijssen, J. G., Ormel, J., van Veldhuisen, D. J., et al. (2004). Prognostic association of depression following myocardial infarction with mortality and cardiovascular events: A meta-analysis. *Psychosomatic Medicine, 66,* 814–822.

Verhaeghen, P., Joorman, J., & Khan, R. (2005). Why we sing the blues: The relation between self-reflective rumination, mood, and creativity. *Emotion, 5,* 226–232.

Vig, E. K., Davenport, N. A., & Pearlman, R. A. (2002). Good deaths, bad deaths, and preferences for the end of life: A qualitative study of geriatric outpatients. *Journal of the American Geriatrics Society, 50,* 1541–1548.

Virmani, R., Burke, A. P., & Farb, A. (1999). Plaque rupture and plaque erosion. *Thrombosis and Haemostasis, 82*(Suppl. 1), 1–3.

Wadden, T. A., Sarwer, D. B., Womble, L. G., Foster, G. D., McGuckin, B. G., & Schimmel, A. (2001). Psychosocial aspects of obesity and obesity surgery. *Surgical Clinics of North America, 81,* 1001–1024.

Walker, J. G., Manion, I. G., Cloutier, P. F., & Johnson, S. M. (1992). Measuring marital distress in couples with chronically ill children: The Dyadic Adjustment Scale. *Journal of Pediatric Psychology, 17,* 345–357.

Waller, G., Ohanian, V., Meyer, C., & Osman, S. (2000). Cognitive content among bulimic women: The role of core beliefs. *International Journal of Eating Disorders, 28,* 235–241.

Waltz, M. (1986). Marital context and post-infarction quality of life: Is it social support or something more? *Social Science & Medicine, 22,* 791–805.

Wannamethee, S. G., & Shaper, A. G. (1998). Alcohol, coronary heart disease and stroke: An examination of the J-shaped curve. *Neuroepidemiology, 17,* 288–295.

Watson, C. G., Detra, E., Fox, K. L., Ewing, J. W., Gearhart, L. P., & DeMotts, J. R. (1995). Comparative concurrent validities of five alcoholism measures in a psychiatric hospital. *Journal of Clinical Psychology, 51,* 676–684.

Weinstein, N. D. (1982). Unrealistic optimism about susceptibility to health problems. *Journal of Behavioral Medicine, 5,* 441–460.

Weinstein, N. D. (1998). Accuracy of smokers' risk perceptions. *Annals of Behavioral Medicine, 20,* 135–140.

Wenger, N. K., Speroff, L., & Packard, B. (1993). Cardiovascular health and disease in women. *New England Journal of Medicine, 329,* 247–256.

Whang, W., Albert, C. M., Sears, S. F., Jr., Lampert, R., Conti, J. B., Wang, P. J., et al. (2005). Depression as a predictor for appropriate shocks among patients with implantable cardioverter-defibrillators: Results from the Triggers of Ventricular Arrhythmias (TOVA) study. *Journal of the American College of Cardiology, 45,* 1090–1095.

Wilcox, S., & Stefanick, M. L. (1999). Knowledge and perceived risk of major diseases in middle-aged and older women. *Health Psychology, 18,* 346–353.

Wilk, C., & Turkoski, B. (2001). Progressive muscle relaxation in cardiac rehabilitation: A pilot study. *Rehabilitation Nursing, 26,* 238–242.

Willems, D. L., Hak, A., Visser, F., & van der Wal, G. (2004). Thoughts of patients with advanced heart failure on dying. *Palliative Medicine, 18,* 564–572.

Williams, R. B. (2000). Psychological factors, health and disease: The impact of aging and the life cycle. In S. B. Manuck, R. Jennings, B. S. Rabin, & A. Baum (Eds.), *Behavior, health and aging* (pp. 135–151). Mahwah, NJ: Erlbaum.

Williams, R. B., Barefoot, J. C., Blumenthal, J. A., Helms, M. J., Luecken, L., Pieper, C. F., et al. (1997). Psychosocial correlates of job strain in a sample of working women. *Archives of General Psychiatry, 54,* 543–548.

Williams, R. B., Barefoot, J. C., & Schneiderman, N. (2003). Psychosocial risk factors for cardiovascular disease: More than one culprit at work. *Journal of the American Medical Association, 290,* 2190–2192.

Williams, R. B., & Williams, V. (1993). *Anger kills.* New York: Harper.

Winston, A., Pinsker, H., & Rosenthal, R. N. (2004). *Introduction to supportive psychotherapy.* Washington, DC: American Psychiatric Publishing.

Winzelberg, A., & Humphreys, K. (1999). Should patients' religiosity influence clinicians' referral to 12-step self-help groups? Evidence from a study of 3,018 male substance abuse patients. *Journal of Consulting and Clinical Psychology, 67,* 790–794.

Wise, F. M., Harris, D. W., & Carter, L. M. (2006). Validation of the Cardiac Depression Scale in a cardiac rehabilitation population. *Journal of Psychosomatic Research, 60,* 177–183.

Wittchen, H. U., Kessler, R. C., Beesdo, K., Krause, P., Hofler, M., & Hoyer, J. (2002). Generalized anxiety and depression in primary care: Prevalence, recognition, and management. *Journal of Clinical Psychiatry, 63*(Suppl. 8), 24–34.

Witte, D. R., Grobbee, D. E., Bots, M. L., & Hoes, A. W. (2005). A meta-analysis of excess cardiac mortality on Monday. *European Journal of Epidemiology, 20,* 401–406.

Yalom, I. D. (1980). *Existential psychotherapy.* New York: Basic Books.

Yalom, V. (2000). *An interview with James Bugental, PhD.* San Francisco: Psychotherapy.net. Retrieved from http://www.psychotherapy.net/interview/James_Bugental

Yan, L. L., Liu, K., Matthews, K. A., Daviglus, M. L., Ferguson, T. F., & Kiefe, C. I. (2003). Psychosocial factors and risk of hypertension: The Coronary Artery Risk Development in Young Adults (CARDIA) study. *Journal of the American Medical Association, 290,* 2138–2148.

Yingling, K. W., Wulsin, L. R., Arnold, L. M., & Rouan, G. W. (1993). Estimated prevalences of panic disorder and depression among consecutive patients seen in an emergency department with acute chest pain. *Journal of General Internal Medicine, 8,* 231–235.

Young, E., Eddleston, J., Ingleby, S., Streets, J., McJanet, L., Wang, M., et al. (2005). Returning home after intensive care: A comparison of symptoms of anxiety and depression in ICU and elective cardiac surgery patients and their relatives. *Intensive Care Medicine, 31*, 86–91.

Young, L., & Little, M. (2004). Women and heart transplantation: An issue of gender equity? *Health Care for Women International, 25*, 436–453.

Zemore, R., & Eames, N. (1979). Psychic and somatic symptoms of depression among young adults, institutionalized aged and noninstitutionalized aged. *Journal of Gerontology, 34*, 716–722.

Zhao, Y., & Encinosa, W. (2007). *Bariatric surgery utilization and outcomes in 1998 and 2004* (Rep. No. Statistical Brief No. 23). Rockville, MD: Agency for Healthcare Research and Quality.

Zigmond, A. S., & Snaith, R. P. (1983). The Hospital Anxiety and Depression Scale. *Acta Psychiatrica Scandinavica, 67*, 361–370.

Zimet, G. D., Powell, S. S., Farley, G. K., Werkman, S., & Berkoff, K. A. (1990). Psychometric characteristics of the Multidimensional Scale of Perceived Social Support. *Journal of Personality Assessment, 55*, 610–617.

Zlotnick, C., Shea, M. T., Pilkonis, P. A., Elkin, I., & Ryan, C. (1996). Gender, type of treatment, dysfunctional attitudes, social support, life events, and depressive symptoms over naturalistic follow-up. *American Journal of Psychiatry, 153*, 1021–1027.

INDEX

Atherosclerosis Risk in Communities Study, 92
Atria, 15–16
Atrial fibrillation, 19
Atrioventricular (AV) mode, 16
Attachment, 45
Attachment anxiety, 42
Autonomic nervous system, 40, 43, 70, 105–106
Avoidance motivation, 41–42

Baby boom generation, 3
Baecke Questionnaire of Habitual Physical Activity, 179–180
Bariatric surgery, 175–178, 182–184
BDI (Beck Depression Inventory), 54–55, 134, 221. *See also* BDI–II
BDI–II, 54–55, 58
Beck, Aaron, 60
Beck Depression Inventory for Primary Care, 55
Behavioral activation, in CBT, 60
Behavioral cardiology, 4, 47
    and collaborative care, 220–221
    defining, 4–5
    future of, 225–229
    identifying target subgroups, 7–8
    practice settings for, 217–220
    rewards and pitfalls of, 224–225
    seminal works of, 5–6
    soliciting referrals for, 221–224
    training in, 216–217
Behavioral cardiology research, 109, 225
Behavioral factors, for morbidity and mortality, 53
Behavioral health, 215
Behavioral medicine, 4, 215. *See also* Behavioral cardiology
Behavior change, 36–38, 159, 166
    for heart failure patients, 136–139
    motivating, 166–169
Bell, A., 167
Benzodiazepines, 192–193
Bereavement issues, 153–154
Berkman, L. F., 104, 116
Beta-blockers, 194
Binge-eating disorder, 174, 176, 183
Biofeedback, 82–83
Biological differences, gender and, 200–202
Biopsychosocial approach, 134–136
Birks, Y., 55
Blood pressure, 30

Blum, D., 106
Bly, Robert, 213
Body image, improving, 180–182
Bowen, Murray, 135
Bradycardia, 19–20, 26
Brain, 41–42, 187–188
Brain plasticity, 43
Breathing, 80
Brummett, B. H., 103–104
BSI (Brief Symptom Inventory), 56, 134
Bugental, James, 11, 150
Bupropion hydrochloride (Zyban), 195–196
Bureau of Labor and Statistics, U.S., 204
Burg, Matthew, 5
Buss, A. H., 94
Bypass surgery, 24–25

Cabeza, R., 100
CABG (coronary artery bypass graft), 24–25, 52, 68, 90–91
CAGE Questionnaire, 164
Canadian Cardiac Randomized Evaluation of Antidepressant and Psychotherapy Efficacy (CREATE), 58–59, 90, 189–190
Cannon, Walter, 40
Cantor-Cooke, R., 120
Cardiac arrest, 20
Cardiac catheterization, 68
Cardiac counseling
    for anxiety, 77–78
    in RCPP, 89–92
Cardiac cycle, 16–17
Cardiac denial, 34, 74–75
Cardiac disease, major classes of, 17–23
Cardiac intensive care unit, 131, 218
Cardiac mortality. *See* Mortality
CARDIA (Coronary Artery Risk Development in Young Adults), 207
Cardiac psychology, 4, 215. *See also* Behavioral cardiology
Cardiac recurrence, and RCPP, 89–92
Cardiac rehabilitation, 82, 98–99, 201, 206, 219, 223–224
    and adherence, 35–36
Cardiac resuscitation training, 131
Cardiac resynchronization therapy, 71–73
Cardiac syndrome X, 74
Cardiac transplant surgery. *See* Heart transplant surgery
Cardiologist, 147, 224
"Cardiology College," 217

Heart transplant surgery, 143
Heather, N., 167
Hedonic well-being, 41–42
Help-seeking behavior, 209, 229
HERS (Heart and Estrogen/Progestin Re-
placement Study), 96, 201
High blood pressure, 30
Hippocrates, 88
Homocysteine, 32
"Hook" technique, 97–99
Hormone replacement therapy, 201–202
Hormones, and risk of heart disease, 201–
202
Hospital Anxiety and Depression Scale
(HADS), 55, 76–77
Hospitals, as practice setting, 217–220
Hospital stay, length of, 19, 61
Hostility, 87
assessment of, 94–96
and gender differences, 206–207
identifying, 97–98
and morbidity/mortality, 89, 92–93
HPA (hypothalamic–pituitary–adrenal) axis,
40
Humanistic–existential therapy, for end-stage
heart disease, 149–150
Hyperglycemia, 31
Hypertension, 30

ICD (implantable cardioverter defibrillator),
26, 68, 70–73, 77, 93, 152–153
ICD storm, 26
IIP-32 (Inventory of Interpersonal Problems–
32), 114
Immunity, 45–46
Impulse control, 97–98
IMT (intima–media thickening), 107
Independent practice, 226
soliciting referrals, 222–224
Inflammation, 45–46, 70, 105–106, 192
Information
emotional, 100
neutral, 100
Inpatient cardiology, 222
Inpatient referrals, 222
Insulin, 30–31
Insulin resistance, 31, 74
Integrated practice model, 226
INTERHEART trial, 69
Internet, as resource for education and sup-
port, 116, 171–172
Interpersonal circumplex, 111

Interpersonal relationships, and morbidity/
mortality, 103–106
Interpersonal therapy (IPT), 7, 56–59, 115
Interviews, use of, 5–6
Intima–media thickening (IMT), 107

Inventory of Interpersonal Problems–32 (IIP-
32), 114
Ischemia, 18
Ischemic heart disease, 17. *See also* Coronary
heart disease

Janicki, D. L., 107
Jarvik artificial heart, 142
Jennings, Peter, 37–38
Job stress, 203–205
Johnson, Susan, 119
Johnston, M., 77
Jones, K., 55
Jordan, J. V., 112, 213
Journal of the American Medical Association,
189

Kalarchian, M. A., 176
Kaplan, M., 208
Klein, S., 47
Kramer, P., 191

LaBar, K. S., 100
Lane, D. A., 134
LDL (low-density lipoprotein), 30
Leary, Timothy, 111
Lett, H. S., 108
Levant, Ronald, 5, 68, 125–126, 151, 210–
211
LHFQ (Minnesota Living With Heart Fail-
ure Questionnaire), 133
Lifestyle change, 35. *See also* Adherence;
Transtheoretical model
Light, K. C., 105
Lip, G. Y., 134
Lipoprotein A, 32
Long-term view, importance of, 220–221,
224
Lorazepam (Ativan), 192

Macrovascular disease, 31
Magnavita, J. J., ix, x, 90, 99, 123, 210
Maintenance, as stage in change, 37, 138,
166
MAO (monoamine oxidase) inhibitors, 188
Marfan's syndrome, 204

Marital quality, 106–107, 130, 212–213
Marital therapy, 7, 56, 62. *See also* Couples therapy
Masculinity, 210–212
May, Rollo, 150
McCullough, Leigh, ix, x, 42, 84–86, 99, 101, 121, 182
McDaniel, Susan, 134
Medical care system, U.S., 226
Medical disability, 126–127
Medical family therapy, 132, 134–136
Medical psychology, 4, 215. *See also* Behavioral cardiology
Medical social worker, 218, 223
Medical technology, 142–143, 152–153. *See also* ICD; VAD
Medical University of South Carolina, College of Nursing, 137
Medications. *See also* Adherence; Antidepressants; *Names of drugs*
   classes of, 6
   in conjunction with psychotherapy, 196–197
Meditation, 43, 80
Men, psychotherapy with, 210–212. *See also* Gender differences
Mended Hearts, 115
Mentor, role of, 217, 220
Metabolic syndrome, 32, 174
M-HART (Montreal Heart Attack Readjustment Trial), 107
Michigan Alcohol Screening Test, 158–159
Microvascular disease, 31
Miller, J., 212
Miller, W. R., 96, 166
Mind–body connection, 82
Mindfulness, 81
MIND–IT (Myocardial Infarction and Depression–Intervention Trial), 190
Minnesota Living With Heart Failure Questionnaire (LHFQ), 133
Mirtazpine (Remeron), 190
Mitral valve, 17, 21, 25
MMPI (Minnesota Multiphasic Personality Inventory), 96
Modifiable risk factors, 29. *See also* Risk factors
Montreal Heart Attack Readjustment Trial (M-HART), 107, 208
Morbidity
   and anger/hostility, 92–93
   and anxiety, 68–70

and depression, 52–53
and marital quality, 106–107
and obesity, 173–174
and social support, 103–106
Morbid obesity, 173, 176
   and psychological assessment, 178–180
   and psychological distress, 174–175
   psychotherapy for, 180–184
   and weight loss surgery, 175–178
Mortality, 19, 148–154, 161
   and anger/hostility, 89, 92–93
   and anxiety, 68–70
   and depression, 52–53
   and heart failure, 128–130
   and marital quality, 106–107
   and obesity, 173–174
   and social support, 103–106
Motivation, use of term, 166
Motivational interviewing, 7, 166–170
Motivational self-statements, 167, 169
MSPSS (Multidimensional Scale of Perceived Social Support), 113
Multigenerational transmission process, in family therapy, 135
Mutuality, 112–113, 212–213
Myocardial Infarction and Depression–Intervention Trial (MIND–IT), 190
Myocardial infarction (MI), 18, 24, 68–69, 160–161, 192, 194
   and depression, 52–53, 206
   and RCPP, 89–92
Myocardial ischemia, induced, 93

Narcotics Anonymous, 169
National Cancer Institute, 172
National Coalition for Women with Heart Disease, 34, 116
National Heart, Lung, and Blood Institute, 34, 54, 60
National Institute of Mental Health Treatment of Depression Collaborative Research Program, 58, 115, 208
National Institutes of Health, 8
National Network of Tobacco Cessation Quitlines, 172
Negative affect, and addictive behaviors, 162–164
Neuropsychology, 42–43, 47
New England Journal of Medicine, 69
New York Heart Association, 22, 133
Nicotine Anonymous, 169
Nicotine inhaler, 195

Nicotine lozenge, 195
Nicotine nasal spray, 195
Nicotine polacrilex gum, 195
Nicotine replacement therapy (NRT), 195
Nicotine transdermal patch, 195
Night-eating syndrome, 174–176, 184
Nonadherence to medical regimens, 136–139
Nonmodifiable risk factors, 29. *See also* Risk factors
Nontricyclic antidepressants, 188
Normative male alexithymia, 210–212
Nortriptyline, 190

Obesity, 31, 173–174. *See also* Morbid obesity
Obsessiveness, 122
Occupational change, 73, 127. *See also* Job stress
Oncology, 90
Open-heart surgery, 24–25
Optimistic bias, 33
Orth-Gomer, K., 106
Overinhibition, 87
Overweight, 31. *See also* Morbid obesity
Oxygen supply, 17
Oxytocin, 105

Pacemaker, 26
Panic disorder, 67–68, 73–74, 193
Paradoxical approaches, in motivational interviewing, 168
Parasympathetic nervous system, 40, 43, 80
Park, Crystal, 149
Paroxetine (Paxil), 188, 190
Patient, use of term, 4–5
Patient acceptance, 73
Paul, S., 137
Pearsall, P., 146
Pedersen, S. S., 110
Pediatric behavioral cardiology, 6
Pennebaker, James, 150
Perceived Social Support Scale, 113
Perfectionism, 122
Perry, M., 94
Personal computer, and biofeedback, 82–83
Personality change, and donor heart, 145–146
Personality factors, and social support, 107–111
Personality traits, altering, 89–92
Pfizer company, 60
Pharmacotherapy. *See Names of medications; Types of medications*

Physical exercise, 20, 31–32, 83
in assessment of morbid obesity, 179–180
Physician variables, and gender differences, 202–203
Pittsburgh Healthy Heart Project, 107
Posttransplant adjustment, 144–145
Posttraumatic stress disorder (PTSD), 67, 144
Poverty, 203
Powell, Linda, 98
Practice settings, for behavioral cardiology, 217–220
Precontemplation, as stage in change, 36, 137, 166
Pregnant women with heart disease, 131
Preparation, as stage in change, 36, 137, 166
Preventive cardiology, 226
as practice setting, 219
Preventive medicine, 226
Prognostic uncertainty, for congestive heart failure, 127–130
Progressive muscle relaxation, 81–82
Prolongation of dying, 152–153
Psych, use of term, 4
Psychiatric distress, in weight loss surgery candidates, 176–177
Psychocardiology, 4
Psychodynamic psychotherapy, 7, 56, 62–64, 98–100
Psychological distress, in morbidly obese cardiac patients, 174–175
Psychological factors, in gender differences, 205–207
Psychosomatic medicine, 4, 215. *See also* Behavioral cardiology
Psychosomatic Medicine, 88, 108
Psychotherapy
for adaptive expression of anger, 96–101
for addiction/dependence, 165–172
for anxiety, 77–86
in conjunction with medications, 196–197
for end-stage heart disease, 149–154
gender-specific effects, 207–209
for heart transplant candidate, 144
to improve coping with chronic heart disease, 134–139
to improve interpersonal functioning, 114–123
informed by gender differences, 209–213
with men, 210–212

for morbid obesity, 180–184
sequencing of modalities, 122–123
to treat depression, 56–64
use of multiple approaches, 7
with women, 212–213
Psychotherapy research, 7–8
PTCA (percutaneous transluminal coronary angioplasty), 24
PTSD (posttraumatic stress disorder), 67, 144
Public awareness, of risk perception, 34–35
Public education campaigns, for risk perception, 34–35
Public outreach, 224
Pulmonary vein, 17
Pulmonic valve, 17
Pump head, 25

Race issues, 6
RCPP (Recurrent Coronary Prevention Project), 89–92
Reciprocal determinism, principle of, 111–112
Recurrent Coronary Prevention Project (RCPP), 89–92
Referrals, soliciting, 221–224
Reflective listening, in motivational interviewing, 168–169
Relapse, 37–38, 157–158
Relapse prevention, 172
Relational competence, 212
Relational model, 112–113
Relational psychotherapy, 7, 212–213
Relationship Support Program, 62
Relaxation response, 40, 80
Relaxation therapy, 7, 79–82, 97
Religion, 149
Resistance, 168–169. See also Nonadherence to medical regimens
Restenosis, 24
Rigotti, N. A., 196
Risk assessments, relative or absolute, 33
Risk factors
    for arrhythmia, 20
    for cardiovascular disease, 29–32
    for CHD, 18
    for congestive heart failure, 22
    genetic, 46
    multiple, 31
    for valve disease, 21
Risk perceptions, for CHD, 32–35
Roebuck, A., 55
Role playing, 182

Rollnick, S., 96, 166–167
Rosenman, R. H., 88
Roux-en-Y gastric bypass surgery, 175
Ruiz, J. M., 111–112
Rumination, 64–65
    angry, 92

SADHART (Sertraline Antidepressant Heart Attack Randomized Trial), 189
Sadness, and cardiac output, 44
Sapolsky, Robert, 45
Scheidt, S., 5, 98
SCL–90–R (Symptom Check List), 56
Screening system, and referrals, 221–222
Seaburn, D. B., 220
Sears, S. F., 5, 70, 142, 153
Sedentary behavior, 31–32
Self-efficacy, and stages of change, 37
Self-help, for anger management, 97
Self-help groups, 115–117, 123
Self-report measures. See Assessment
Selye, Hans, 40
Sequencing
    of therapy modalities, 122–123
    of treatments, 197
Serotonin, 46
Serotonin dysregulation, 188
Serotonin transporter polymorphism, 46
Sertraline Antidepressant Heart Attack Randomized Trial (SADHART), 189
Sertraline hydrochloride (Zoloft), 60, 188–189
Sexual functioning, 120
Short-term dynamic psychotherapy (STDP), 99–100
Sick sinus syndrome, 19
Siegman, A. W., 108
Sinoatrial (SA) node, 16
SI (Structured Interview), 206–207
Skala, J., 5
Sleep medication, 193–194
Smith, Bob, 170
Smith, T. W., 92
Smokers, and risk perception, 33
Smoking cessation, 30, 171
    medications for, 194–196
Sneed, N. V., 137
Social class, and gender differences, 203–205
Social dominance, 108–109
Social inhibition, 108–111
    assessment of, 113–114

Social isolation, as risk factor, 44–45, 103–106

Social support, 103
    assessment of, 113–114
    and gender differences, 106–107
    and morbidity/mortality, 103–106
    and personality factors, 107–111
    psychotherapy for, 114–123

Sotile, W. M., 5, 120, 138
Specialization, in behavioral cardiology, 225
Spiegel, D., 90
Spirituality, 148–149
Spitz, René, 105
SSRIs (selective serotonin reuptake inhibitors), 60, 188–192
STAI (State–Trait Anxiety Inventory), 76
State anger, 95
State anxiety, 76
STAXI–2 (Spielberger State–Trait Anger Expression Inventory—2), 95–96
Stents, drug-eluting, 24
Stephanik, M. L., 34
Stiver, I., 212
Stockholm Female Coronary Risk Study, 106
Stone Center model, 112–113, 212–213
Stonewalling, in communication pattern, 117
Stress, 67, 69–73, 203–205. See also Anger; Anxiety; Hostility
Stress management therapy, 7, 97
Stress-related growth, 149
Stress response, 40, 45
Stroke, 6, 18n
Structured Clinical Interview for DSM–IV, 176
Study visits, 61
Substance abuse. See Alcohol abuse; Cocaine use; Tobacco use
Sudden Arrhythmia Death Syndromes Foundation, 115–116
Sudden cardiac death, 27, 70, 75, 120, 129, 131
Suicide, 206
Support
    functional, 108
    to improve body image, 180–181
    structural, 108
Support groups, 116–117
    for social support, 115–117
    12-step, 169–171
Supportive psychotherapy, 180–181
Surgery. See Heart transplant surgery; Weight loss surgery

Sympathetic nervous system, 40–41, 43, 70, 105–106
Synapse, 188
Systematic deesensitization, 84–85
Systems approach to therapy, 135
Systole, 16

Tachycardia, 20, 26. See also Ventricular tachycardia
Tafrate, R. C., 95
Tako-Tsubo syndrome, 69
Taylor, Shelley, 107
Telephone hotlines, 172
Telephone quitlines, 172
Tend-and-befriend model, 107
Therapeutic alliance, 182, 197
Therapeutic alliance research, 213
Therapist, gender of, 208
Therapist, role of
    and affiliation research, 111–113
    and morbidly obese patient, 177–178
    and patient's decision about return to work, 126–128
    and psychological assessment of heart transplant candidates, 146–148
    and support groups, 116–117
    and working with clients who are controlling, 120–122
Therapist–client relationship, 120–122. See also Therapeutic alliance
Thompson, D. R., 55
Thompson, Paul D., ix, x, 219
Thrombosis, 31
Time-limited therapy, 63, 99–100, 119–120
Tobacco use, 30, 161. See also Nicotine replacement therapy (NRT)
Tolerance, use of term, 162
Townsend, S. T., 108
Traditional mental health settings, 226–229
Training, in behavioral cardiology, 216–217
Training sites, for behavioral cardiology, 216
Trait anger, 95
Trait anxiety, 76
Trait Anxiety Scale, 114
Transplant coordinator, 147
Transtheoretical model, 36–38, 165–166
Treatments, for cardiovascular disease, 23–27
    gender differences in, 200–201
Triangles, in family therapy, 135
Tricuspid valve, 17
Tricyclic antidepressants (TCAs), 188

ABOUT THE AUTHOR

Ellen A. Dornelas, PhD, is director of behavioral health programs for the Henry Low Heart Center at Hartford Hospital in Hartford, Connecticut, and an associate professor of clinical medicine at the University of Connecticut School of Medicine in Farmington. Dr. Dornelas received her doctoral degree in the health psychology program at Ferkauf Graduate School of Psychology, Yeshiva University, New York, and postgraduate psychotherapy training through the Connecticut Center for Short-Term Dynamic Psychotherapy in Glastonbury. Dr. Dornelas has devoted her career to adapting psychotherapeutic approaches to meet the needs of the cardiac population by providing direct service, training psychologists in the practice of behavioral cardiology, and conducting clinical research focused on behavioral approaches to cardiac risk-factor reduction.